# TREATING ARTICULATION DISORDERS

*To Charles Van Riper—*
*through his teachings, writings, and*
*clinical practices a profession has been shaped.*

Cover portrait of Charles Van Riper, by Ghulam Hassan Ahmed of
Baltimore.

# FOR CLINICIANS BY CLINICIANS
## Harris Winitz, Series Editor

This book, **Treating Articulation Disorders**, is the second volume in the
**FOR CLINICIANS BY CLINICIANS** series of texts on the diagnosis and clinical management of speech, language, and voice disorders. Each text provides a contemporary perspective of one major disorder or clinical area, and
is designed for use in clinical methodology courses and continuing education programs. Authors have been selected who represent a broad spec-
trum of clinical interests and theoretical postions, but who hold the common
belief that their viewpoints, experiences, and successes should be shared in
order to provide a forum **FOR CLINICIANS BY CLINICIANS**.

Already published is **Treating Language Disorders**, and volumes are
planned on cerebral palsy, cleft palate, aphasia, apraxia, dysarthria, voice,
and stuttering.

# TREATING ARTICULATION DISORDERS

## FOR CLINICIANS BY CLINICIANS

Edited by
**Harris Winitz, Ph.D.**
Professor of Communication Studies and Psychology
University of Missouri–Kansas City

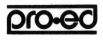

5341 Industrial Oaks Boulevard
Austin, Texas 78735

**Library of Congress Cataloging in Publication Data**
Main entry under title:
Treating articulation disorders.
Includes bibliography and index.
1. Articulation disorders—Treatment.   2. Speech therapy.
I. Winitz, Harris, 1933—   . [DNLM: 1. Articulation
disorders—Therapy. WL 340   W772t]
RC424.7.T74     1984      616.85'5      83-14657
ISBN 0-936104-97-X (previously 0-8391-1814-7)


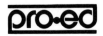

5341 Industrial Oaks Boulevard
Austin, Texas 78735


10   9   8   7   6   5   4   3        85   86   87   88   89

# Contents

# Contributors

**Nicholas W. Bankson, Ph.D.**
Professor and Chairman
Department of Communication
  Disorders
Sargent College of Allied Health
  Professions
Boston University
Boston Massachusetts 02215

**John E. Bernthal, Ph.D.**
Professor, Speech Pathology and
  Audiology
Barkley Memorial Center
University of Nebraska–Lincoln
Lincoln, Nebraska 68583

**Gloria Borden, Ph.D.**
Associate Professor
Temple University
Philadelphia, Pennsylvania 19122
and
Research Associate
Haskins Laboratories
New Haven, Connecticut 06510

**James M. Caccamo, Ph.D.**
Director of Special Education
Independence School District
Independence, Missouri 64005

**Frederic L. Darley, Ph.D.**
Consultant in Speech Pathology
Mayo Clinic
Rochester, Minnesota 55901

**William M. Diedrich, Ph.D.**
Professor of Speech Pathology
Hearing and Speech Department
University of Kansas Medical
  Center
Kansas City, Kansas 66103

**James Paul Dworkin**
Department of Communicative
  Disorders

San Diego State University
San Diego, California 92182

**Mary Elbert, Ph.D.**
Associate Professor, Speech and
  Hearing Sciences
Indiana University
Bloomington, Indiana 47401

**Barbara Hartmann, M.A.**
Clinic Instructor, Speech-
  Language-Hearing Clinic
University of Utah
Salt Lake City, Utah 84112

**Barbara Williams Hodson, Ph.D.**
Associate Professor of
  Communicative Disorders
San Diego State University
San Diego, California 92182

**Edwin A. Leach, Ph.D.**
Meyer Children's Rehabilitation
  Institute
University of Nebraska Medical
  Center
Omaha, Nebraska 68131

**Jeri A. Logemann, Ph.D.**
Professor, Communicative
  Disorders
Northwestern University
Evanston, Illinois 60201

**Lorraine M. Monnin, Ph.D.**
Professor, Speech-Language
  Pathology
California State University,
  Los Angeles
Los Angeles, California 90032

**Hughlett L. Morris, Ph.D.**
Professor of Speech Pathology
Department of Otolaryngology—
  Head and Neck Surgery

University Hospitals and Clinics
The University of Iowa
Iowa City, Iowa 52242

**Donald Mowrer, Ph.D.**
Professor, Department of Speech
and Hearing Science
Arizona State University
Tempe, Arizona 85287

**Elizabeth Prather, Ph.D.**
Associate Professor, Speech and
Hearing Science
Arizona State University
Tempe, Arizona 85287

**John E. Riski, Ph.D.**
Assistant Professor of Speech
Pathology
Department of Surgery
Duke University Medical Center
Durham, North Carolina 27710

**Barbara K. Rockman, Ph.D.**
Clinical Supervisor, Speech and
Hearing Sciences
Indiana University
Bloomington, Indiana 47401

**John C. Rosenbek, Ph.D.**
Chief, Audiology and Speech
Pathology
William S. Middleton Memorial
Veterans' Hospital
Madison, Wisconsin 53705

**Marilynn Schmidt, Ph.D.**
Professor of Speech Pathology
Central Missouri State University
Warrensburg, Missouri 64093

**Susan J. Shanks, Ph.D.**
Professor of Communicative
Disorders
California State University, Fresno
Fresno, California 93740

**Patricia Whaley, M.Ed.**
Clinic Director
Speech and Hearing Clinic
Arizona State University
Tempe, Arizona 85287

**Harris Winitz, Ph.D.**
Professor of Communication
Studies and Psychology
University of Missouri–Kansas
City
Kansas City, Missouri 64110

# Preface

*Treating Articulation Disorders* is the second book in the *For Clinicians by Clinicians* series. As with each volume in this series, the purpose of this text is to provide a forum for clinicians to describe their clinical approach for treating speech and language disorders. This particular text emphasizes articulation disorders.

Recently, Shriberg and Kwiatkowski (1982) proposed that the term *phonological disorders* be substituted for the term *articulation disorders*, although the latter is the standard clinical term replacing dyslalia more than half a century ago. The term articulation disorders, as it has been used, carries at least four meanings. First, it designates the locus of the speech and language disorder as that involving incorrect or non-standard articulatory patterns. In this regard the term articulation disorder references only one type of speech and language disorder. Causes of the disorder or specific behavioral characteristics remain unspecified when the term is used in this way.

Second, the term articulation disorders has been used as a cover term for a broad range of disorders that show different social and organic etiologies, but for which the primary clinical behavior is that of incorrect or nonstandard articulation. For example, the articulation disorder observed in young children, the cleft palate individual or the cerebral palsied patient may be somewhat different, but are regarded as varying along a common continuum. These disorders are distinctly different from disorders of fluency, voice, syntax, or vocabulary. Of course, sometimes there is room for disagreement as to whether a particular speech and language disorder, such as cluttering, can be rightly called an articulation disorder.

The third way in which the term articulation disorders is used by speech-language pathologists is to distinguish troublesome areas in treatment. For example, one can refer to difficulty in carryover as a type of articulation disorder. Or one can cite a patient's difficulty to articulate certain sounds or to use them correctly in running speech at a normal to rapid rate as a type of articulation disorder. Even the categories that are used for identifying sound errors are sometimes referred to as types of articulation disorders when they are regarded by theoreticians as different clinical symptoms as, for example, when individuals with misarticulations are designated as "distorters," "omitters," or "substituters."

Last, the term articulation disorders has been used to distinguish the point at which the breakdown occurs in the speech process. There are several potential points at which a breakdown in the process of articulation may occur of which the first is the sensory or perceptual level. For example, children may have difficulty discriminating between speech sounds. It will have the effect of causing the underlying phonological system to be defective. Of course, the phonological component can be defective for other reasons, such as when a child's conceptual processes are retarded. Motivational and social factors can also delay the development of speech and language, and therefore cause the underlying phonological system to be impaired.

Under some circumstances, the underlying phonological representation for vocabulary items may be correct, but the phonological rules that operate on base lexical forms may be defective. According to this formulation, the breakdown may occur at any point beyond the underlying form up to the point at which an instruction is provided to the speech mechanism. Thus, for example, a child who stores the word *rabbit* correctly with an initial /r/, but because of certain constraints changes the /r/ into a [w] sound, has provided an additional input into the articulatory system. Of course, as we will see below, the output of the phonological rules may be correct, but the articulatory system may be unable to use this information correctly. In any event, when the breakdown occurs in either the base representation or in the rules that operate on this base representation, investigators have referred to this type of articulation disorder as a phonological disorder.

Finally, as is generally known, the breakdown may occur after the instructions have been received by the speech mechanism either at the motor programming stage or at the next lower level, the motor control stage. Traditionally, the disorder of apraxia has been identified as a breakdown in motor programming, and dysarthria as a breakdown in motor control. This distinction has sometimes been applied to children with functional articulation disorders. Children who, for example, can articulate single sounds but cannot articulate these sounds consistently in strings of sounds or in running speech, and in some cases additionally demonstrate other motor deficits in the organization of coordinated motor movements, would be regarded as showing a breakdown at the motor programing stage. On the other hand a child may be unable to articulate single sounds. This inability might be regarded as a breakdown in motor control.

The articulation process from sensation to production is complex. Along the chain of events that mark this process, a breakdown may occur at any point. At this time these potential sites of breakdown are largely hypotheses that are used by clinicians and investigators to guide them in their work. In this regard the term phonological disorder is particularly apt when applied to certain points at which the process of articulation fails to operate correctly. This term has no functional value, however, when it is employed to refer to the entire articulation process. This viewpoint is recognized by Shriberg and Kwiatkowski (1982) when they insist that the application of the term phonological disorders is in reality nothing more than a "cover term" to describe the range of disorders usually implied by the term articulation disorders. We see no heuristic value in trading a new cover term for an old one, especially when the term phonological disorders currently is used to designate special types of articulation disorders.

The contributors of this text have addressed a multitude of issues in the clinical treatment of articulation disorders that reflect the broad scope and variety of articulation disorders. In the first two chapters Monnin and Winitz discuss the role of auditory discrimination in the treatment of articulation disorders. Borden focuses on feedback processes and treatment procedures in Chapter 3. Chapters 4, 5, and 6 address treatment procedures for the child with multiple articulation disorders. Schmidt introduces this topic, and Hodson and Mowrer provide procedures for analysis and treatment within a phonological framework. In Chapter 7, Prather and Whaley present strategies of articulation training based on the theory of coarticulation. Chapters 8 and 9 are concerned with general principles of acquisition and generalization. In Chapter 8, Bernthal and Bankson discuss individual differences in speech sound acquisition that fall within general laws of development, and Rockman and Elbert review generalization principles that apply to the teaching of speech sounds. The next three chapters are concerned primarily with carryover. In Chapter 10, Leach presents a procedure called the *Semantic Conflict Approach.* Shanks, in Chapter 11, demonstrates the use of media to teach carryover skills. In Chapter 12, Hartman reviews research studies on carryover and presents principles for teaching carryover. How computers may be used for writing individualized educational programs is illustrated by Caccamo in Chapter 13.

The focus of the remaining chapters is on the organic disorders. Morris, in Chapter 14, and Riski, in Chapter 15, provide guidelines for the diagnosis and treatment of articulation disorders for individuals with cleft palates. Diagnostic goals and options for treatment are provided by Logemann in Chapter 16 for patients with degenerative and nondegenerative vocal tract impairments. The next two contributors, Rosenbek in Chapter 17, and Dworkin in Chapter 18, indicate the several clinical procedures for treating patients with dysarthria. In Chapter 19, assessment and treatment procedures for apraxia of speech are outlined by Darley. In the final chapter, Diedrich distinguishes the disorder of cluttering from other speech and language disorders, and presents methods of treatment.

## REFERENCE

Shriberg, L. D., and Kwiatkowski, J. 1982. Phonological disorders. I: A diagnostic classification system. J. Speech Hear. Disord. 47:227–241.

## CHAPTER 1

# Speech Sound Discrimination Testing and Training: Why? Why Not?

*Lorraine M. Monnin*

*An analysis of the relationship between articulation errors and speech sound discrimination for children with functional misarticulations is provided by Monnin. Her analysis shows that the discrimination deficits of these children are selective to the sounds they misarticulate, and on this basis she suggests procedures for treatment.*

1. *How does Monnin define speech sound discrimination? What is the distinction between discrimination and identification?*
2. *Monnin comments on the Weiner report which investigated the relationship between articulation errors and speech sound discrimination. What conclusion did Weiner draw regarding this relationship?*
3. *Distinguish between a general and specific speech sound discrimination deficiency. According to research findings, which deficiency do individuals with functional articulation errors have? What are some experimental factors that may influence the research findings with regard to the relationship between articulation errors and speech sound discrimination?*
4. *Review and contrast the several discrimination tests described by Monnin. How do they differ and what are the limitations of each test?*
5. *Monnin concludes that, although children may evidence a deficit in speech sound discrimination, treatment should be directed to production practice rather than to discrimination practice. Why does she draw this conclusion? Do you agree with her position? What clinical procedures does she recommend to teach auditory skills through production?*

MANY PRACTICING SPEECH-LANGUAGE PATHOLOGISTS use speech sound discrimination activities as an integral part of their assessment and remediation procedures for individuals with articulation disorders.

For more than 50 years the relationship between speech sound discrimination ability and articulatory proficiency has been studied by researchers. After all these years the literature still appears to be contradictory and inconclusive on the existence of a relationship between speech sound discrimination ability and articulation disorders. Researchers continue to collect and analyze data in an attempt to resolve these apparent contradictions. In the meantime, clinical speech-language pathologists are fulfilling their responsibilities to their clients on the basis of their professional interpretation of information currently available.

It may be that the results of the studies are not inconclusive and contradictory, but rather that the research has not been analyzed from a perspective that focuses on the similarities and explains the differences of the reported studies.

There are several facets of the speech sound discrimination controversy which may be explored and analyzed and some conclusions drawn. This chapter discusses:

1. The relationship between articulation proficiency and speech sound discrimination ability.
2. Clinical implications of speech sound discrimination testing and training.

Articulation disorders constitute the greatest proportion of defects of speech for all ages (Powers, 1971). Because only a small percentage of articulation disorders have a known organic cause, functional articulation defects account for a large proportion of disorders in the field of speech-language pathology.

The terms *organic* and *functional* refer not so much to the symptomatology as to the presumed etiology of the disorder. Many articulatory cases may have an etiology of a subtle organic base but are classified as functional on the basis of factors in evidence at the time of diagnosis. For the purpose of this chapter, the term *functional articulation disorder* implies no known or observable organic anomaly or impairment which contributes to deficient speech sound production.

Speech sound discrimination must not be confused with hearing acuity. Discussion of speech sound discrimination in the context of this chapter assumes normal hearing and refers to the individual's ability to distinguish between closely related speech sounds. This discussion will focus on young children up to the age of 8 and older children between the ages of 9 and 14.

As traditionally defined, speech sound discrimination is an attempt to measure the perceptual ability of a subject to distinguish speech sounds in his linguistic system. If listeners had a total inability to discriminate, all phonemes would sound the same and speech and language should be impossible (Eisenson et al., 1963, p. 105).

Two basic procedures are utilized to measure this perceptual ability: discrimination and identification.

*Discrimination* implies a comparative judgment between two stimuli which are presented simultaneously or in rapid succession to a subject who is instructed to report if the two stimuli are the same or different. Under optimal testing conditions, small differences between test items can be detected. Speech sound discrimination tasks are based on two fundamental assumptions: 1) the listener can detect relevant phonemic feature differences when two different phonemes are presented, and 2) the listener will generalize intraphonemic differences and place these phones into the correct phonemic category.

*Identification* requires the individual to categorize the stimuli. Speech sound identification requires a more sophisticated response than a discrimination task because the subject must not only determine if there is a difference between the stimuli presented, but must categorize them according to adult phonemic standards. "An appropriate response to an identification task implies an appropriate selection of phoneme categories. Conversely, an inappropriate response to an identification task would imply an inappropriate selection of phoneme categories which may be attributable to defects of discrimination or inappropriate labeling or both" (Monnin and Huntington, 1974, p. 353).

When a child is asked to respond to a discrimination task, it is difficult for the examiner to evaluate the child's response in a meaningful way. The examiner must be aware that a child's acceptable range for a given phoneme may not be the same as that used by adults. Even though a child may judge correctly two unlike phonemes to be different, it is not known if he perceives and classifies either of these stimuli according to acceptable adult phoneme categories. Two contrasting phonemes presented to a child may be perceived by him or her as being two allophones of the same phoneme. A child's response to a discrimination task provides evidence only of the ability to perceive similarities and differences based on his or her own individual criteria. If the ability to discriminate between similarities and differences of two stimuli is relevant, then a discrimination task may be appropriate.

Perceptual tasks required in most daily activities are that of recognition which requires the use of all modalities: auditory, visual, tactile, sensory, and proprioceptive. In most clinical situations the clinician is interested in a child's ability to use his or her auditory modality to recognize verbal phoneme stimuli and then categorize them according to the adult phonemic system. When this is the objective, then an *identification* task is appropriate to achieve the desired objective.

Researchers studying children's ability to respond to verbal stimuli have utilized both the speech sound discrimination paradigm and the identification technique. In the literature both methods are included under the umbrella term *speech sound discrimination.*

## RELATIONSHIP BETWEEN ARTICULATION
## PROFICIENCY AND SPEECH SOUND DISCRIMINATION

Of all the variables that have been studied to establish a relationship with functional articulation disorders, speech sound discrimination ability has been an area of ongoing interest. Travis and Rasmus published a speech sound discrimination test in 1931 which has served as the prototype for the development of other tests and the base for further research in this area. It is not the intent of this chapter to review in detail the research relating articulation and speech sound discrimination abilities; however, those studies pertinent to the topic will be discussed.

Studies conducted over the years have tested subjects of all ages ranging from young children through young adults. They have included subjects with minimal articulation errors to those with severe articulation disorders. A variety of testing procedures has been used from standard speech sound discrimination tests to tasks designed for individual research projects. Research techniques have included live presentation of stimuli, recorded stimuli, and distortion of the speech signal. The tasks most frequently required of the subjects were 1) to respond "same" or "different" to two paired stimuli; 2) to point to the correct picture of the stimulus items presented; or 3) to monitor and evaluate their own productions, both live and recorded. Most of the studies explored the concept of a general discrimination impairment although a few investigated the relationship of speech sound discrimination ability to the specific sound or sounds the subjects misarticulated.

The results of the majority of the studies showed that children with articulation disorders made significantly more errors on speech sound discrimination tasks than normal speaking children; however, there are investigators who have failed to support this premise (Powers, 1971). Some of the ambiguous results may be attributed to the fact that the studies differed in criteria for selecting subjects, research design, and methods utilized. The one exception was the study conducted by Cohen and Diehl (1963) replicating an earlier study by Kronvall and Diehl (1954). In both of these studies children with functional articulation disorders made significantly more errors than normal speakers.

Although the results of the studies in this area appear to be inconsistent and inconclusive, a pattern has been shown which supports a relationship between articulation and speech sound discrimination abilities. Weiner (1967) reviewed the literature and came to the conclusion that the factor of age seemed most important in determining results. A positive relationship was found in almost every study involving children below the age of 9 and seldom in studies with subjects older than 9. According to Weiner, of particular importance was the generally consistent findings of a positive relationship between speech sound discrimination ability and the more severe articulation impaired subjects when they were below the age of 9 years. He states that the inconclusive results are primarily attributable to a failure to keep the effects of age and severity of defect delineated.

## Why Studies Are Inconsistent

*General versus Selective Discrimination Deficiency*     It has been suggested that children with severe articulation disorders have a generalized discrimination deficiency, whereas children with mild articulation disorders have difficulty in discriminating only their own sound errors (Johnson, 1980, p. 53). However, an analysis of the literature fails to support this statement.

The majority of studies have explored the concept of children with articulation disorders having a *general deficiency* in speech sound discrimination. These studies have contributed to the observed inconsistencies reported in the literature.

Studies that investigated the possibility of a *specific discrimination deficiency* found children have greater difficulty in correctly discriminating their misarticulated sounds than sounds they articulate correctly (Anderson, 1949; Aungst and Frick, 1964; Monnin and Huntington, 1974; Prins, 1963; Wolfe and Irwin, 1973). Conclusive and consistent results are seen in these studies which have focused on relating the specific sounds subjects misarticulate to their ability to discriminate those sounds.

In a study conducted by Monnin and Huntington (1974), an in-depth approach was utilized for measuring discrimination skills of young children. The experimental group consisted of 15 kindergarten children, 5 years old, who misarticulated /r/ in the initial, medial, and final positions. Fifteen children of the same age who articulated correctly all the phonemes, including /r/, comprised the control group. The developmental group was composed of 15 4-year-old children who articulated the /r/ phoneme correctly and were in the top 25% of articulation production for their age group according to Templin's norms (1957). The test items consisted of: 1) /r/-/w/ contrasts; 2) acoustically similar contrasts; 3) acoustically dissimilar contrasts, and 4) vowel contrasts. The task was composed of pointing to the correct picture on four tests containing 15 contrasting word pairs in which the two words differed from one another by one phoneme—test 1: read-weed, rich-witch, rake-wake, run-one; test 2: meat-beet, ship-chip, save-shave, tub-cub; test 3: bead-feed, dig-pig, tame-name, gun-sun; test 4: beet-boot, kick-cook, gate-goat. The 15 subjects in each group were presented with 32 contrasts for each test. Of a total of 480 /r/-/w/ responses per group: the control group made 6 errors, mean (M) = 0.40; the experimental group made 73 errors, M = 4.87; and the developmental group made 19 errors, M = 1.27. The experimental group made significantly more errors on this task than either of the other two groups. No significant differences between groups were found on the other tasks which tested sounds subjects in the experimental group could articulate correctly. These children did not exhibit a general speech sound discrimination deficiency, but showed a deficiency specific to their misarticulations. These data are consistent with the results of other research which investigated speech sound discrimination from a specific rather than a general or global perspective.

On the basis of the preceding information, let us operate on the premise that discrimination impairment is selective to the sounds children misarticulate, that is, they do not have difficulty discriminating sounds they produce correctly, but they do have difficulty discriminating stimuli containing their error sounds. Operating from this premise, it is possible to explain the inconsistencies reported in the literature.

When given a discrimination test that incorporates most or all the consonants, the child with the greatest number of articulation errors would be expected to score the largest number of discrimination errors and, conversely, the child with a minimal number of articulation errors would make fewer discrimination errors. For example, if children in Group A have consistent substitutions for five or six sounds, they could be expected to make several errors on the discrimination test. When these subjects are compared with a control group who have normal articulation, a significant difference between the groups on their discrimination abilities would be expected. If, however, children in Group B have consistent substitutions for one or two sounds only, they could be expected to make few errors on the discrimination test. Thus, subjects in Group B would not be expected to show a significant difference from a control group of normal children.

Very few children misarticulate all the phonemes; therefore, even severely involved children articulate some sounds correctly. A child with a severe articulation disorder will respond correctly to some speech sound discrimination items. His total number of errors may be large, but he has shown some ability to perform the task; therefore, to say he has a generalized discrimination deficiency is an assumption that is difficult to support. The use of research paradigms that test for general deficiencies almost certainly assures the results we have seen: children with severe articulation disorders will differ significantly from normal speakers, whereas, mildly impaired subjects will not.

*Selection of Subjects*   A factor that has made the research difficult to evaluate is that many studies are vague in explaining criteria for inclusion of subjects in experimental groups. Frequently, subjects are identified as having mild, moderate, or severe articulation disorders. This tells the reader very little. One individual's definition of a moderate articulation disorder may not—in all probability is not—the same as another person's definition. This makes it difficult for the reader to make precise evaluations of the studies. In addition, some studies have included children with one or two articulation errors in the control group of normal speaking children. Although the researchers justify the inclusion of such children in the control group by stating they did not skew the results, it is unfortunate that this variable was introduced.

*Older Children*   As discussed by Weiner (1967) in his review of the literature, studies using older subjects, those 9 years old and older, seldom showed a positive relationship between functional articulation errors and speech sound discrimination abilities. This observed inconsistency between studies of younger and older children may be explained by looking at the number and type of misarticulations made by older children.

The frequency of many children's misarticulations decreases with age and most older subjects would probably be classified as having mild articulation disorders. The number of older children who maintain severe functional articulation disorders is relatively small in comparison with the younger population. Often it is difficult to identify a sufficient number of children 9 years old and older with severe misarticulations to conduct a meaningful study, therefore, experimental groups of older children are usually composed of subjects having one or two errors. As discussed earlier, children with mild misarticulations do not show a significant discrimination impairment when subjected to a task designed to test for a general discrimination deficiency. Failure to take this into account would contribute to the generally accepted statement that research results are inconsistent, whereas, a distinct pattern could exist if viewed from the context of discrimination ability being related to specific articulation errors.

Many older children do not use specific substitutions of one phoneme for another but rather an approximation toward the target sound which is a distortion of the intended phoneme. The young child who uses a definite substitution of one phoneme for another often is unaware there are two distinct phonemes, that is, won/run. It is believed that habitual use of an incorrect sound obscures perceptual differences (Winitz, 1975, p. 48). However, if an older child distorts the /r/ sound, he is aware there is a difference between the /w/ and /r/ sounds. The /r/ sound he is attempting is different, at least to him, from his production of /w/. Being aware of phonemic differences, he may recognize in the speech of others some differences between the two phonemes. Hence, it is not unexpected that he may categorize correctly his own production and the production of other speakers on a speech sound discrimination task.

Children between the ages of 6 and 8 years have been found to differentiate between their own production of /w/ and /r/ even though listeners do not perceive an acoustic difference. Kuehn and Tomblin (1977) used high-speed, lateral-view cineradiography to compare articulatory positioning and movement characteristics between /w/ and intended /r/ productions of three 6-year-old children exhibiting /w/-/r/ substitutions with one normal control subject. Based on articulatory positioning and movement, the data suggest a lack of phonetic differentiation between correct /w/ and /w/-like phones which are substituted for /r/, however, the observed variability of articulatory positioning suggest different physiological behaviors for the two consonant elements. The authors state that ". . . differences in articulatory variability between /w/ and intended /r/ reflect different entities in each experimental subject's phonology" (Kuehn and Tomblin, 1977, p. 471).

In a study conducted by Metcalf (1963), 22 second- and third-grade children who misarticulated /r/ in the initial position were matched with a control group of normal speaking children. Paired stimulus words containing /r/-/w/ contrasts were produced by the children themselves, their peers and adult speakers. No differences in speech sound discrimination ability were found between the groups when the stimulus items were uttered by adult speakers. It was found, however, that the speech defective children who substituted /w/ for /r/ in their speech perceived their own recorded misarticulations as /r/ more often than other listeners did. It would appear that speech defective children were attending to some cues which differentiated for them the /w/ from the /r/. The fact that normal speaking individuals did not perceive the subtle differences does not negate the fact that the children in the experimental group were conscious of making a distinction in their own productions.

The idea that children may be capable of making a distinction between slight variations in their production has been generally overlooked by adults. Consider how adults chuckle when they recount an episode such as the following: Adult: "Say 'red.'" Child: "wed." Adult: "Not wed, red." Child: "I didn't say 'wed,' I said 'wed.'" The perception of the child saying "wed" is in the ear of the listener. The child is saying he has made a distinction in his production.

The literature states older children have not shown a consistent relationship between articulation deficiency and speech sound discrimination impairment. This perceived inconsistency may be due to one or more of the previously discussed factors:

1.  Most older children exhibit mild to moderate articulation disorders rather than severe articulation disorders.
2.  Generally, older children are approximating the target sound by producing distortions rather than direct substitutions, therefore, they may be aware of the existence of phonemic differences.
3.  Some children perceive their substitutions as different from their production of the intended phoneme.

It must be remembered that most research discusses group means but does not show how individuals within the group performed on the task required.

## CLINICAL IMPLICATIONS OF SPEECH SOUND DISCRIMINATION TESTING AND TREATMENT

### Evaluation of Discrimination Tests

This section discusses speech sound discrimination tests frequently used for clinical assessment and research studies. Those involved in clinical procedures should be knowledgeable of the benefits and limitations of speech sound discrimination tests. They should understand what the test results are telling them about the children assessed. Clinicians should keep in mind these tests are assessing a global ability or attempting to identify a general speech sound discrimination deficiency. They are not designed to relate specific articulation errors to speech sound discrimination responses of misarticulated sounds.

The Templin Speech-Sound Discrimination Test for Six to Eight Year Old Children (1957) and the Wepman Auditory Discrimination Test (1973) both use the same basic approach, that of discrimination between two paired stimuli. The majority of the paired stimuli differ by one phoneme, whereas the remaining pairs are the same. The Templin test utilizes nonsense syllables such as *sa-sha* and *az-az*. The Wepman test follows the same design using meaningful words, such as *thread-shred* and *chap-chap*. The use of nonsense syllables is considered a more abstract task than the word approach.

These two tests tell the clinician how the child responds to an auditory task requiring same-different responses; however, the clinician should be cognizant of the limitations of this type of testing procedure.

1. These two tests require a subject to state if the two stimuli are the "same" or "different," therefore, the subject must have the concept of same-different. Before administering these tests, the clinician must be assured the child understands the task. Children below the age of 6 and those with language disabilities may not have this concept.

2. When a child responds correctly to two unlike stimuli, the examiner assumes the child can differentiate between the two phonemes being tested. The child may be responding to allophonic differences without perceiving them as separate phonemes. The clinician does not know the basis for the child's response.

3. The child may be responding to variables other than phonemic differences. These two tests are administered live. Anyone who has administered this type of test knows how difficult it is to avoid unwanted variables. When a child responds "same" to two like stimuli, the response is accepted as correct. When his response is "different" to two unlike stimuli, the examiner does not know to what cues the child is attending. The examiner may make the erroneous judgment that the child can differentiate phonemes, when, in fact, he or she may be responding to variations in pitch, stress, intensity, or duration. Informal observations have shown many clinicians are unaware of the variations in their presentations. Both inter-examiner and intra-examiner variability have been observed when administering live tests. Brandy (1966) found intra-examiner variability was sufficiently great that repeated readings of a list of words by the same speaker did not necessarily give equivalent results on a speech sound discrimination test. When clinicians administer a test live they must a) be careful to diminish variations in their presentation; and b) be aware the child may respond to variables other than phonemic differences.

4. A major limitation of both the Templin test and the Wepman test is that each paired combination is presented one time only and

requires a choice between two stimuli. The child has a 50% chance of giving a correct response based solely on a correct guess.
5. These tests are constructed to measure a child's global discrimination ability. As discussed previously, it may be more appropriate to test speech sound discrimination relative to the sound or sounds misarticulated.

Three tests, the Templin Speech-Sound Discrimination Test for Three to Five Year Old Children (Templin, 1957), the Boston University Speech Sound Discrimination Test (Pronovost, 1974), and the Goldman-Fristoe-Woodcock Test of Auditory Discrimination (Goldman et al., 1970), require identification responses. An identification task, as discussed previously, tests the child's ability to make categorical judgments based on phonemic differences.

In the Templin test one word is presented at a time and the child chooses one of two pictures, such as sail-pail, chairs-stairs, mouse-mouth. Some combinations include a sound frequently substituted for another, that is, /s/ for /θ/; others have several feature differences, that is, /tʃ/ for /st/ and do not represent paired sounds normally substituted by young children. The scoring method used attempts to reduce the level of chance in recording and evaluating responses. The number of presentations for specific phonemic combinations is limited, however, and once again, a general speech sound discrimination disability is being investigated.

The Boston test introduced an interesting design. Three pairs of pictures are presented and the child's task is to identify which pair is named, for example, cat-cat, cat-bat, or bat-bat. The test is administered live, and the difficulties of live presentations of paired stimuli have been discussed. The paired stimuli are not consistent with the substitutions children frequently use, that is /b/ for /k/ is not a common substitution (Snow, 1963). The test is not testing the child's ability to discriminate between his substitution and the correct phoneme. Each phoneme combination is presented one time only so the level of chance for a right or wrong response is one in three. Again, a general speech sound discrimination ability is being tested.

The Goldman-Fristoe-Woodcock Test of Auditory Discrimination is also a picture identification task. The stimulus items are recorded so that consistency of presentation is maintained. Each plate contains four pictures; each of the presented stimuli differs from the other by one phoneme. The chance of guessing is decreased as the child must select the correct picture from four possible choices. However, many of the possible responses are not commonly substituted sounds or have feature differences children normally would not confuse with the test phonemes. Of specific interest is the fact that only 17 phonemes are tested; five in the initial and final positions, 10 in the initial position only, and two in the final position only. The /s/, a frequently misarticulated sound, is presented two times in the initial position. The /m/ is presented three times, the /b/ four times, and the /w/ two times, all in the initial position. Children seldom misarticulate the /m/, /b/, and /w/ phomenes. It is understandable that the authors of this test were under serious constraints to find test stimuli that could be represented by pictures and were within the vocabulary of young children. However, astute clinicians must be cognizant of the limitations of this test: 1) it tests only 17 phonemes; 2) many of the pictures presented as alternate choices to the test word have feature differences most children do not use in their substitutions and would not confuse with the test phoneme; 3) test phonemes presented more than once, with the exception of /s/, are phonemes not usually misarticulated by children; and 4) the purpose of this test is to investigate general speech sound discrimination ability or disability.

The discrimination tests discussed give the clinician very little information. Locke (1980) discusses in detail inherent difficulties encountered in the conventional procedures for testing speech perception. According to Winitz (1975), it is important to discover the contexts as well as the phonemes the child may have difficulty discriminating.

Tasks requiring the child to give one or two discrimination responses between his substitution and the correct phoneme do not test the limit of the subject's ability. The subjects in one study (Monnin and Huntington, 1974) misarticulated /r/ and made significantly more errors on the /r/-/w/ contrasts than normal speaking children; however, they responded correctly to many of the /r/-/w/ stimuli. In-depth testing revealed these children could not maintain a consistently correct response level. When these children were required to make numerous decisions for sounds they misarticulated, they were significantly less proficient than their normal speaking peers. When the task involved sounds they articulated correctly they had no difficulty in maintaining a correct response level; therefore, factors other than requirements of the task must have been operating.

It would seem that an appropriate method of testing speech sound discrimination ability would be to concentrate on the phonemes the child misarticulates and to conduct in-depth testing of these sounds. Having the child respond to many paired stimuli containing the sound substitution and the correct phoneme in different phonetic environments would provide a meaningful evaluation of the child's ability. Good assessment instruments and procedures incorporate a range of stimuli. Why does speech sound discrimination assessment tend to be superficial? If speech sound discrimination assessment were more extensive using an in-depth evaluation, this would give the clinician useful information.

### Motor Theory of Speech Perception

Children with functional articulation disorders often show selective speech sound discrimination ability. They can discriminate sounds they produce correctly but do not discriminate with the same proficiency sounds they misarticulate. If correct responses are based on acoustic information only, it is difficult to explain how discrimination can be selective, that is, how the child perceives correctly some acoustic information but not other acoustic information.

Studies cited previously have endeavored to establish a relationship between speech sound discrimination and articulation production; however, the direction of a causal relationship is seldom stated. It is generally assumed that children cannot produce phonemes they cannot discriminate. It may be, however, that the relationship goes from production to discrimination. It could be stated that articulation and discrimination are related to the extent that articulatory experience may affect discrimination. In other words, children do not discriminate what they do not produce.

The above statement that production precedes discrimination is based on the motor theory of speech perception. The motor theory of speech perception, as developed by researchers at Haskins Laboratories, states that speech is perceived by reference to production, that is, there is mediation of higher order articulatory correlates which contributes to the perception of the acoustic stimulus. Perception may be mediated by neuromotor correlates of gestures that are similar to those used in production. These researchers (Liberman et al., 1967) found a marked lack of correspondence between acoustic cue and perceived phoneme. They found listeners more easily discriminated between sounds to which they habitually attach phoneme labels than they did between sounds that they normally include in the same phoneme class. The conclusion reached was that listeners discriminate these sounds only to the extent that they can identify them as different phonemes.

Sokolov (1961) stated that in the process of speech perception, an activity of the muscles of speech had been observed and this muscle activity for some reason seemed to be of importance to perception. Subvocal laryngeal muscle activity has also been observed in adults during a reading task and such movement aided subjects in their comprehension ability. Subvocal speech was found to be a useful stimulus input capable of mediating a cognitive response (Hardyck and Petrinovich, 1970). In one speech sound discrimination study (Monnin and Huntington, 1974), the examiner observed that when stimuli were subjected to distortion and became more difficult to identify many children used verbal responses in conjunction with pointing to the picture. These subjects appeared to need verbalization to assist them in making their discrimination decisions.

A study conducted by Briere (1966) supports the concept that ability to produce differences between sounds often comes before the ability to hear these differences. A group of adult students were taught phonological contrasts of another language which were not part of their English linguistic system. Usually, there was a stage when subjects could produce correctly the new contrasts but could not hear the differences when they were produced by the native speaker. This stage, however, did not last long. As soon as subjects became adept at producing the contrasts they began to make correct identifications more consistently.

Clinical observations of adults learning English as a second language show they have difficulty in discriminating sounds not in their native phonological systems. For example, Spanish speakers evidence difficulty between /ʃ/ and /tʃ/, both in production and discrimination. They state the two phonemes sound the same to them. This comment frequently is made after extensive speech sound discrimination training, but before achieving correct production of the sound. It cannot be said these adults have a general speech sound discrimination deficiency as they have mastered production and recognition of the sounds in their native language. Their poor discrimination performance is related specifically to sounds not yet within their phonological system.

If articulatory experience affects the discrimination ability of adults learning new phonemes, then it is conceivable that children are similarly affected. *If discrimination depends on articulation, then it follows that the most prudent treatment approach would start with production rather than discrimination training.*

There are, of course, critics of the motor theory of speech perception. To date, however, there have been no other theories offered or rationale given for selective discrimination of phonemes.

## Production Training and Self-Evaluation

The goal of articulation training is to help children produce phonemes they have not mastered. In the traditional approach for children with functional articulation errors, the first step is speech sound discrimination training. The rationale is that before the child can produce the new sound he or she must first discriminate between his or her substitution or distortion and the correct phoneme as produced by an external model. According to this premise, once the child responds to the acoustic cues given by the clinician, the child then should be able to produce the sound being remediated. If this premise is valid, why then is it necessary to introduce the second step? Why is it necessary to teach production using descriptions and directions for the placement of the articulators in order to achieve the desired acoustic results? Why are so many techniques for teaching production described in texts and in the literature? Williams and McReynolds (1975) have shown through their research that production training alone is sufficient to remediate articulation errors. The authors found production training was effective in changing both articulation and discrimination, whereas, speech sound discrimination training changed only discrimination responses to an external model. The effects of speech sound discrimination training have not given the child the tools he or she needs to produce the sound. Speech sound discrimination training is not a substitute for production training. In fact, what is accomplished as a result of speech sound discrimination training is not known. Perkins states, "In practice, it [speech sound discrimination training] does no harm. The worst that could be said is that it may be inefficient, possibly to the extent of doubling the number of therapeutic steps" (1977, p. 388).

Using the traditional approach, the clinician spends a considerable period of time having the child judge and evaluate the production of an external model. When the clinician is satisfied the child has developed some expertise in the speech sound discrimination tasks, then production training of the desired phoneme is introduced. The clinician models the sound and asks the child to repeat it. When the child's response is incorrect, the clinician gives directions for placement of the articulators and asks the child to produce the sound. When the child's response remains incorrect, we need to ask why. The child has been given speech sound discrimination training, verbal models by the clinician, and excellent instructions for placement of the articulators, but is still unable to produce the desired sound.

Given these tools for correct production, why does the child continue to produce his or her substitution or distortion? The following scenario often takes place. A child and a clinician are working on production. The child will, no doubt, after many attempts produce the sound correctly. The clinician is delighted and says so. The clinician has the child try again and after several more attempts the child is successful once again. The clinician asks, "Did you hear what a good sound you made?" The child is puzzled and asks, "Oh, is that the sound you want?" The clinician may be bewildered by this response and thinks, "We've been working on this sound for hours and you didn't even know that was the correct sound?" Now the child is aware of the difference, and now has a model for discrimination. It is an internal model, not an external one. Aungst and Frick (1964) found a difference in how children perceive the phonemes of a speaker in relation to how they perceive their own production of the same phoneme. The children were using an internal model to evaluate their own production.

How is it possible for a child or adult to be given directions for placement of a specific phoneme and still continue to produce the same substitution or distortion? A simple exercise tried with a large number of graduate students may offer an explanation. The students described the tongue position they used to produce a vocalic /r/. Some reported using the retroflex position, others the bunched position with tongue tip down. They were all asked to produce the vocalic /r/ using four different tongue positions: retroflex, bunched with tongue tip down, tip of the tongue pointing toward the right cheek, and tip of the tongue pointing toward the left cheek. They were able to make an acoustically acceptable /r/ using all four positions. Why were they able to place the tongue into unfamiliar and unconventional positions and still produce the sound? They were making compensatory adjustments of their vocal tracts so their production would match their internal auditory image for an /r/ sound.

What happens when children who misarticulate the /r/ are given verbal directions and auditory stimuli to change their production? They respond in the same way the graduate students did, they change their tongue position but they modify their vocal tract so they can continue to match their acoustic output to their respective internal images of their distorted /r/. The acoustic characteristics for a correct /r/ are not yet part of their internal monitoring systems.

Rather than presenting the children with an auditory stimulus that may evoke their internal auditory image, it may be more appropriate to use "verbal play." Verbal play may consist of various activities such as making sounds heard in their environment, imitating the sound of an engine starting, making as many "funny sounds"as they can, and so forth. The children may emit the desired sound by "accident" because they are not trying to avoid it by matching it to an established internal model. If the use of verbal play is not successful, it may be necessary to pursue other, more direct approaches; giving directions for placement of the articulators; or having the children move their tongues to the target position using a phoneme that is in their systems which contain articulatory features common to the target sound (Shriberg, 1975 and 1980). Many frustrations for both the child and the clinician could be avoided if the clinician is aware of the dynamics involved in having the child incorporate a new sound into his or her established phonological and self-monitoring systems.

After the child correctly produces the sound and has established an internal auditory model, the clinician should capitalize on this accomplishment and incorporate it into treatment. Although the child has developed an internal model, it is not yet firmly established and the phonetic parameters of this new sound are unknown to him or her. He or she needs help in establishing the acoustic limits of the range of acceptability for the phoneme. At first the clinician will act as the child's monitor by telling him or her when a production is correct or incorrect. This stage should be short. When the clinician acts as a monitor, the child depends on an outside source for feedback. This arrangement has only limited value for the child. In some instances clinicians have acted as the child's sole monitor. When the child achieved a predetermined level of success, the clinician instructed him or her to use the "new sound" outside the clinical setting, but he or she was not given the means to be successful. The child was not able to evaluate his or her own production, but was still dependent upon the clinician to be the monitor.

As soon as the child shows the ability to produce the phoneme correctly several times, the clinician should teach the child to use his or her own feedback system to monitor and evaluate the productions. Each time the child produces the intended phoneme, whether it is in a syllable, word, or phrase, the clinician should ask him or her to evaluate the production of the phoneme. The role of the clinician is to agree or disagree with the child's evaluation. The child will not always be correct during this early self-evaluation period, but the clinician is helping him or her to establish and internalize acceptable phonemic boundaries for the newly acquired sound.

The clinician is teaching speech sound discrimination and self-evaluation so that the child can serve as his or her own monitor and judge. The child is learning self-evaluation so that he or she will not be dependent upon an outside source to be a monitor. The clinician's goal is not to have the child be dependent, but to become independent and assume responsibility for his or her own speech production.

The clinician has the responsibility to make available to the child the tools for success. It is particularly important for the child to have self-monitoring skills because they are the means to self-sufficiency and independence. Generalization and carryover will not be successful if the child is unable to evaluate his or her production. As with any skill, the performer must be capable of making an evaluation of what he or she has produced. The goal set for the child may be to produce the correct sound in a given number of words, phrases, or sentences.

The goal for the clinician, however, should be to make the child as self-sufficient and independent as possible as quickly as possible.

## SUMMARY

For more than 50 years the relationship between speech sound discrimination ability and articulation proficiency has been researched, studied, and discussed. That so much time and effort have been devoted to this area attests to the fact there are no easy answers. Many authors describe the results of the research as inconsistent and inconclusive. The concept that children with functional articulation disorders have a general or global speech sound discrimination deficiency has contributed to the research being described as "inconsistent." When speech sound discrimination performance is viewed as being specific or selective to the sound or sounds the child misarticulates, then a positive, consistent relationship can be established.

Clinicians frequently use speech sound discrimination tests as part of their assessment procedure; however, these tests have limitations: 1) they are designed to measure a general deficiency, not one that is specific to sounds misarticulated; 2) the number of paired stimuli contrasting the child's substitution with the correct phoneme may be presented one or two times only, and in some tests, not at all; 3) frequently, they do not present paired sounds normally substituted by young children; 4) when a same-different task is used, the clinician does not know what variables influenced the child's response. Unfortunately, current speech sound discrimination tests are not designed to provide adequate information for assessment and remediation purposes. To obtain meaningful information, clinicians should use in-depth speech sound discrimination testing of the misarticulated sound or sounds.

The focus of articulation treatment should be on production training of phonemes needing remediation. The viability of using an external model for speech sound discrimination training is questionable on the basis of present evidence. Speech sound discrimination training is valuable, however, when it is used to help the child process his or her own articulatory performance. Training the child to use his feedback system will enable him or her to develop self-monitoring and self-evaluation skills. Dependency on the clinician is fostered when the clinician acts as the child's monitor. An emphasis on self-monitoring and self-evaluation makes it possible for the child to become independent of outside sources. This procedure helps the child acquire the skills necessary for generalizing correct phoneme production and increasing carryover, both of which are essential if implementation of remediation procedures into everyday activities is to be achieved.

## REFERENCES

Anderson, P. 1949. The relationship of normal and defective articulation of the consonant /s/ in various phonetic contexts to auditory discrimination between normal and defective /s/ production among children from kindergarten through fourth grade. Master's thesis, State University of Iowa, Iowa City.

Aungst, L., and Frick, J. 1964. Auditory discrimination ability and consistency of articulation of /r/. J. Speech Hear. Disord. 29:76–85.

Brandy, W. 1966. Reliability of voice tests of speech discrimination. J. Speech Hear. Res. 9:461–465.

Briere, E. 1966. An investigation of phonological interference. Language 42:768–796.

Cohen, J., and Diehl, C. 1963. Relation of speech-sound discrimination ability to articulation-type speech defects. J. Speech Hear. Disord. 28:187–190.

Eisenson, J., Auer, J. and Irwin, J. 1963. The Psychology of Communication. Appleton-Century-Crofts, New York.

Goldman, R., Fristoe, M., and Woodcock, R. 1970. Goldman-Fristoe-Woodcock Test of Auditory Discrimination. American Guidance Service, Circle Pines, MN.

Hardyck, C., and Petrinovich, L. 1970. Subvocal speech and comprehension level as a function of the difficulty level of reading material. J. Verbal Learn. Verbal Behav. 9:647–652.

Johnson, J. 1980. Nature and Treatment of Articulation Disorders. Charles C Thomas, Springfield, IL.

Kronvall, E., and Diehl, C. 1954. The relationship of auditory discrimination to articulatory defects of children with no known organic impairment. J. Speech Hear. Disord. 19:335–338.

Kuehn, D., and Tomblin, B. 1977. A cineradiographic investigation of children's w/r substitutions. J. Speech Hear. Disord. 42:462–473.

Liberman, A., Cooper, F., Shankweiler, D., and Studdert-Kennedy, M. 1967. Perception of the speech code. Psychol. Rev. 74:431–461.

Locke, J. 1980. The inference of speech perception in the phonologically disordered child. Part I: A rationale, some criteria, the conventional tests. J. Speech Hear. Disord. 45:431–444.

Metcalf, J. 1963. An investigation in certain aspects of speech discrimination in children. Doctoral dissertation, Stanford University, Stanford, CA.

Monnin, L., and Huntington, D. 1974. Relationship of articulatory defects to speech-sound identification. J. Speech Hearing Res. 17:352–366.

Perkins, W. 1977. Speech Pathology: An Applied Behavioral Science. 2nd Ed. C. V. Mosby Co., St. Louis, MO.

Powers, M. H. 1971. Functional disorders of articulation—Symptomatology and etiology. In: L. Travis (ed.), Handbook of Speech Pathology and Audiology. Appleton-Century-Crofts, New York.

Prins, D. 1963. Relations among specific articulatory deviations and responses to a clinical measure of sound discrimination ability. J. Speech Hear. Disord. 28:382–388.

Pronovost, W. 1974. Boston University Speech Sound Discrimination Test. Go-Mo Products, Cedar Falls, IA.

Shriberg, L. 1975. A response evocation progam for /ɚ/. J. Speech Hear. Disord. 40:92–105.

Shriberg, L. 1980. An intervention procedure for children with persistent /r/ errors. Lang. Speech Hear. Serv. Schools 11:102–110.

Snow, K. 1963. A detailed analysis of articulation responses of 'normal' first grade children. J. Speech Hear. Res. 6:277–290.

Sokolov, A. 1961. Studies on the problem of the speech mechanisms of thinking. In: Psychological Science in the USSR, Publication no. 11, p. 466. Joint Publications Research Service, Washington, DC.

Templin, M. 1957. Certain Language Skills in Children. University of Minnesota Press, Minneapolis, MN.

Travis, L., and Rasmus, B. 1931. The speech sound discrimination ability of cases with functional disorders of articulation. Q. J. Speech 17:217–226.

Weiner, P. S. 1967. Auditory discrimination and articulation. J. Speech Hear. Disord. 32:19–28.

Wepman, J. 1973. Auditory Discrimination Test. Language Research Associates, Chicago.

Williams, G., and McReynolds, L. 1975. The relationship between discrimination and articulation in children with misarticulations. J. Speech Hear. Res. 18:401–412.

Winitz, H. 1975. From Syllable to Conversation. University Park Press, Baltimore.

Wolfe, V., and Irwin, R. 1973. Sound discrimination ability of children with misarticulation of the /r/ sound. Percept. Motor Skills 37:425–420.

CHAPTER 2

# Auditory Considerations in Articulation Training

*Harris Winitz*

*The relationship between auditory discrimination and artic-
ulation performance for children with articulation errors is
considered by Winitz. He concludes that auditory discrimination is an important component in articulation training,
and provides a plan of treatment that emphasizes intensive
auditory experience as preliminary to training in articulation
production.*

1.  *Discuss the reasons given by Winitz as to why some re-
    search studies fail to demonstrate a relationship between
    articulation performance and auditory discrimination.
    Do you agree with his analysis?*
2.  *Winitz suggests that when children fail to discriminate
    between phonemes of the community language, their un-
    derlying phonological structure for these phonemes is
    incorrect. He also comments that when they have no
    difficulty distinguishing between phonemes, their un-
    derlying phoneme system may also be defective. Why
    does he make these claims? What experimental proce-
    dure would you suggest that might be used to affirm or
    deny his conclusions?*
3.  *Why does Winitz suggest the use of intensive auditory
    discrimination training before production practice? How
    does this approach differ from several traditional meth-
    ods?*
4.  *Do you prefer the informal or formal method of auditory
    discrimination training? Why?*

WHEN PHONOLOGICAL ANALYSES WERE FIRST APPLIED to the study of articulation disorders by Haas in 1963, the primary aim was to determine the underlying phonemic unit for each of the several sound errors. Within the framework that Haas was working, the phonemes of the child with an articulation disorder were regarded as not necessarily the same of those for the community language.

That the underlying phonological representation of children's articulation disorders may be different from the community language was suggested also by several investigators whose focus of interest was the relationship between auditory discrimination and articulation errors (Locke, 1968; Winitz, 1969; Winitz and Bellerose, 1962, 1963). They made this inference on the basis of fairly strong evidence that indicated that children with articulation errors had difficulty discriminating between target sounds and their respective error sounds (Spriestersbach and Curtis, 1951). As an illustration, when children produce [w] for the consonantal segments of the /w/ and /r/ phonemes, and also do not discriminate between these two phonemes, a reasonable interpretation is that the underlying mental representation is the same for each phoneme.

As a result of recent interest in the relationship between phonological development and articulation disorders, the study of auditory discrimination is now attracting increased attention. The purpose of this chapter is to reconsider the relationship between auditory discrimination and articulation disorders, to indicate reasons why a relationship is not always found, and finally to recommend procedures for articulation training that have an auditory focus. There is now theoretical interest in this relationship as it may provide important information on the phonological structure of children's articulation errors.

### COMPARATIVE STUDIES

In 1967, Weiner, and later Winitz (1969), reviewed the results of studies on the relationship between auditory discrimination and articulation performance. These results, and more recent findings (Monnin and Huntington, 1974; Strange and Broen, 1981) indicate, with few exceptions, that children with functional articulation disorders show lower discrimination scores relative to children who do not have articulation disorders. These few exceptions have led some investigators (Locke, 1980a,b; McReynolds et al., 1975) to conclude that the results of studies on the relationship between auditory discrimination and articulatory performance are largely inconsistent, and that no definitive conclusions can be drawn regarding the auditory capabilities of children with articulation disorders.

In the following section, several studies that failed to yield a relationship between articulation performance and auditory discrimination will be reviewed in order to cite circumstances under which children with functional articulation errors will not necessarily evidence poor performance on tests of auditory discrimination. Four primary conditions and others of lesser consequence will be described for which a positive relationship between articulation performance and auditory discrimination is not to be expected. These conditions establish the boundary conditions for the relationship between auditory discrimination and articulation.

## CONDITIONS THAT MAY FAIL TO PROVIDE A POSITIVE RELATIONSHIP BETWEEN ARTICULATION AND DISCRIMINATION

### Relevant Discrimination Test Items

In auditory discrimination testing, a distinction is often made between general and specific discrimination tests (Winitz, 1969, 1975). The purpose of a general auditory discrimination test is to assess general auditory functioning, whereas the purpose of a specific auditory discrimination test is to assess only those auditory distinctions that relate to a child's specific misarticulations.

These two types of auditory tests reflect two respectively different theoretical positions. General discrimination tests, such as the Wepman (1958) Auditory Discrimination Test, are designed to examine an individual's auditory capacity to distinguish among speech sounds. The term *general* is used because these discrimination tests include a large number of English sounds in a variety of phonetic contexts in order to assess one's overall ability to process speech sounds.

A specific discrimination test is used to assess the auditory discrimination of sounds for which an individual demonstrates articulatory errors. The term *specific* is used because it denotes a specific assessment in auditory processing, that which is associated with a child's articulation errors. For example, a child who misarticulates [w] for [r] and who has difficulty discriminating between [r] and [w] is regarded as having a specific disability in auditory functioning when the difficulty lies only with these two sounds and not with other sounds.

In many of the investigations in which the speech sound discrimination of children with articulation errors was compared with that of normal speaking children, general discrimination tests were used. The children in these investigations frequently had multiple articulation errors and, in addition, the severity of their articulation disorders ranged from mild to severe (Weiner, 1967; Winitz, 1969). It was pointed out by Weiner (1967), and subsequently by others (Locke, 1980a; Winitz, 1969, 1975) that one reason children with articulation errors will not always show a deficiency in auditory discrimination is because the paired items of general discrimination tests are not always relevant. Often the sounds of the paired items and those which an individual child misarticulates are not the same. This lack of equivalence in the sounds of the two assessments is to be expected when a standard general discrimination test is applied to all children regardless of their articulation performance. For example, when the same general discrimination test is administered to a child who misarticulates /r/, and to a child who substitutes stops for fricatives, it is unlikely that the discrimination test will contain a sufficient number of items in these two cases to provide for a valid assessment of auditory discrimination. Furthermore, a recent investigation by Bountress and Laderberg (1981) has shown that general discrimination tests do not provide comparable assessments of auditory discrimination. Bountress and Laderberg compared the performance of young children on the Wepman Auditory Discrimination Test (Wepman, 1958) and the Goldman-Fristoe-Woodcock Test of Auditory Discrimination (Goldman et al., 1970) and found that these two tests failed to provide similar results.

Weiner (1967) indicated that children with few articulation errors often do not evidence a deficiency in auditory discrimination. He concluded that when children have few articulation errors, the target sounds, in the context in which they are misarticulated, are not represented adequately in the general discrimination test. On the other hand, when children have a great number of sounds in error, the chances are greater that the target sounds will be represented on tests of general auditory discrimination. Therefore, the greater the number of articulation errors the more likely the sounds will be represented on the general discrimination test. Additionally, the longer the general discrimination test, the greater the likelihood that the target sounds will be represented. Conversely, when a specific discrimination test is restricted to a few items, or in some cases, to only a single sound pair even though it is relevant, a consistent and positive relationship between auditory discrimination and misarticulation is not always observed (for example, Locke, 1980b).

## CONSIDERATION OF THE CHILD'S
## SPECIFIC ARTICULATION ERRORS

Several years ago I (Winitz, 1975) observed a young child who substituted a [k] sound produced substantially more forward in the mouth than the standard English /k/ phoneme. The child's clinician reported that the child made a /t/ for /k/ substitution, and she had begun to treat this error by trying to teach the child to articulate a dorsovelar [k]. My perceptual impression was that the gestural components for this [k] sound were more forward than those usually observed for the English fronted [k̟] as in *key* or *kit*. Most likely this child's fronted [k], symbolized by [k̟], was made by bringing the dorsum of the tongue into contact with the hard palate. Further testing indicated that the child was able to discriminate between /k/ and /t/, but unable to discriminate between the target sound [k] and the error sound [k̟].

Spriestersbach and Curtis in 1951 after reviewing the results of several research studies on articulation and discrimination were the first to conclude that children frequently will show a deficiency in auditory discrimination when each contrasting item pair is composed of the child's sound error(s) and its respective target sound. They additionally remarked that the child's sound errors sometimes are nonstandard sounds.

Usually the term distortion is applied to an articulation error when it involves a nonstandard production or one intermediate between two sounds, such as a lateralized [s], a partial flattening of the tongue for [r], or a forward [k]. Investigators (Kornfield, 1971; Spriestersbach and Curtis, 1951; Winitz, 1975) have speculated that children who produce distortions can give the impression that their auditory discrimination is normal because they perform well when the discrimination test involves two target sounds. These same children may have difficulty in auditory discrimination tasks when their nonstandard or intermediate sound is contrasted with the target sound that it has replaced. For example, children whose tongue placement for [r] is intermediate between the [r] and [w], often give the impression of substituting a [w] sound. When the auditory discrimination test includes only [r-w] pairs, they may not show a disorder in auditory discrimination, but they may have difficulty when their nonstandard [r] is contrasted with the standard [r].

In one investigation McReynolds and her associates (McReynolds et al., 1975) came to the conclusion that children with articulation errors, in general, do not show an impairment in auditory discrimination. The focus of that study was not on distorted sounds, but its methodology is pertinent to the issue of relevant item sound pairs. In their investigation McReynolds et al. (1975) examined normal speaking and articulatory defective children on their ability to distinguish between a fairly large number of sound pairs, such as [w-r] and [d-n]. The same test was used for all children regardless of their particular articulation errors. Additionally, some item pairs included sounds that are usually not misarticulated (such as [d-n] and [z-v]) in the speech of children. The results of this investigation by McReynolds and her associates indicated that children with misarticulations performed about the same on the auditory discrimination test as the children without articulation errors. This negative result largely can be attributed to methodological considerations as the investigators generally did not take into account the specific articulation errors of each child nor were the items necessarily relevant for each child.

Sometimes it is difficult to test the specific speech sound discrimination of children because some sound substitutions cannot be simulated easily. For example, the many /s/-type distortions that children produce are difficult to imitate. Yet, for these distortions to be used as contrasting items in a discrimination test, it is necessary for the clinician in each case to imitate the child's particular type of /s/ distortion correctly. If the distortion is not imitated correctly, as in the example given above with regard to the child who produced a forward [k], an accurate assessment of a child's ability to distinguish between the standard sound and his or her distorted sound will not be made.

In only a few studies on the relationship between auditory discrimination and articulation is each child's specific articulation error directly taken into consideration. As Spriestersbach and Curtis (1951) originally remarked, this factor is an important consideration in auditory discrimination testing and should be considered when developing the item pairs of a discrimination test.

## PHONETIC CONTEXT

A third consideration in discrimination testing is phonetic context, also discussed by Spriestersbach and Curtis (1951). The investigations of Spriestersbach and Curtis (1951), Templin (1957), Eilers and Oller (1976), and Locke (1980b) indicate that phonetic context may contribute substantially to the relationship between auditory discrimination and articulatory performance. This consideration cannot be overlooked in auditory discrimination testing. For example, for a child who misarticulates /s/ in clusters and in final word position, and for which the discrimination test includes only initial /s/ sounds, the correct phonetic contexts are not being used to assess auditory discrimination. Similarly, auditory perception is not being assessed adequately for a child who misarticulates front stops when they precede back vowels, as in *pony, took, boot*, and *door*, but for which the auditory test only includes front stops before vowels, as in *pen, tea, beat* and *dip*.

This consideration of phonetic context is sometimes overlooked. Specific discrimination tests may include several instances of paired items for an individual sound, but may not reflect reliably the phonetic contexts in which a child's articulation errors occur. When phonetic context is not adequately controlled for, the relationship between auditory discrimination and articulation performance may not be apparent or may be diminished considerably.

This factor becomes clear to adult speakers of American English when asked to distinguish between /t/ and /tʃ/ in the context of words that begin with /tr/ cluster as in *train* and *tree*. Some speakers use the cluster /tʃr/ and others use /tr/, and because each is an acceptable and frequently heard pronunciation as an initial cluster, many native speakers of English cannot hear the difference between them.

## PRIOR EMERGENCE OF DISCRIMINATION SKILLS

If you have ever listened to the sounds of a foreign language that are distinctly different from English, you know that they are difficult to hear and even more difficult to imitate correctly. With sufficient auditory experience, the ability to imitate the foreign sounds correctly usually improves.

In this regard there is an interesting phenomenon that occurs in second language learning that is difficult to explain at this time. It has generally been observed that when individuals learn a second language after the age of puberty (Lenneberg, 1967) they have an accent. In many cases, however, these individuals have achieved nativelike fluency in all other aspects of language usage (Carroll, 1961) in that their use of grammar across the dimensions of syntax, semantics, and pragmatics is on a par with the native speaker. Some display extraordinary literate talent as exemplified by the writer Joseph Conrad, the linguist Roman Jakobson, and the former United States secretary of state Henry Kissinger, even though their English pronunciation would not be regarded as nativelike.

Still there are other individuals whom we meet occasionally that have acquired English after pubescence who exhibit not the slightest trace of a foreign accent. Unfortunately, to my knowledge, the circumstances which led to their native-like pronunciation are unknown. For example, we have little information on the educational and social backgrounds of these individuals.

One possible difference in the background between individuals who have accents and those who do not may lie in their communicative experiences. When the communicative mileau demands production of speech, individuals will most likely utilize whatever resources are available to them. They will make the best effort possible to communicate even if it means that they will have to say words for which they are unsure as to their pronunciation. Young children, on the other hand, are not forced to speak as they are acquiring their native language. They can remain silent until they understand or partially understand a particular grammatical construction.

It has been recognized that immigrant children often remain silent for several months when they are first placed into an English speaking environment. They go through what is called the silent period (Newmark, 1981), during which time their utterances usually consist of one or two words and a few formulaic expressions. This silent period, of course, usually takes place in the school where the child is suddenly plunged into a totally strange language environment, but in one instance the parents of a very young preschooler reported to me that their child spoke neither the first language nor the second language for a period of almost 5 months after arriving in the United States. On further questioning of the parents, I learned that both spoke English well, and had made a decision to speak mostly English at home. One would expect this situation to be totally baffling to a young child who would have no choice but to remain silent until the new language could be understood.

I have also observed the speech of immigrant children who were integrated into the regular class for a certain part of the day, and also received special instruction in English outside the classroom, although the type and intensity of the instruction varied considerably from teacher to teacher. Some stressed imitative modeling and dialogue practice, others reading, and still others taught comprehension of language through the use of commands. These different methods of instruction, the time spent in the classroom, and the child's communicative responsibilities in these two settings no doubt have an effect on a child's acquisition of English. In this regard I have observed children who have acquired English with a foreign accent, a finding also reported by Asher and Garcia (1969), and Snow and Hoefnagle-Höhle (1977). Possibly they spoke English with a foreign accent because the environmental conditions did not provide sufficient auditory experience with the sounds of English before speaking was demanded.

It is generally recognized that perceptual processes play an important role in the acquisition of language. Initially, all information about a language is perceived through the senses. Children make use of linguistic and nonlinguistic context to guess the meaning of utterances, and use this information to derive the underlying grammar and lexical units of the language. Speaking serves only to increase the communicative interaction of children and to broaden their verbal milieu (Winitz, 1981a, 1983; Winitz and Reeds, 1975). As their verbal environment increases in complexity the language directed to them also increases in complexity. Speaking, then, provides the kinds of language experiences that are essential for learning a language. Speaking, however, does not contribute directly to the underlying knowledge that one must acquire to use a language.

In this regard, the silent period of native language acquisition is probably not restricted to the early phases of language learning. At this early point, to be sure, the silent period is more obvious, as children remain mostly silent as they strive to comprehend fundamental properties of their native language. Beyond this point, when children seem to talk endlessly, the silent period of the first language is not directly apparent, although it no doubt continues throughout the formidable language learning period.

Similarly, in the phonological dimension it has been suggested (Menyuk and Anderson, 1969) that knowledge about the phonemes and their articulatory correlates begins with perception. According to Menyuk and Anderson (1969), there are three stages in the development of perception and articulation. These stages, supported, in part, by recent research investigations (Eilers and Oller, 1976; Winitz et al., 1981), are as follows:

1.  Perception and articulation have not developed.
2.  Perception has developed, but articulation has not developed.
3.  Both perception and articulation have developed.

All three stages are regarded as developmental events and should be taken into account when analyzing the relationship between auditory discrimination and articulation performance. The usual procedure, however, is to regard stages 1 and 3 as providing legitimate evidence for the existence of a positive relationship between discrimination and articulation, and stage 2 as evidence that no relationship exists between these two functions (Locke, 1980a,b). When analyzed in this way stage 2 is not recognized as a normal developmental event. Rather, it is viewed as evidence that a relationship does not exist between auditory discrimination and articulation performance. We believe this conclusion to be incorrect as the percentage of children in each investigation who fall within stage 2 is unknown, but nonetheless their presence attenuates the correlation between articulation and discrimination when traditional statistical tests are applied. An alternate experimental procedure involves a determination of the number of children who fall within each of the three stages identified above (Eilers and Oller, 1976; Winitz et al., 1981). When children are classified according to subgroups there is less chance that the relationship between discrimination and articulation will be obscured.

## ADDITIONAL REASONS THAT MAY CONTRIBUTE TO
## THE INCONSISTENT CORRELATION BETWEEN
## AUDITORY DISCRIMINATION AND ARTICULATION PERFORMANCE

### Effect of Clinical Training

There are a number of other possible conditions that may reduce the correlation between articulation and auditory discrimination. One involves the amount of experience subjects have had in a clinical setting. For example, in one investigation (Wilcox and Stephens, 1982) in which the results were equivocal, the age of the subjects was 7.5 years, and there was no indication as to whether or not they had received or were receiving speech instruction. From the details provided in that investigation, which involved six children with /s/ errors, we do not know whether the children were receiving speech instruction. It is generally recognized, however, that auditory discrimination directly or indirectly plays a significant role in articulation training. In the standard imitation-production training procedure, clinicians provide auditory stimulation of the target sound several times, and frequently contrast it with the error sound. Below we discuss a training method called the *minimal pair approach* and indicate that discrimination practice is a major component of this articulation training procedure. Therefore, children who receive clinical training are not appropriate candidates to assess the relationship between articulation and discrimination as they receive, no doubt, a considerable amount of practice in auditory discrimination during the course of articulation instruction.

### Accuracy of Children's Performance

Poor test taking performance may sometime account for the inconsistent relationship between auditory discrimination and articulation performance. Usually, the traditional testing format involves a response of same or different by the child to the presentation of two sounds. In some cases the child's task is to select, from two or more pictures, the picture named by the clinician. Some children may respond in a random fashion in these testing situations. This consideration is particularly noteworthy when a small number of subjects is studied or subjects serve as their own control.

Locke (1980b) recommended that a neutral set of sounds be added to the discrimination test to assess the reliability of a child's performance. This procedural approach was followed in a recent investigation in our laboratory for which the results are currently being prepared for publication (Winitz et al., 1983). In that investigation we tested whether or not kindergarten children with [w] for [r] errors performed unreliably when tested on the discrimination between [w] and [r]. The standard format was used in which the child heard one of three experimental pair types in varying vowel contexts, namely /w-r/, /w-w/ and /r-r/, and was to indicate whether the items of each pair were the same or different. The control phonemes were /k/ and /v/, that is /k-v/, /k-k/ and /v-v/ interspersed throughout the discrimination list. In both the control group (children without /r/ errors) and in the experimental group (children without /r/ errors) the children scored close to perfect on this neutral sound contrast, and yet the experimental children's score on the /r/-/w/ items was considerably below that of the control children. These results indicate that the children in both groups understood the task required of them and performed reliably.

Of interest is the finding that one or two children in both groups performed poorly on the neutral sounds. One might conclude that these children did not understand the task or that they were unable to discriminate between /k/ and /v/. The latter explanation is unlikely. Almost certainly their scores reflect inattentiveness rather than an inability to discriminate accurately among the neutral sounds which they articulated correctly.

Also of interest is the finding that for the normal speaking children the discrimination between /r/ and /w/ proved to be more difficult than between the /k/-/v/ items. Possibly, /r/-/w/ discrimination is an inherently difficult perceptual task, and that native speakers utilize extraphonetic cues in making /r/-/w/ distinctions in natural speech.

Linguistic extraphonetic cues include expectancies about grammatical units, phonotactic sequences, and words as they occur in running speech. With regard to /r/, a few examples of each are given. Grammatical units involve elements such as the prefix *re*, as in *redo* and the agentive *er* as in *reporter*; phonotactic sequences are *pr* in *print* and *rd* in *board*; illustrative words are *rest* in the context of *sleep, exhaustion*, and *sickness*, and *print* used in the context of *sentence, paper*, and *writing*. Thus, for example, a young child who does not hear the difference between /r/ and /w/ will no doubt respond appropriately to the sentences "You're tired, I want you to *rest* now," and "Put the *wing* on the airplane" as linguistic context provides little choice here. Additionally, with young children, situational cues that involve objects and events in the immediate environment are usually prominent.

The fact that young children may vary in performance on sound discrimination pairs when different sounds are involved points up an important clinical issue. Control sound pair items may be used to assess the reliability of children's attentiveness; however, they cannot be used as a measure against which discrimination performance can be compared. The reason is that there are no doubt different performance levels of achievement for different sounds when used as items in discrimination tests. For example, performance on /r/-/w/ pairs and control pairs may differ substantially, but there is no way to know whether this difference is meaningful without information from control subjects, as the difference in performance between the control items and the experimental items may lie in the inherent difference in difficulty of the two types of items. For example, a child who obtains a score of 95% on the neutral items and only 80% on the test items (e.g., /r/-/w/ or /s/-/θ/) may be performing this way because the test items are inherently more difficult than the neutral items. Without testing control subjects, the relative difference in difficulty between neutral and test items is unknown. It is not difficult to test control groups, although it is time consuming because paired items for each specific discrimination test must be evaluated, and should include norms for several age levels.

Although Locke (1980b) was the first one to employ neutral sound pairs as control items, his procedures did not take into account the inherent difference in difficulty between the experimental items and the neutral items. Therefore, it is difficult to interpret the auditory discrimination scores of the children in his study without knowing the relative difference in difficulty between experimental and neutral items.

## Type of Item and Context in Which It Occurs

A wide range of linguistic items currently is used in discrimination testing. They include words, syllables, and sentences. Each of these units of expression may affect differentially the performance of children as each may be correlated with other factors such as age, type of sound error, overall level of severity and amount of clinical training. Thorough attention should be given to the linguistic units of the test item in discrimination testing, in order to determine their influence on test results.

## Age

The factor of age and its effect on the relationship between articulation and discrimination deserves considerable investigation. As indicated by Weiner (1967), the relationship between articulation and discrimination decreases as age increases. However, this interpretation is based on a small number of studies of older children and adults (Winitz, 1969). Yet if this observation by Weiner is correct, then the effect of age on the discrimination performance of children who evidence misarticulations deserves attention. Conceivably, there are some children who may achieve normal auditory discrimination (Stage 2 above), but may be unable to achieve normal articulation (Stage 3). It is important to understand the factors that contribute to their delay in articulation development. In particular, they should be compared with children who also have below average auditory discrimination skills, but who acquire normal articulation.

### UNDERLYING PHONOLOGICAL STRUCTURE

Auditory discrimination tests examine a client's ability to distinguish between sounds. In this regard they are largely tests of perceptual performance. They do not indicate whether the source of the difficulty is sensory or the result of a phonological system that processes sounds differently from the adult system. In any event, when children fail to distinguish reliably between two sounds a reasonable inference is that the phonologic structure for these two sounds is not the same as that for mature speakers of the language. For example, when children do not discriminate between [r] and [w] one can assume that the phonological structure for these two sounds is not the same as for the adult language user.

On the other hand, when children demonstrate that their auditory discrimination is normal we know that they can capably make the perceptual distinctions between sounds that their language requires. It does not necessarily follow, however, that they *utilize* these distinctions in speech. They may only attend to certain perceptual distinctions when asked to do so in a formal testing situation.

The next step is to do a thorough phonological analysis in order to gain some insight as to the underlying phonological structure of children who misarticulate. A number of procedures is available, but one recommended by Weismer et al. (1981) is useful. They advise that a large number of phonological contexts be examined for consistency in production. For example, the medial and final contexts are useful for the examination of the /r/ phoneme, as in the following hypothetical illustration:

| Final  | hear    | /hɪ/    |
| Medial | hearing | /hɪrɪŋ/ |
| Final  | tear    | /tɛ/    |
| Medial | tearing | /tɛrɪŋ/ |
| Final  | care    | /kɛ/    |
| Medial | caring  | /kɛrɪŋ/ |

On the basis of the child's use of /r/ in the medial position of the words *hearing, tearing* and *caring*, it may be assumed that the child's underlying phonologic structure for the words *hear, tear*, and *care* contains a final /r/ phoneme. The reason for the deletion of the [r] sound in the final word position and not in the medial position cannot be determined from this analysis.

The deletion of /r/ in word final position can be described by using a linguistic rule that specifies the sounds or distinctive features that are omitted, but the linguistic rule does not provide the reason for this psychological behavior. It only states the conditions under which it takes place. For the example given immediately above, it would be helpful to know whether the child discriminates between /r/ and omission of /r/ in word-final position. This information may provide additional understanding of the child's underlying phonological structure, and may suggest at what point in the articulatory process the breakdown occurs.

Conceivably, the breakdown may occur at one of several levels. For example, the child may not discriminate the /r/ from omission of the /r/ in word final position. Or the child may make this discrimination, but has acquired a special phonological rule which specifies that /r/ is to be deleted in word-final position. Other hypotheses may be generated also for the use of the phonological deletion rule. Possibly, there are articulatory constraints associated with the [r] consonantal sound in word-final position. Or possibly, the child's personal implicit learning strategy is that /r/ in final position conveys little information, as in English /r/-less dialects, and that other language units require more attention (Winitz, 1969).

Consider one more example. Two children who evidence the process of cluster reduction for frequent double /s/ clusters have the following errors:

| Target word | Child 1's response | Child 2's response |
|---|---|---|
| smell | /wɛl/ | /dɛl/ |
| snow | /dou/ | /dou/ |
| swim | /bɪm/ | /dɪm/ |
| spin | /bɪn/ | /dɪn/ |
| step | /dɛp/ | /dɛp/ |
| skip | /gɪp/ | /dɪp/ |

From this analysis we can infer that the first child's underlying phonological representation is not the same for each /s/ cluster. We can further guess that the child's discrimination is probably normal, although discrimination testing is still recommended to determine whether the child's auditory discrimination is normal. The responses of the second child indicate that the underlying structure for each double /s/ cluster is probably the same. However, we cannot be confident of this conclusion without testing the child's auditory discrimination for these clusters. Conceivably, this child may be able to distinguish among the several /s/ clusters, and between each /s/ cluster and /d/. We might then conclude that the second child's errors have a phonological and/ or articulatory basis rather than a perceptual basis.

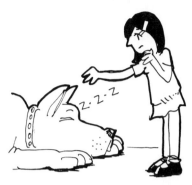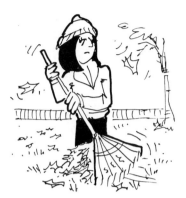

Figure 1.    Phonological Performance Analysis Test.
I was to rake it up.
I didn't want to rake it up.
Finally I was told to rake it up.

I was to wake it up.
I didn't want to wake it up.
Finally I was told to wake it up.

It should be recognized that a phonological analysis provides only a starting point for understanding a particular child's articulation errors. It must be supplemented by other types of information. We have recommended that auditory discrimination testing may provide an important source of information. Additionally, we would like to propose another source of information that we have found to be useful in understanding children's articulation errors.

We have entitled this approach "phonological performance analysis." The purpose of this analysis is to determine whether contrastive test sounds in the ambient language which are perceptually distinctive for a child are regarded as functionally equivalent. The procedure is as follows. The clinician tells the child to listen to three sentences, and when they are completed two pictures will be presented. At that time the clinician tells the child to select the picture which best represents the meaning of the three sentences. In each sentence the same word (e.g., rake) from a single minimal pair is used. At a later point of the testing, the contrastive word (e.g., wake) is examined for the same three sentences.

In Figures 1–3 sentences for three different test items are given. In each sentence the target word begins with /r/ or /w/. For example, for the first item each subject is presented in an individual testing session with the following sentences in which the word *rake* occurs:

I was to *rake* it up.
I didn't want to *rake* it up.
Finally I was told to *rake* it up.

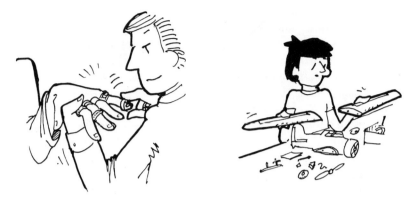

Figure 2.    Phonological Performance Analysis Test.
He said to put the rings on.
I didn't want to put the rings on.
But he said the rings should be put on.

He said to put the wings on.
I didn't want to put the wings on.
But he said the wings should be put on.

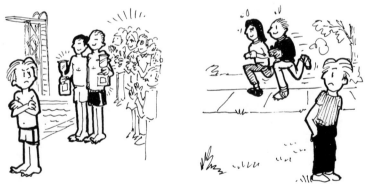

Figure 3.    Phonological Performance Analysis Test.
They've always run.
I've never run.
But they've always run.

They've always won.
I've never won.
But they've always won.

At this point the subject is presented with the two pictures illustrated in Figure 1, and is told to select the picture which the three sentences describe best. If /r/ and /w/ are conceptualized as the same phoneme, then, when contextually free sentences, as illustrated above, are heard, the meaning of the sentences should be ambiguous. In other words, when words beginning with /r/ or /w/ are conceptualized as the same then a child's performance on this task should be random or 50% with a forced choice two picture task. The child may perform randomly on the phonological performance test even though he or she can discriminate between /r/ and /w/, presumably, because the underlying phonological representation is the same for these two sounds.

Experiments are now being carried out in our laboratory with this instrument and with a number of others similar in design, in order to gain an understanding of where the breakdown in articulation occurs. The preliminary results indicate that children whose auditory discrimination for /r/-/w/ is impaired find phonological performance tasks (Winitz et al., 1983) to be somewhat difficult. If these results prove to be reliable, then it may be said that a deficiency in auditory discrimination reflects a breakdown in underlying phonological structure. Additionally, phonological performance testing must be done with children who misarticulate sounds, but who show normal auditory discrimination.

## CLINICAL IMPLICATIONS

The evidence as reviewed above strongly suggests that auditory discrimination is an important consideration in the treatment of children with articulation disorders. A number of issues surface, however, when clinical application becomes the primary objective. Each of several issues is considered separately.

### Single Sound Errors

When a child has only one or two sounds in error, and these errors seem to be unrelated, as when both /r/ and /s/ errors are present, one approach is to provide discrimination training for each sound separately. According to this approach, the child is asked to make distinctions between paired sound contrasts that involve the error sound and the target sound, or between /w/ and /r/, and /s/ and /θ/, for example. Units of training may involve syllables, words, and sentences. The objective is to teach the child to react quickly and correctly to the appropriate phonetic distinctions.

## Related Sound Errors

When multiple sounds are in error and the sound errors cluster into a pattern, as determined by a phonological analysis, the sounds for a particular pattern may be grouped together in discrimination training. For example, when children substitute stops for fricatives, all appropriately paired stop-fricative distinctions are selected for training. According to this approach, stopping is regarded as an underlying phonological process or pattern which should be treated as a unitary disorder, and not as a collection of unrelated errors.

Two options for treating disordered phonological patterns are available to clinicians. The first is to select one contrast from the group of potential discrimination contrasts and initially train this one in discrimination. As soon as the child is successful with this single pair, all other pairs are introduced. For example, for the stopping pattern the clinician may select the t/s substitution first, and train discrimination between /t/ and /s/. When the child can capably discriminate the items of this pair, all other pairs involving stop errors are introduced according to some preformulated schedule of generalization.

The selection of the initial sound pair may be based on a number of factors. Although these factors have not been tested at this time, some that may be useful are the magnitude of the phonetic difference between the target sound and the error sound, the frequency of the sound contrast in the language, and the person's use of already acquired distinctions in a limited number of linguistic or phonetic contexts.

The second option is to train all sound contrasts at the same time. For example, the clinician may select a single phonological process, such as stopping, and train all or a large number of representative samples of stop fricative distinctions in each lesson. As yet we do not know whether this approach provides for greater generalization than the first procedure (Hodson, 1982).

## INTRODUCTION OF PRODUCTION PRACTICE

Another decision the clinician has to make is when to introduce production practice in articulation. I have observed three approaches which may be regarded as three points on the same continuum. According to Winitz (1975, 1981c), one approach is to provide intensive discrimination training before production practice in order to ensure that the child has acquired the difference between the appropriate contrasting sound units, and has internalized this difference as part of his or her underlying phonological structure.

Intensive discrimination may be conducted over several months and usually includes a comprehensive program of instruction. The target sound is contrasted with the error sound in a great number of phonetic contexts and linguistic units. There is no attempt at any point to force articulation production. During this time the child may show spontaneous improvement in articulation performance, and there may be no need to conduct formal training in articulation. Winitz (1981a) likens this process to that of learning a first language, where the child is given the opportunity to acquire grammatical rules through experience in comprehending the language. In this approach the child is not prohibited from talking. In fact, as described below, the discrimination activities are designed to elicit the spontaneous use of target sounds.

When the clinician is firmly convinced that auditory discrimination training produces no further progress in articulation improvement, practice in articulation production is begun. This decision is not an easy one to make. Often children require a fairly long period of listening experience before spontaneous progress in articulation production is observed. It is often tempting to step over the auditory discrimination preparatory stage because progress in articulation performance is usually gauged by achievement in production rather than by listening. In a similar vein Robbins Burling (1982) raises this issue when he notes that traditional teaching practices in foreign language education stress how one should sound rather than how one should listen. Listening, it seems, is yet to be recognized as an important dimension of language and speech training.

A more traditional approach is to provide auditory discrimination training in combination with practice in articulation. The clinician provides some minimal practice in auditory discrimination either by stimulating the child with the correct sound or by presenting contrasting pairs. Sometimes the discrimination training is relatively brief and occurs only occasionally throughout the training session. At other times it can be fairly extensive. Van Riper (1939–1978), throughout his career, has recommended that auditory discrimination training should be extensive, systematic, and presented before production practice. He does not indicate, however, how intensive the discrimination practice should be, and when to begin production practice. Additionally, he recommends that discrimination and production training should be mixed across four sequentially presented linguistic levels by providing training in both these skills for each level. The four levels are: the sound in isolation, in syllables, in isolated words, and in words in sentences. Thus, Van Riper advocates discrimination training first in isolation followed by production practice in isolation, and then discrimination training followed by production practice again for each of the next three linguistic levels.

A third approach is to provide almost no formal discrimination practice (Ingram, 1976; Weiner, 1981), and to introduce minimal pair contrasts through training in articulation. This approach has been called the "minimal pair approach" although it should be recognized that minimal pair contrasts are used in discrimination routines which involve contrasting items. In the minimal pair approach, the target sound and the error sound are introduced simultaneously into the training session. A number of different procedures has been used, but essentially they involve practice in saying the error sound and the target sound together as a way to change a child's underlying phonological structure and to improve articulation.

It is interesting to speculate why articulation practice is often regarded by linguists and speech pathologists as the primary procedure to effect change in phonological structure (Compton, 1970; Ingram, 1976; Weiner, 1981). The reason may be in the way they conceptualize phonological disorders. There are at least two ways that are of immediate interest to us: (1) the underlying phonological structure is different from the community language; and (2) the underlying phonological structure is correct, but the output from this base component, as explained below, is incorrect.

Articulatory practice, although used frequently, is not necessarily an obvious procedure for correcting underlying phonological structure that is different from the community language. As a first step, attention to discrimination training and auditory experience would seem to be the most reasonable approach to take, as the problem involves a breakdown in the conceptualization of underlying phonological structure. This approach is consonant with our earlier remarks in that a major purpose of discrimination training is to provide perceptual experiences that will help a child develop a normal phonological system.

When a child's underlying phonological representation is regarded as correct, the use of articulation production training as the primary method of treatment is common. This approach is taken because the breakdown in the articulation process is believed to be due to "natural processes" that simplify or change correct underlying phonological representations to developmentally less mature articulatory forms (Shriberg and Kwiatkowski, 1980; Smith, 1973). For example, the /r/ may be represented correctly in a child's mental dictionary in that all words which contain an /r/ in the adult language are represented by an /r/ phoneme in the child's language, yet the child may utilize also a phonological rule beyond this point to change the [r] to a [w] or to omit it. Thus, according to the natural process theory the child, in effect, implicitly knows that /r/ is correct, but because of certain constraints imposed on the phonological or articulatory systems, changes the /r/ to an incorrect phonetic form. These constraints are not well explained. One explanation is that certain articulatory forms are more natural or simpler than others, and are likely to occur more readily or earlier in development.

In standard English there are many examples of phonological simplification. Speakers alter underlying phonological representation as a matter of course. For example, almost all English speakers delete the /f/ in the word *of* in phrases such as *cupa coffee* and *glassa milk*. This perfectly normal alteration does not mean, of course that speakers of English do not know implicitly that *a* is a replacement for the word *of*. Another example, one given by Belasco (1981), is the unit *amina* which when said is isolation many individuals are unable to recover easily the appropriate underlying phonological form. Yet in the sentence: *amina go home* all native speakers recognize that *amina* means *I am going to*. When pressed, native English speakers also admit that *amina* cannot be used in the context *amina New York*. The syntactic usage of the word *to* in the second sentence is a preposition and not part of the infinitive construction. We see, then, that although simplification is common in adult speech, its use is governed by complex linguistic rules. In this particular example the correct underlying representation for *anima* is *I am going to* + (verb).

What should be the primary treatment procedure for children when the underlying phonological representation is correct? Consider children whose articulation is regarded as defective because [w] is substituted for consonantal [r]. Furthermore, let us assume that the children's mental dictionary contains the /r/ and /w/ as distinct phonological units. In this situation we would expect that the children would be able to discriminate easily between /r/ and /w/. It does not necessarily follow, however, that procedures of training should start with articulatory production practice (Compton, 1970; Ingram, 1976; Weiner, 1981), especially if articulatory constraints are still in force when articulation training is begun. These constraints are not necessarily released by practicing articulatory movements. Perhaps it may be more advantageous to teach children to recognize that they are doing something that is different from the standard patterns of the community speakers which they need to change.

More than likely, when articulation practice is used, children soon learn, either directly through instruction or indirectly through untutored experience, that certain changes are to be made in the way sounds are conceptualized. Conceptual understanding of these changes may not necessarily come about because the production of sounds is practiced, but rather because through production practice there is the constant reminder that sounds are used incorrectly as Weiner (1981), in fact, suggests. Therefore, our recommendation is that auditory experience be the initial and sole focus of training in order to demonstrate to children with this type of disorder that their pattern of behavior is different from the community norm. At some later time articulatory practice may be necessary to correct articulatory errors, but initially the training should emphasize the teaching of correct sound patterns through auditory experience within communicative contexts (Winitz, 1975).

## RELATIONSHIP BETWEEN AUDITORY EXPERIENCE AND ARTICULATION

When auditory discrimination is recommended as a primary procedure in articulation training, two questions are usually asked. First, the question is raised as to whether or not discrimination training alone can produce a change in articulation performance, and second, clinicians want to know the conditions under which auditory training is to be recommended.

The research results indicate that there are circumstances under which auditory discrimination training will result in improvement in articulation without production practice (Winitz and Preisler, 1965). Winitz (1975, 1981c) has speculated that auditory training will probably effect a change in articulatory production for those sounds for which the underlying phonological structure is correct or becomes correct through training, and whose articulatory features appear as correct elements of other sounds. For example, for a child who substitutes t/n auditory training of the contrast /n/-/t/ may result in the spontaneous articulation of /n/ if the child learns from this training that /n/ and /t/ are independent phonemes in the underlying structure of the adult language, and the articulatory features of *nasal* and *voice*, as in /m/ or /ŋ/, are correctly articulated, and therefore, generalize to /n/ through discrimination training. A study which supports this conclusion is an investigation of children with /r/ errors for whom intensive discrimination training produced no improvement in articulation performance (Winitz and Bellerose, 1967). None of the children had acquired previously the gestures of partial retroflexion or bunching that are required in the production of /r/, although through training they had learned that /r/ and /w/ are different phonological elements. Our conclusion, then, is that auditory training without articulation practice will produce a change in articulation only when children can capably make the articulatory features required of the sounds that are defective (Winitz, 1975).

This particular finding that discrimination training may not result in correct articulatory production when articulatory features are not present in a child's sound repertoire does not demonstrate that discrimination experience is unimportant. Rather auditory discrimination training is regarded as a necessary, but not a sufficient condition for sound learning. The reason auditory discrimination training is regarded as necessary is because it enables a child to acquire the phonological distinctions of the language and to conceptualize correctly its phonological structure without undue emphasis on articulatory production.

An interesting clinical issue is whether the goal of training is to teach correct underlying structure for all sounds that are misarticulated or only certain sounds or sound groups. Hodson (1982), for example, approaches this issue by treating certain patterns of errors (phonological processes) first while delaying treatment of others. Her motivation for taking this point of view may be that she places emphasis in treatment almost entirely on practice in articulatory production. When auditory experience is regarded as a primary approach, however, it does not seem unreasonable to take the point of view that training should be directed to a child's entire sound system. If this approach is taken, auditory training, as described below, will probably extend over a period of many months. It would not be unusual, in severe cases, to last a full year.

## IMITATION TRAINING AND AUDITORY DISCRIMINATION

Auditory discrimination training is not necessarily restricted to paired items. Auditory experience with single sound input also can be regarded as a form of auditory discrimination training.

The traditional clinical format consists of stimulus-imitation cycles in which the clinician says the target sound and then requests that the child repeat it. Usually the clinician says the target sounds several times in each stimulus-imitation cycle. This clinical approach involves a large amount of stimulus input. The child hears the target sound many times during the course of training. More important, the child knows that he or she will be asked to repeat the sound, and for this reason listens attentively.

It is not clear at this time what listening dimensions are brought to bear when persons know in advance that they will be asked to repeat a sound. Under this circumstance they probably do their best to track the acoustic properties of the target sound carefully in order to replicate the sound correctly. Part of this process may involve internal mental comparisons between the target sound and other sounds with which the child is familiar. In this regard, the single stimulus input approach may provide the same auditory function as paired item discrimination training, but in a less effective way.

In the early phases of articulation training, children may utilize their own error productions in this comparative process. They may hold in temporary memory each error response and compare it with the immediately preceding production of the target sound provided by the clinician. This comparative process has been called internal auditory monitoring in contrast to external auditory monitoring which involves comparisons between two sounds produced by another speaker. Some investigators have speculated that children with articulation errors may be able to discriminate between sounds presented externally, although unable to discriminate between an externally produced target sound and an internally produced error sound.

If indeed internal auditory monitoring is difficult for children in the early stages of articulation training, then they may need to rely on the clinician's evaluation as to the correctness of their production. It may take many clinical sessions before they can evaluate correctly their own articulatory responses.

The motorical activity involved in making an articulatory production may not directly contribute to the process of internal monitoring. Forced production may provide a situation in which children are encouraged to make internal auditory evaluations, often before they are able to make external auditory evaluations. It is unknown as to whether internal auditory monitoring takes place before or after correct articulation is achieved, and whether experience in external monitoring is necessary for internal auditory monitoring. Our position is that external auditory training is critically important for the development of internal auditory monitoring. In order to accelerate the process of internal auditory monitoring some clinicians have children listen to their own tape recorded error productions. Also, some clinicians use tape delay recording systems so that a child may compare his or her production with the target sound a fraction of a second after it is produced.

The traditional clinical format of stimulus-imitation cycles provides extensive auditory input that is no doubt an important part of the articulation acquisition process. In fact, in this regard it is difficult to separate the auditory component from the production component. For example, in one study (Williams and McReynolds, 1975) an attempt was made to assess the relative effect of auditory discrimination training on articulatory production. However, those children who received no discrimination training were given extensive auditory input as part of the production training task. The effect of auditory input on improvement in articulation was not assessed in that investigation, but no doubt it was an important contributing factor in the way we have speculated above.

## FORMAL AND INFORMAL METHODS OF AUDITORY TRAINING

Auditory discrimination training has been administered traditionally as a formal or conscious activity. Usually, the clinician tells the child to listen carefully and to try to distinguish between certain speech sounds. The child is often told that this activity is an important part of learning how to say a sound correctly.

There is another procedure that can be used to teach children to listen attentively and appropriately. It involves informal methods of auditory training (Winitz, 1975). Here the clinician does not direct the child's conscious attention to the auditory discrimination activities. Instead, the discrimination training is part of more general language training activities.

In the informal approach, the clinician selects items and objects that represent minimal pairs, and utilizes these in highly motivating, goal directed activities. The term *goal directed* means that each activity has as its purpose the completion of an objective or goal. For example, if the /k/ and /t/ phonemes are selected for training, the clinician will select a variety of items for which /t/ and /k/ contrast. Some word pair contrasts are *key*: *tea, tape*: *cape, cable*: *table*, and *tar*: *car*. Each of these pairs is used in game-like activities that have specific objectives. For example, the clinician may wish to help the child make a small paper table, and use small cable like wires in another craft activity.

The activities should be regarded as authentic by the child. When the clinician, for example, requests, "Give me that part over there for the table," the child is being told to respond appropriately by bringing the correct item to the clinician. If instead a part that goes with the cable activity is brought over, the clinician may respond, "No this is for the cable, that is for the table." As far as the child is concerned the activities of table building and the use of cables are real, have a purpose, and involve careful listening in order to participate.

A large number of activities can be developed that include games, arts and crafts, painting, grooming, and miniature work sessions. At no time is the child directly told to listen. Instead, the child listens in order to participate in the activity. It is a procedure that I have found to be personally satisfying and one in which I find children to be highly attentive. Some of the specific activities that we have used are hand tracing, sorting rocks into various sizes, playing darts, blowing bubbles, preparing for snack time, potting plants, and feeding fish. It is important to remember, however, that certain specific items are pre-selected for each task in order to emphasize predesignated phonological contrasts.

This approach is not widely used in discrimination training. However, it teaches the child to listen attentively and to attend implicitly to speech sounds. Conceivably, many of these children may no longer be responding appropriately to many phonetic cues in the language that is directed to them. Children with many articulation errors may appear to discriminate fairly well. However, the language directed to them may be fairly simple in content and may contain situational cues that enable them to understand most of what they hear. Children with few articulation errors may no longer be attending to phonetic cues because linguistic cues readily assign meaning to most words when language is fairly complex. Children, for example, who misarticulate only /r/, and who do not distinguish between /r/ and /w/ will rarely have difficulty understanding language that is directed to them, as /r/ and /w/ contrast infrequently in spoken speech. Usually words that contain /r/ and /w/ as constrastive elements, such as *rag* and *wag*, *wound* and *round*, and *rent* and *went*, represent different parts of speech or different subcategories within each part of speech. For example, it would be rare that the verbs *went* and *rent* would be misunderstood as *rent* contrasts with *go* in present tense, and *rented* with *went* in past tense. Thus, for children with many errors and children with few articulation errors discrimination training is recommended to enable them to refocus their attention on phonetic cues to which they no longer attend.

As children learn to attend to phonetic cues in the context of goal directed activities they will probably extend this process beyond the walls of the clinic. Their natural response will be to listen attentively to these same phonetic cues in other settings. In this way their language and discrimination skills will grow together. In some instances, their articulation may show spontaneous improvement because they are attending to phonetic cues that are communicatively relevant.

## SUMMARY

The importance of auditory discrimination in the treatment of articulation disorders was considered. In the past, the validity of auditory discrimination training has been challenged because in some investigations an inconsistent relationship between articulation and discrimination has been observed. This inconsistency is largely the result of factors, such as the relevancy of the discrimination items, the child's specific error, the phonetic context in which the error occurs, and the relationship between the development of articulation and discrimination. When these factors are controlled for, the relationship between auditory discrimination and articulation performance is fairly strong. When children with articulation errors show a deficit in auditory discrimination skills, their underlying phonological system may also be defective. Clinical procedures which emphasize intensive auditory discrimination training as a way to correct a deficiency in underlying phonological structure or in the use of phonological rules were described.

## REFERENCES

Asher, J. J., and Garcia, R. 1969. The optimal age to learn a foreign language. Modern Lang. J. 53:334–341.
Belasco, S. 1981. Aital cal aprene las lengas estrangièras, Comprehension: The key to second language learning. In: H. Winitz (ed.), The Comprehension Approach to Foreign Language Instruction. Newbury House, Rowley, MA.
Bountress, N. G., and Laderberg, C. M. 1981. A comparison of two tests of speech-sound discrimination. J. Commun. Disord. 14:149–156.
Burling, R. 1982. Sounding Right. Newbury House, Rowley, MA.
Compton, A. J. 1970. Generative studies of children's phonological disorders. J. Speech Hear. Disord. 35:315–335.
Carroll, J. B. 1961. The Study of Language, A Survey of Linguistics and Related Disciplines in America. Harvard University Press, Cambridge, MA.
Eilers, R. E., and Oller, D. K. 1976. The role of speech discrimination in developmental sound substitutions. J. Child Lang. 3:319–329.
Goldman, R., Fristoe, M., and Woodcock, R. 1970. The Goldman-Fristoe-Woodcock Test of Auditory Discrimination. American Guidance Service, Circle Pines, MN.
Haas, W. 1963. Phonological analysis of a case of dyslalia. J. Speech Hear. Disord. 28:239–246.
Hodson, B. W. 1982. Remediation of speech patterns associated with low levels of phonological performance. In: M. Crary (ed.), Phonological Intervention, Concepts and Procedures. College Hill Press, San Diego, CA.
Ingram, D. 1976. Phonological Disability in Children. American Elsevier, New York.
Kornfield, J. 1971. What initial clusters tell us about a child's speech code. Massachusetts Institute of Technology Research Laboratory of Electronics, Quarterly Press Report, 218–221.
Lenneberg, E. H. 1967. Biological Foundations of Language. Wiley, New York.
Locke, J. L. 1968. Discrimination learning in children's acquisition of phonology. J. Speech Hear. Res. 11:428–434.
Locke, J. L. 1980a. The inference of speech perception in the phonologically disordered child. Part I: A rationale, some criteria, the conventional tests. J. Speech Hear. Disord 45:431–44.
Locke, J. L. 1980b. The inference of speech perception in the phonologically disordered child. Part II: Some clinically novel procedures, their use, some findings. J. Speech Hear. Disord. 45:445–468.
McReynolds, L. V., Kohn, J., and Williams, G. C. 1975. Articulatory-defective children's discrimination of their production errors. J. Speech Hear. Disord. 40:327–338.

Menyuk, P., and Anderson, S. 1969. Children's identification and reproduction of /w/, /r/, and /l/. J. Speech Hear. Res. 5:39–52.

Monnin, L. M., and Huntington, D. A. 1974. Relationship of articulatory defects to speech-sound identification. J. Speech Hear. Res. 17:352–366.

Newmark, L. 1981. Participatory observation: How to succeed in language learning. In: H. Winitz (ed.), The Comprehension Approach to Foreign Language Instruction. Newbury House, Rowley, MA.

Shriberg, L. D., and Kwiatkowski, J. 1980. Natural Process Analysis (NPA): A Procedure for Phonological Analysis of Continuous Speech Samples. Wiley, New York.

Smith, N. V. 1973. The Acquisition of Phonology, a Case Study. Cambridge University Press, London.

Snow, C. E., and Hoefnagel-Höhle, M. 1977. Age difference in pronunciation of foreign sounds. Lang. Speech 20:357–365.

Spriestersbach, D. C., and Curtis, J. F. 1951. Misarticulation and discrimination of speech sounds. Q. J. Speech 37:483–491.

Strange, W., and Broen, P. A. 1981. The relationship between perception and production of /w/, /r/, and /l/ by three-year-old children. J. Exp. Child Psychol. 31:81–102.

Templin, M. C. 1957. Certain Language Skills in Children, Their Development and Interrelationships. Institute of Child Welfare, Monograph Series, No. 26. University of Minnesota Press, Minneapolis.

Van Riper, C. 1939–1978. Speech Correction, Principles and Methods. Prentice-Hall, New York.

Weiner, F. 1981. Treatment of Phonological disability using the method of meaningful minimal contrast: Two case studies. J. Speech Hear. Disord. 46:97–103.

Weiner, P. S. 1967. Auditory discrimination and articulation. J. Speech Hear. Disord. 32:19–28.

Weismer, G., Dinnsen, D., and Elbert, M. 1981. A study of the voicing distinction associated with omitted, word-final stops. J. Speech Hear. Disord. 46:320–327.

Wepman, J. M. 1958. Auditory Discrimination Test. Language Research Associates, Chicago.

Wilcox, K. A., and Stephens, M. I. 1982. Childrens identification of their own /s/ misarticulations. J. Commun. Disord. 15:127–134.

Williams, G. S., and McReynolds, L. V. 1975. The relationship between discrimination and articulation training in children with misarticulations. J. Speech Hear. Res. 40:401–412.

Winitz, H. 1969. Articulatory Acquisition and Behavior. Appleton-Century-Crofts, New York.

Winitz, H. 1975. From Syllable to Conversation. University Park Press, Baltimore.

Winitz, H. 1981a. Nonlinear learning and language teaching. In: H. Winitz (ed.), The Comprehension Approach to Foreign Language Instruction. Newbury House, Rowley, MA.

Winitz, H. 1981b. The Comprehension Approach to Foreign Language Instruction. Newbury House, Rowley, MA.

Winitz, H. 1981c. Considerations in the treatment of articulation disorders. In: R. W. Rieber (ed.), Communication Disorders. Plenum Press, New York.

Winitz, H. 1981d. The comprehension approach: An introduction. In: H. Winitz (ed.), The Comprehension Approach to Foreign Language Instruction. Newbury House, Rowley, MA.

Winitz, H. 1983. Use and abuse of the developmental approach. In: H. Winitz (ed.), Treating Language Disorders, For Clinicians By Clinicians. University Park Press, Baltimore.

Winitz, H., and Bellerose, B. 1962. Sound discrimination as a function of pretraining conditions. J. Speech Hearing Res. 5:340–348.

Winitz, H., and Bellerose, B. 1963. Effects of pretraining on sound discrimination learning. J. Speech Hear. Res. 6:171–180.

Winitz, H., and Bellerose, B. 1967. Relation between sound discrimination and sound learning. J. Commun. Disord. 1:215–235.

Winitz, H., and Preisler, L. 1965. Discrimination pretraining and sound learning. Percept. Motor Skills 20:905–916.

Winitz, H., and Reeds, J. 1975. Comprehension and Problem Solving as Strategies for Language Training. Mouton, Hague.

Winitz, H., Reeds, J. A., Burt, C., and Skotak, D. 1983. The effect of rate of speech, phonological performance, and general discrimination ability in assessing the auditory discrimination of children with articulatory errors of the /r/ phoneme. Unpublished manuscript.

Winitz, H., Sanders, R., and Kort, J. 1981. Comprehension and production of the /-əz/ plural allomorph. J. Psycholinguistic Res. 10:259–271.

# CHAPTER 3

# Consideration of Motor-Sensory Targets and a Problem in Perception

*Gloria Borden*

*Borden's chapter concentrates on recent research findings in the perception and production of speech with particular emphasis on feedback processes. Within this framework she discusses remedial techniques and procedures that are certain to gain attention in the future.*

1. *Contrast the three potential levels outlined by Borden at which feedback may be provided to the speech production system. In this regard, what do the terms* internal feedback, external feedback, *and* response feedback *mean?*

2. *Borden suggests that a primary consideration in articulation training is to bring the relationship between perception and production under voluntary control. What feedback procedures does she suggest might be used to achieve this relationship? Identify each remedial approach according to the three types of speech feedback presented by Borden. In particular define the term* conscious self-monitoring. *Do you agree with these procedures for articulation remediation?*

3. *In what ways can laboratory research in speech physiology, speech acoustics, and speech perception contribute to an understanding of the clinical process in treating articulation disorders? Describe areas of research that you feel should be emphasized.*

This chapter is a composite and expanded version of two talks: "Research in Motor Control: Implications for Articulation Therapy," Mt. Sinai Hospital, New York, March 27, 1981 and "Research in Speech Production and Speech Perception with Implications for Clinical Management," Northeast Regional Conference of the American Speech-Language-Hearing Association, Philadelphia, July 24, 1981.

THERE ARE MANY IMPLICATIONS for clinical management of articulation and resonance disorders to be found in the results of recent research in speech science. Speech science, or experimental phonetics, includes the study of the anatomy and physiology of speech, acoustics of speech, and perception of speech. Basic research into the ways in which normal people produce and perceive speech must ultimately relate to a better understanding of the breakdown of normal processes that we witness with speech and language disorders. Recently, many speech scientists have directed their attention to research on clinical populations, so the overlap between the two disciplines is becoming more obvious. Of course, the overlap is furthered when the speech pathologist and the speech scientist are the same person, as when a speech pathologist conducts research. While speech scientists are increasing their interest in the pathologies of speech, students of speech pathology are beginning to receive a comprehensive academic grounding in the physiology, acoustics, and perception of speech. These developments may result in increased research on the part of speech pathologists, an increase in collaborative efforts among researchers and clinicians, and an increase in research findings that will offer new ideas for clinical management.

The purpose of this chapter is to illustrate the relationship between findings from basic research in speech science and possibilities for clinical application by the speech pathologist. Three general areas of investigation will be applied to speech pathology: research on feedback, research on motor physiology, and research on the acoustics and perception of speech.

### RESEARCH ON FEEDBACK APPLIED TO SPEECH PATHOLOGY

Our ideas of how speakers use feedback—information on their performance—during speech have changed substantially between the 1950s and the 1980s due to research in this area. The changes in how we view speech feedback have important implications for clinical management.

There are at least three levels of the speech production system that can receive information about how the system is behaving. One information loop may reside entirely within the central nervous system and be predictive when the person is producing well-learned motor acts. At this level, parts of the brain may simulate the sensory results of motor patterns without having to wait for the actual sensations from the periphery. The cerebellum may "know" what consequences the actions of the cerebrum and the higher brainstem will have. Each of these areas may be informed about the others—an internal central feedback loop. We know (Evarts, 1971; 1979) that before movements occur, increased activity is recorded from the motor cortex, basal ganglia, and cerebellum, and blood flow studies implicate another area of the brain for speech—the long neglected supplementary motor cortex at the superior surface of the frontal lobes. Penfield and Roberts (1959) found by stimulation studies that this area was one of three areas of the cortex important for speech. Twenty years later, Lassen and his Scandinavian colleagues (1978) are suggesting, on the basis of blood flow studies, that the supplementary motor area is involved in the planning of sequential motor tasks. At the same time, speech-language pathologists are beginning to see the planning of speech as separate from its execution, not only in the traditional contrast between apraxia and dysarthria but in viewing other speech disorders. Researchers are investigating the respective roles played by the planning and execution processes in the speech of stutterers, the deaf, and those with articulation disorders. It may turn out that the planning and execution of speech are separated physiologically in the speaker as well as conceptually among theorists.

A second possible level of feedback may operate during speech movement and positional change. It may consist of feedback of our own muscle and joint activities as they are being activated. For speech, this information is primarily sensed by muscle spindles. Muscle spindles are specialized muscle fibers encapsulated and independently innervated, lying embedded in and parallel to the main fibers of the muscle. There are muscle spindles in the intercostal muscles regulating respiration, in the intrinsic muscles of the larynx, and in the intrinsic muscles of the tongue, especially prominent in the flexible part of the tongue just behind the tip. The consensus of scientific opinion at the moment is that muscle spindles transmit information on changes in muscle length that, when integrated with other muscle information, gives the sense of proprioception, the sense of movement and position of oneself. A muscle spindle is a complex sensor, for its activation involves not only afferent neurons, but it is also supplied with motoneurons called *gamma motoneurons* which are distinguished from the alpha motoneurons that supply the fibers of the main muscle. The gamma motoneurons are thought to keep the spindles tuned and maximally responsive.

It is impossible to interrupt proprioception of speech activity in humans short of applying surgical techniques to the spindle afferents, but researchers can investigate it indirectly by unexpectedly perturbing the movements of speech or by restraining movement with a bite block.

Also, researchers can study the deprivation of proprioceptive sensation in animals. One example of this research is a study by Polit and Bizzi (1978). They trained monkeys to point to a light—the lighted one among 10 lights in a row. The monkeys were not allowed to see their own arm pointing. The researchers randomly applied loads to the forearm 20% of the time, but the monkeys could always reach the correct final positions. Then the researchers severed the dorsal roots ($C_1$–$T_3$) thereby eliminating proprioception—verified because no stretch reflex was recorded—yet the monkeys could still point to the light as they had been taught, despite the changes in load placed upon the arm. One interpretation of this research is that learned skilled motor performance can operate without any feedback. Furthermore, it seems that when blocked from proceeding to its target, a limb can store the energy needed, according to some equilibrium point previously set, so that when the load is released, it simply springs forward to the target without reprogramming the gesture.

How about proprioception for speech? Again, normally skilled speakers seem to compensate immediately for any perturbation such as sudden unexpected loading (Folkins and Abbs, 1975) or speaking with a bite block (Lindblom and Sundberg, 1971). Although results from this kind of research are recent and tentative, their implications for articulation treatment are significant. They offer objective evidence of what we have feared—that any articulation strategies that have been well learned, however disordered, are operating largely under central control with little benefit of feedback from the periphery. To break them down in order to establish new strategies, one has to take rather extraordinary measures to force the speaker to experiment and try novel coordinated activities.

One way to facilitate new motor organization is to transduce the movements to visual signals for biofeedback training. Examples of signals that can be visualized on an oscilloscope are electromyography (muscle activity), laryngography (changes in impedance of a signal across the vocal folds), real time spectrography (changes in vocal tract resonances across time), and dynamic palatography (changing patterns of tongue contact with palate) (Borden and Harris, 1980). We look forward to the day when such instruments will be available in many speech-language pathology clinics.

Meanwhile, one can heighten an awareness of the sense of proprioception—the sense of movement and position—without biofeedback instruments, but it is often difficult. *Kinesthesia* is the term for conscious awareness of proprioception. In the clinic, kinesthesia often needs to be enhanced by coupling it with another sense—to watch the tongue tip elevate at the same time as one feels the movement helps to prepare the speaker for the exercise of sensing the movement with eyes closed. In situations for which vision is inappropriate, as for the movements involved in producing [s], the sense of movement can be coupled with touch. For example, a speaker is often unable to report the position of the tongue tip during [s] production unless instructed to pinch the tip of the tongue before producing the gesture. The receptors stimulated by pinching are more likely to be touch receptors than spindles, but they heighten the sense of movement and position by being paired with it. This works even though some speakers do touch the tip of the tongue to the lower gum ridge during [s], whereas others hold it higher not touching anything. The same technique can be used to sensitize the patient to the blade of the tongue.

The third and lowest level of feedback operates as a result of speech processes. This knowledge of results, or *external* feedback, includes taction—feeling the contacts made as a result of the movements—and audition—hearing the audible sound pressure variations produced. External feedback, operating as a result of speech movements, contrasts with *internal* feedback at the highest level that operates before as well as during the speech, and with *response* feedback at the middle level that operates during the movements.

In the 1950s, studies of the effects of delayed auditory feedback (Lee, 1950) and the effects of reduced tactile feedback via nerve blocks (Ringel and Steer, 1963) led researchers to conclude that speakers need to monitor their speech continuously in order to speak; in other words, speech was modeled as a servomechanism (Fairbanks, 1954). Further research, however, led investigators to question the necessity of moment-by-moment monitoring for normally skilled speakers. The findings that the segmental aspects of speech deteriorate very little under masking of auditory feedback (Lane and Tranel, 1971) and that only the most vulnerable consonant clusters were distorted under oral anesthesia (Borden et al., 1973) persuaded investigators that use of external feedback may change with age and be less important for adult skilled speakers (Borden, 1979, 1980) than for children developing language.

The effects of delayed auditory feedback have been studied to investigate whether children rely on auditory feedback more than adults. After years of conflicting results, Siegel and his colleagues (1980) have replicated studies that show adults to be much less affected by the distorted feedback than were 8-year-old children. Five-year-old children were most affected, both in terms of syllables per second and in number of nonfluencies per sentence. Inferences made from this research indicate that adults, who are more skilled than children in speech, produce speech relatively automatically and do not require constant self-monitoring by audition. It is also true that in many instances speech is too fast to correct by audition as you are producing it. By the time you hear a [t] burst, you have already completed it, so that you can only correct it by producing it again. We are left with the view that listening to oneself, however important for babbling infants and for children developing speech, is reserved in adult speech for fine adjustments. For example, second formants of high front vowels are somewhat higher in frequency when speakers hear themselves than when their auditory feedback is masked (Borden et al., 1981), but there is no loss in intelligibility. If adult skilled speakers are so little affected by distortions in self-audition, even though the signal has been amplified and delayed, as in the DAF studies, producing a signal that is difficult to ignore, how much less might we expect them to attend to the sound of themselves speaking with no distortion applied to the feedback signal?

The same principles hold for the sense of touch. The sensation of air pressure changes against the walls of the vocal tract (Stevens and Perkell, 1977) and the sensations of touch afforded by articulator contacts may be used for articulatory refinements, but the basic motor activity for speech succeeds despite impoverished auditory and tactile feedback.

The clear implication for articulation treatment is that the job of bringing the relationship between speech production and these sensory channels of information back under voluntary control from their state of automatic control, and to conscious awareness from their relatively dormant state, is more difficult than we have assumed. Because research findings indicate that some kinds of feedback information are not necessary to skilled speech, speech pathologists must marshal imaginative means to reactivate self-monitoring systems when new gestures are to be learned. We have all experienced the resistance to treatment that some seemingly simple articulation disorders have demonstrated. More extreme measures are required to augment feedback signals. Simultaneous auditory feedback, when amplified sufficiently, becomes salient to a speaker. It can at least be used to self-correct post hoc. Furthermore, one can draw the speaker's attention to certain aspects of the sound by filtering it as it is returned to the speaker. If a speaker is hypernasal, one can low-pass filter the speech and this distortion will cause speakers to decrease nasal resonance (Garber and Moller, 1979) and increase intelligibility. Transducing signals into a visual image may help increase self-awareness. For example, either a nasal bulb attached to a pressure transducer or a small accelerometer held to the side of the nose can be displayed on an ordinary oscilloscope. The client who has ceased to monitor his or her own hypernasality or perhaps hears the relatively strong nasal resonance as acceptable can easily be shown the difference when it is made visual. With practice, the client may learn to associate the desired visual trace with a new kinesthetic sense and interpret the new event as the acceptable target. Tactile awareness is also dulled in skilled speakers, but it takes elaborate equipment to transduce tactile patterns of the tongue against the palate into a visual image. Electropalatographs are not yet widely used in the clinic, but with further simplification and the development of a palatal device that can be adapted to palates of varying shapes and sizes, it may be a useful clinical aid in the future. Speech pathologists in France, called *orthophonistes*, carry around with them a tool kit with all sorts and shapes of oral probes for pushing the tongue around and for increasing awareness of tactile sensation in the mouth. In sum, recent research in the area of feedback during normal speech production points to special problems in making people aware of motor-sensory targets and puts special demands upon the resourcefulness of the speech pathologist.

As a way of summarizing the research in motor control, three models of speech production are presented. They reflect the development of recent thinking, but are merely representative of many current models. First, in the 1950s and 1960s the model of speech as a feedback system or servomechanism was generally accepted (Fairbanks, 1954). Moment-by-moment feedback was not only considered to be the rule but was considered to be essential for the control of speech production. Then, in the 1970s, the target theory of speech production became popular with the paper by MacNeilage (1970) on the serial ordering of speech. This theory is an attempt to account for variations in initial position and in external constraints. For example, a speaker produces [t] automatically whether approaching the stop from a low vowel or high vowel position, so it would be inefficient to have a particular set of muscle commands for [t]. The idea here is that speakers have stored the x-y coordinates of the vocal tract in the brain, and they feed forward the target commands in terms of vocal tract configurations, not specific muscles. There is only an occasional need for feedback in the target model.

The third view conceives of motor control as operating under simple mechanical principles intrinsic to the set of muscles and articulators that coordinate with one another. This concept of motor control emerges from work among Soviet physiologists. Fowler and Turvey (1978, 1980) have applied this model to speech production and hold that groups of muscles, called *coordinative structures*, control themselves automatically, without further control from higher centers. Feedback is not mentioned but information flows among the components of the cooperating muscles. Basically, the system acts like a series of mass-spring vibrators, so that if one part of the system is constrained another part will automatically compensate.

The mass-spring model fails to account for learning, but explains how the organism adapts so quickly and successfully to ecologic change. A complete model of speech control should be flexible enough to operate under central regulation in some circumstances and under feedback control in other situations.

In addition to amplifying and transducing feedback signals for the speaker, the charge of the speech pathologist may be to take advantage of the compensatory properties of the coordinative structures. In situations in which the jaw and lip cooperate, for example, constraint of the jaw will force increased lip movement.

## RESEARCH ON MOTOR PHYSIOLOGY
## APPLIED TO SPEECH PATHOLOGY

Recent findings gleaned from research in the physiology of respiration, laryngeal-supralaryngeal timing, velopharyngeal activity, and even in the relationship between speech and hand movements will follow as examples of laboratory results that can be applied in the clinic.

In the control of respiration for speech, we have learned that speakers typically use only 25% of their vital capacity when speaking at normal conversational intensity (Hixon, 1973). Vital capacity is the maximum volume of air that one can exhale after a maximum inhalation. For conversational speech, a speaker may inhale up to perhaps 60% of vital capacity and speak until lung volume is down to about 35% or 40% of vital capacity, thus using only one quarter of the air available. We have found, too, that a speaker controls the exhalation phase of the cycle by continuing to contract muscles of inhalation during exhalation, letting the inspiratory muscles relax only gradually during speech in order to conserve the breathstream (Draper et al., 1959). These findings have directly shaped clinical management in that the procedures used to train better respiration for speech are rarely aimed at providing more air—little is needed—rather, the emphasis is on speaking at the onset of exhalation, not after much air is wasted, and on letting it out gradually instead of suddenly. Recent evidence from research in respiratory physiology (Hixon et al., 1976) indicates that when in an upright position, speakers activate the abdominal muscles during both inspiratory and expiratory parts of the cycle. Previously, it was thought that abdominal activity was only expiratory. The theory is that continued contraction of the abdomen during speech keeps the diaphragm elevated so that it can be maximally responsive to perform the rapid inhalations required in speech. This theory justifies the "support of tone" concept that good teachers of voice and speech have imparted to their students for years. Making singers and speakers aware of abdominal activity has not only been an effective device for displacing tension from the larynx, but we also think now that it has acted to tune the respiratory system and make it optimally responsive.

In the interaction of phonation with articulation, the timing of some articulatory adjustments in the oral cavity relative to the onset of voicing is critical in distinguishing voiced-voiceless contrasts, and furthermore, that the timing is linguistically determined, as it varies across languages (Lisker and Abramson, 1964, 1967). Voice onset time (VOT) is the measured time represented on a sound spectrogram between the burst of noise that accompanies the release of an occlusion for a plosive and the beginning of glottal pulses at the onset of the voicing for the following vowel. Voice onset time is longer for voiceless stop vowel combinations than for those with voiced stops, and voice onset time increases as the place of occlusion moves back in the mouth from labial /p,b/, to alveolar /t,d/, to palato-velar /k,g/ positions. These findings have direct clinical applicability. Voicing confusions are common among children with articulation disorders, deaf speakers, speakers with dysarthria, or those with verbal apraxia. Freeman et al. (1978) found that the VOT measures of voiced-voiceless cognates in the speech of a patient with verbal apraxia overlapped instead of being distinct as they are for speakers with normal timing. In addition to auditory training, real time spectrographic equipment would aid the speaker by making the contrast visible, but lacking that, the speech pathologist can have the patient feel the glottal vibrations as they are accurately timed with the release of the stop. Also, VOT can be measured periodically during the course of treatment as an objective record of improvement.

Work on normal velar movement and muscle activity indicates that the levator palatini muscle is the prominent force for velar elevation. Knowledge of this finding will do little help to someone having difficulty in activating it, but such research has also revealed that normally there are interactions between laryngeal and velo-pharyngeal mechanisms and between tongue and velar movements that are useful to know when prescribing exercises for increasing velar activity. Velar movement is maximum when going from a nasal consonant to an oral consonant, such as a fricative. For example, phrases such as "ten zero" or "one seat" demand rapid and extensive elevation of the velum. For some speakers, the velum is higher for voiced consonants than for voiceless consonants. This difference in velar elevation increases the volume of the supralaryngeal cavity which is necessary to maintain the pressure drop across the glottis during voicing. Also, the velum is higher for high or close vowels than for low or open vowels, and is, of course, lowest for nasals. The height of the velum for a particular consonant depends more upon the vowel following the consonant than the vowel preceding the consonant. Thus, because the velum is higher for [i] than for [a], it is higher for the consonant in /aCi/ than for /iCa/ (Bell-Berti, 1980).

Finally, speech movements relate to hand movements in ways that may be applied to clinical procedures. Some basic research (Kinsbourne and Hicks, 1978) indicates that certain activities that one can do with one's hands can suffer due to interference from speech, for example, balancing a dowel on one finger while speaking suffers more when the cortical control for the speech and the hand are presumed to be in the same cerebral hemisphere (that is, when the finger used is on the right hand) than when separated. Speech interferes less with balancing a dowel on a finger of the left hand. These studies are designed to test theories of cerebral hemispheric interference, and they indicate that speech interferes with the hand activity. In other studies designed to test theories of motor control, hand movements and speech have been shown to have a tendency to be rhythmically locked and they are seen to influence one another (Kelso et al., 1983). Thus, hand movements and speech movements may be mutually facilitative or interfere with one another, depending on the degree of movement similarity. When a client produces hand movements that track the rhythms or intonation patterns of speech models, it may facilitate those patterns in the speaker. These findings are applicable when, for example, one is working on prosody in deaf speakers.

## RESEARCH ON SPEECH ACOUSTICS AND
## SPEECH PERCEPTION APPLIED TO SPEECH PATHOLOGY

Research in acoustics of speech also has direct application to clinical procedures. An important work by Fant that helped establish the acoustic theory of speech production was first published in 1960. Simply stated, it holds that the sounds of speech are the product of a sound source initiated at the vocal folds or in the vocal tract and the selective amplification and filtering of the sound offered by the resonances of the vocal tract. Kuhn (1975) has further demonstrated that for most of the sounds of speech, the second formant ($F_2$) reflects the resonance of the front cavity. To the degree that this is true, the speech-language pathologist can make inferences about changes in oral cavity configuration as a result of treatment by making sound spectrograms of a standard passage containing the speech sounds of interest. For example, a member of a speech science seminar at Temple University,

Lefton-Greif, measured formant changes in a patient undergoing therapy after a glossectomy, and was able to document the acoustic results of the compensatory adjustments adopted by the patient. Whereas the spectrographic display was essentially flat immediately postoperatively, more appropriate formant spacing and more formant movement were evident after speech remediation, which indicates that the patient had discovered ways of modifying vocal tract shape to take the place of her former strategies of tongue movement. Also, observation of the gradually improving movements of the second formant might act as both a motivating and reinforcing influence on the patient.

Finally, the wealth of research on speech perception has shown us the importance of context, of expectations, and of our particular linguistic experiences upon how we interpret the speech we hear. Researchers may not agree upon size of the perceptual units that people process when they perceive speech, and they may not agree on the stages or levels of processing involved, but there is agreement that listeners tend to group speech sounds into categories according to the phoneme classes of their particular language.

One fact of categorical perception is that when you present people with speech-like sounds that are varied in equal increments of some acoustic dimension—for example, the starting frequency of the second formant transition—people label the stimuli in the continuum categorically. In this case, some of the stimuli are heard as /b/, some as /d/, and some as /g/. Equally important to the definition of categorical perception is the second finding that when listeners are asked whether pairs of the stimuli are the same or different, they report differences between stimuli that lie at the boundaries between the phonemes they have identified, but they fail to report a distinction between the same amount of acoustic difference when the compared stimuli lie within the phoneme category (Liberman et al., 1957). Furthermore, speakers fail to identify and discriminate such stimuli categorically when the particular phoneme contrast tested is not distinctive in their language. For example, English speaking listeners perceive an /r/ to /l/ continuum categorically, whereas Japanese speaking listeners do not (Miyawaki et al., 1975). That is, there is a point along the /r/ to /l/ continuum at which English listeners differentiate /r/ from /l/, whereas Japanese listeners do not identify or discriminate the phoneme contrast in the same way, because there is no /r/-/l/ distinction in the Japanese language.

The significance of categorical perception to clinical treatment is that the tests of identification and discrimination used in research provide a method of tracking small allophonic changes in perception as efforts are made in the clinic to change the production of phoneme confusions. By periodically testing speech perception in people learning a new phoneme contrast in a second language or in others learning to modify misarticulations, the speech-language pathologist could track subtle shifts in phoneme boundaries during treatment. Also, in the cases of misarticulation, one could identify at the outset those misarticulators whose perception is normal. By testing production and perception in detail (the usual clinical tests of speech perception test only phoneme identification, not which allophones belong to which class), we may discover more about how perceptual changes interact with changes in speech production.

The second application of the findings of categorical perception in speech research to the practice of speech pathology centers on the speech perception of the clinician instead of the client. The tendency to categorize speech sounds into the phoneme classes of one's own language is so strong that speech pathologists are in danger of perceiving misarticulations incorrectly, because phonemic expectations often override one's ability to discriminate phonetic differences. Thus it is important to listen carefully and watch speakers closely to extract the exact phonetic details. We who are concerned with training speech-language pathologists must counteract the tendency toward categorical perception by explicit and extensive training of clinicians in the discrimination of allophonic variations and distorted speech productions. Currently, clinicians learn to make broad phonetic transcriptions. We may not be well enough trained to make accurate narrow phonetic transcriptions, and our training is too often restricted to the English phonetic system.

To conclude, we can discover ideas in research findings in speech perception as well as speech production that will apply to clinical procedures in the treatment of articulation problems. In speech perception research, we are reminded of how vulnerable we are as clinicians to the dulling of allophonic discrimination due to the categorical nature of perceptual processes. At the same time, we can take advantage of the effects of linguistic experience upon perception by adopting speech perception tests in the course of treatment to track perceptual change in people learning new phoneme contrasts in their first or second language. In the application of speech production research findings, we can maximize the effectiveness of speech exercises by understanding better the motor coordination of the different muscle groups involved. Finally, we are reminded by research on speech feedback of how important it is to awaken the latent information loops by amplification, by selective filtering, or by transducing the output into visual displays for biofeedback training.

In talking to researchers and in reading about speech production and perception, one finds that the results of studies seem to be rather consistent, but the production and perception models that the researchers posit to explain their findings vary. One reason for these varying points of view is that the training of the researchers differs, resulting in difference in focus. It is like looking out a window: one sees both the window pane and the distant scene but chooses which to focus upon. Investigators tend to view their findings with the particular focus that their discipline provides. One way of viewing speech is as a product of linguistic processes and another way is to view it as the result of neurophysiological events. These views are not mutually exclusive; both views capture the whole picture, but the emphasis is different. This change of focus is not unlike the ways in which speech-language pathologists approach articulation disorders—some with more emphasis on phonological rules, some concentrating on distinctive features, and some focusing on motorsensory relationships and the coordination of muscle groups. The clinical outcome may not vary significantly with the particular focus, but using every perspective you have is probably healthy. It seems advantageous for a speech-language pathologist to be flexible enough to change focus as the need demands. It may be a good sign that the linguistic features detailed by Chomsky and Halle in 1968 are much more physiological in their definitions than the previous (1952) Jakobson, Fant, and Halle features. We may be moving toward a synthesis of linguistic and neurophysiological views.

Whether one emphasizes the linguistic or neurophysiological aspects of speech, it behooves speech-language pathologists to keep abreast of basic research findings reported in such journals as the *Journal of the Acoustical Society of America, Journal of Phonetics*, and the *Journal of Speech and Hearing Research*. This chapter is directed to an exploration of ways in which speech science can be applied to speech pathology. We can cross the bridge from the other side as well. There are many ways in which the experiences of a speech pathologist in the clinic can lead to both clinical and laboratory research—so it behooves speech scientists to keep abreast of the clinical questions studied and reported in such journals as the *Journal of Speech and Hearing Disorders, Journal of Communication Disorders*, and the many journals devoted to specific disorders. In that way, the laboratory and the clinic will reinforce one another more directly and more effectively.

## REFERENCES

Bell-Berti, F. 1980. Velopharyngeal function: A spatial-temporal model. In: N. Lass (ed.), Speech and Language: Advances in Basic Research and Practice, Vol. 4, pp. 291–316. Academic Press, New York.

Borden, G. J. 1979. An interpretation of research on feedback interruption in speech. Brain Lang. 7:307–319.

Borden, G. J. 1980. Use of feedback in established and developing speech. In: N. Lass (ed.), Speech and Language: Advances in Basic Research and Practice, Vol. 3, pp. 223–242. Academic Press, New York.

Borden, G. J., and Harris, K. S. 1980. Speech Science Primer: Physiology, Acoustics, and Perception of Speech. Williams & Wilkins, Baltimore.

Borden, G. J., Harris, K. S., and Catena, L. 1973. Oral feedback II. An electromyographic study of speech under nerve-block anesthesia. J. Phonet. 1:297–308.

Borden, G. J., Harris, K. S., Fitch, H., and Yoshioka, H. 1981. Producing relatively unfamiliar speech gestures: A synthesis of perceptual targets and production rules. Status Report on Speech Research SR-66, pp. 85–117. Haskins Laboratories, New Haven, CT.

Chomsky, N., and Halle, M. 1968. The Sound Pattern of English. Harper & Row, New York.

Draper, M., Ladefoged, P., and Whitteridge, D. 1959. Respiratory muscles in speech. J. Speech Hear. Res. 2:16–27.

Evarts, E. V. 1971. Feedback and corollary discharge: A merging of the concepts. Central Control of Movement: Neurosci. Prog. Bull. 9:86–112.

Evarts, E. V. 1979. Brain mechanisms of movement. Sci. Am. 241:164–179.

Fairbanks, G. 1954. A theory of the speech mechanism as a servosystem. J. Speech Hear. Disord. 19:133–139.

Fant, G. 1970. Acoustic Theory of Speech Production. Mouton, The Hague.

Folkins, J. W., and Abbs, J. H. 1975. Lip and jaw motor control during speech: Responses to resistive loading of the jaw. J. Speech Hear. Res. 18:207–220.

Fowler, C. A., and Turvey, M. T. 1978. Skill acquisition: An event approach with special reference to searching for the optimum of a function of several variables. In: G. E. Stelmach (ed.), Information Processing in Motor Control and Learning. Academic Press, New York.

Fowler, C. A., and Turvey, M. T. 1980. Immediate compensation in bite-block speech. Phonetica 37:306–326.

Freeman, F., Sands, E., and Harris, K. S. 1978. Temporal coordination of phonation and articulation in a case of verbal apraxia: A voice onset time study. Brain Lang. 6:106–111.

Garber, S. R., and Moller, K. T. 1979. The effects of feedback filtering on nasalization in normal and hypernasal speakers. J. Speech Hear. Res. 22:321–333.

Hixon, T. 1973. Respiratory function in speech. In: F. D. Minifie, T. J. Hixon, and F. Williams (eds.), Normal Aspects of Speech, Hearing, and Language. Prentice-Hall, Englewood Cliffs, NJ.

Hixon, T. J., Mead, J., and Goldman, M. D. 1976. Dynamics of the chest wall during speech production: Function of the thorax, rib cage, diaphragm, and abdomen. J. Speech Hear. Res. 19:297–356.

Jakobson, R., Fant, C. G. M., and Halle, M. 1963. Preliminaries to Speech Analysis. MIT Press, Cambridge, MA. (Originally published in 1952 as Technical Report No. 13, Acoustics Laboratory, MIT.)

Kelso, J. A. S., Tuller, B., and Harris, K. S. 1983. A 'dynamic pattern' perspective on the control and coordination of movement. In: P. F. MacNeilage (ed.), The Production of Speech. Springer-Verlag, New York.

Kinsbourne, M., and Hicks, R. E. 1978. Mapping cerebral functional space: Competition and collaboration in human performance. In: M. Kinsbourne (ed.), Asymmetrical Function of the Brain, pp. 267–273. Cambridge University Press, New York.

Kuhn, G. M. 1975. On the front cavity resonance and its possible role in speech perception. J. Acoust. Soc. Am. 58:428–433.

Lane, H. L., and Tranel, B. 1971. The Lombard sign and the role of hearing in speech. J. Speech Hear. Res. 14:677–709.

Lassen, A. R., Ingvar, D. H., and Skinhoj, E. 1978. Brain function and blood flow. Sci. Am. 239:62–71.

Lee, B. S. 1950. Effects of delayed speech feedback. J. Acoust. Soc. 22:824–826.

Liberman, A. M., Harris, K. S., Hoffman, H. S., and Griffith, B. C. 1957. The discrimination of speech sounds within and across phoneme boundaries. J. Exp. Psychol. 54:358–368.

Lindblom, B., and Sundberg, J. 1976. Acoustical consequences of lip, tongue, jaw, and larynx movement. J. Acoust. Soci. Am. 50:1166–1179.

Lisker, L., and Abramson, A. 1964. A cross-language study of voicing in initial stops: Acoustical measurements. Word 20:384–422.

Lisker, L., and Abramson, A. 1967. Some effects of contexts on voice onset time in english stops. Lang. Speech 10:1–28.

MacNeilage, P. F. 1970. Motor control of serial ordering of speech. Psychol. Rev. 77:182–196.

Miyawaki, F., Strange, W., Verbrugge, R., et al. 1975. An effect of linguistic experience: The discrimination of [r] and [l] by native speakers of Japanese and English. Percep. Psychophysics 18:331–340.

Penfield, W., and Roberts, L. 1959. Speech and Brain-Mechanisms. Princeton University Press, Princeton, NJ.

Polit, A., and Bizzi, E. 1978. Processes controlling arm movement in monkeys. Science 201:1235–1237.

Ringel, R. L., and Steer, M. 1963. Some effects of tactile and auditory alterations on speech output. J. Speech Hear. Res. 6:369–378.

Siegel, G. M., Fehst, C. A., Garber, S. R., and Pick, H. L., Jr. 1980. Delayed auditory feedback with children. J. Speech Hear. Res. 23:802–813.

Stevens, K. N., and Perkell, J. S. 1977. Speech physiologgy and phonetic features. In: M. Sawashima and F. S. Cooper (eds.), Dynamic Aspects of Speech Production, pp. 323–345. University of Tokyo Press, Tokyo.

CHAPTER **4**

# Intelligibility and the Child with Multiple Articulation Deviations

*Marilynn Schmidt*

*For children with many articulation errors, Schmidt advises
that intelligibility be the primary consideration in treatment.
She provides the rationale for this approach and outlines a
set of clinical procedures.*

1. *Why does Schmidt's approach to articulation training
   center around the concept of intelligibility? What phonological processes seem to effect most the intelligibility
   of children's speech? What procedures does Schmidt
   recommend to assess and evaluate intelligibility?*
2. *According to Schmidt, what is the goal in the treatment
   of children who are highly unintelligible?*
3. *The order in which phonological constituents are to be
   treated is provided by Schmidt. Do you agree with this
   order?*
4. *In what way does Schmidt's approach differ from a distinctive feature approach?*

CHILDREN WITH MULTIPLE ARTICULATION ERRORS pose special problems for the speech clinician. Often we find that these children do not respond well to treatment. This chapter emphasizes an approach that may be especially useful in working with the young child with multiple articulation deviations. In addition, reasons why there is often a lack of progress in traditional programming practices are suggested. This chapter concentrates on early aspects of articulation training.

Success in articulation intervention, especially with children with multiple articulation errors, may be more easily achieved if the following procedures and approaches are considered:

1. A complete phonological assessment should be obtained.
2. As complete a resumé of the child's expressive vocabulary as possible should be obtained.
3. The sentence complexity used by the child should be determined through a language sample.
4. The child's level of intelligibility should be determined.

The initial goal in treatment should be intelligible utterances, not correct articulation, for the child with multiple articulation errors. A hierarchy for establishing intelligibility is presented in this chapter.

## PHONOLOGICAL PROCESSES ASSESSMENT

Obviously, the child with multiple articulation errors needs to have a complete phonological processes assessment. This assessment is often a difficult task because of the child's reluctance to participate in conversation or produce words when he is aware of his unintelligibility. Considerable research and investigation presently stresses the importance of this assessment and describes specific procedures (Compton, 1970; Hodson, 1978, 1980; Ingram, 1976).

Intelligibility in children with severe phonological disorders seems to be most affected by the following processes (Hodson, 1980):

1. The child either omits syllables in words, or produces the final syllables weakly.
2. Consonant clusters or blends are reduced by omitting a consonant in the cluster, for example, /tr/ for /str/.
3. The consonants may be omitted before or after the vowel; postvocalic omissions are most common.
4. The child omits sounds containing the strident feature, for example, /pun/ for "spoon." This is considered one of the most common contributing factors to unintelligibility.

5.  Many sound substitutions are produced anteriorly in the mouth instead of posteriorly, for example, /t/ for /k/; this process is called *fronting*.
6.  Children substitute glottal stops for post vocalic consonants; most severely involved children do this.
7.  Children substitute velar phonemes for anterior phonemes; this "backing" seriously affects intelligibility.

### ASSESSMENT OF THE CHILD'S EXPRESSIVE VOCABULARY AND THE LANGUAGE SAMPLE

In cases of multiple misarticulation, a critical area of assessment that must be provided to the clinician is information on the developing language system and the vocabulary of the child. Formal and informal testing of receptive language assesses the understanding of the speech of others. An assessment of expression evaluates the spoken use of language. In particular, this evaluation should indicate whether an abbreviated syllable is used for a given word.

The expressive language of children with multiple articulation errors is difficult to assess. Much critical time can be used in learning what children are saying because they are so unintelligible. Often weeks or months can be spent in painstaking effort to decipher whether a child really has names for basic concepts or even has a developing language system. Asking children questions about themselves, their environment, and their families when the answer is unknown is not efficient use of clinical time. Additionally, it is frustrating to the child.

Included in Figure 1 is a form that has proved to be helpful in determining what a child may be trying to say. This form can be completed by the family or by the clinician when interviewing the parents. The parents should be aware that this method of eliciting information is not an attempt to secure "private information," but merely a procedure to prevent needless frustration on the part of a young child who cannot, for example, produce his own sister's or brother's name well enough to be responded to appropriately. The parents should be asked to provide the approximations that the child uses for the adult form of the word. We suggest that the clinician continue to make use of this form at each clinical session. Equally useful is a phonic spelling of each word that is provided by the parents. For example, it would be helpful for the clinician to know that the child's use of /o ma/ means "grandma." This process of identifying the child's vocabulary should be on a continuous basis, with constant updating being provided by the family and the clinician perhaps weekly.

---

SPEECH/LANGUAGE INFORMATION SHEET FOR CHILDREN

Child's name _____Age _____Birthdate _____
Name of father/mother _____
Name/s of other child/ren _____
    and age/s _____
    Nicknames (if appropriate) _____
Names of other close relatives and where they live (grandparents)
_____

Occupation of father _____Place of work _____
Occupation of mother _____Place of work _____
Favorite foods (dessert, beverage, dishes) _____
Food dislikes _____
Favorite colors _____
Color of family car/s, child's bicycle, truck, etc. _____
TV and radio programs watched _____
Favorite movie and TV stars _____
Pets of family (names also) _____
Favorite pastimes _____
Books the child likes to have read _____
Chores the child does _____
Daily routine (appointments, lessons, groups in which they partic-
    ipate—Brownies, Cubs, Sunday School) _____
_____

Music likes and dislikes (songs) _____
Names of close friends/playmates _____
_____

Vacation Trips taken or planned (who, when, where, etc.) _____
_____

Additional information _____
Street and number _____
Telephone number _____
What words in the following categories does your child have?

Animals

Body parts

Furniture

Clothing

Colors

Numbers

Places

Toys

Words dealing with the house

Words dealing with a city, buildings, vehicles

Please indicate in spelling how your child might actually say any of
these words. Provide us with the child's word, not some adult form.

---

Figure 1.   Speech-language information sheet for children.

The phonetic form of a word can serve as a guide in planning treatment, especially for determining words which require initial treatment. Included in this information gathering procedure should be those responses that parents "wish" their child could produce more intelligibly (Rieke et al., 1977). Parents often have very specific suggestions. For example, their child's name might be said so unintelligibly that others do not understand it. Time could be spent in teaching an intelligible rendering of the child's name so that strangers will reinforce the child's pronunciation instead of looking puzzled and directing all questions to his or her parents. In one case, a young child named Jeff learned to say /ʒɛf/ for /dɛf/. This pronunciation of his name, although not completely correct, enabled Jeff to respond to questions more readily. Also his pronunciation of his name was sufficiently intelligible to enable others to relate to him on a first name basis.

**USE OF WORDS AS STIMULI**

Young children, under 5, often do not respond to traditional programming beginning with the sound in isolation or in nonsense syllables because these stimuli lack meaning. Beginning clinical sessions should concentrate on words that are actually produced by the child at home. These words can be selected from categories that the child produces, such as food (meat, milk, more, bread, spoon) or family names (mama, daddy, Betty, Bobby).

**LEVEL OF INTELLIGIBILITY**

Weiss (1978) describes a procedure for quantifying intelligibility in articulation. A sample of the child's speech is obtained and taped in conversation. The clinician or some other person who is not familiar with the child's speech transcribes a continuous sample of 100 words spoken by the child in the taped conversation. The criterion of evaluation is intelligibility, not correct articulation. A percentage of 100 words that have been transcribed will provide a measure that can be used as baseline data. This procedure is used at a later time to determine improvement. Weiss includes data on intelligibility in children, age 18 to 48 months.

**INTELLIGIBILITY AS AN INITIAL GOAL**

One of the principal clinical goals for the child with multiple articulation errors is the improvement of intelligibility. Improvement is often gradual with traditional articulation programming procedures in which only one phoneme is treated at a time. Our intention here is to teach the child to talk so that listeners know what the child is saying. The primary focus is not on the correct production of speech sounds.

The clinician should concentrate on words that the child is actually using and should try to improve their intelligibility. Because words, not sounds in isolation or nonsense syllables, are being modeled, pictures and/or objects should be used along with the appropriate verbal input in order to make the task meaningful and interesting. Procedures that we have found to be effective are given below. The following list is a working hierarchy in which attention is given initially to vowels and syllable structure and later to consonants.

1.  Monosyllabic words from the child's own vocabulary are modeled; the child is reinforced when the vowel clearly resembles the vowel of the targeted word. For example, the clinician models the word "dog," and accepts the vowel /ɔ/ as a correct response. We have found that most children are able to produce the vowels in some words. This is probably why it is recognized by the parent as the word.

2.  Bisyllable words are modeled by the clinician by emphasizing the vowel in each syllable. Approximations of the vowels and syllable structure are acceptable responses for this step, for example, /e o/ for "table," /aɪ i/ for "ice cream." In some cases, bisyllable words are accompanied by a hand tap to demonstrate the individual syllables to the child, for example, /te bo/.

3.  Monosyllabic words in which the initial consonants are stressed are then modeled. Initially, any attempt at constriction is accepted; later consonants that share several consonantal features are accepted, such as /te/ for "cake." Intelligibility rather than correct articulation is the criterion; therefore, this approximation is accepted until training for the final consonant begins. Many young children produce words with consonant phonemes which resemble target phonemes except for one or two features, such as place or voicing, /dɔ/ for "dog"; /bɪ/ for "pig." Place seems to be one of the last features to be mastered (Menyuk, 1971).

4.  Next the words are modeled so that the child can add the final constriction where required. We have found that most children understand the concept that each word is to have an ending. Initially, any constriction or evidence of consonantal ending satisfies as criterion. Eventually a final consonant with common consonant features is accepted /bæf/ for "bath."

5.  The next step is to have the child reach the criterion level of being able to produce the correct initial phoneme in the modeled word (CVC).
6.  The final stage involves having the child produce the entire word, including final consonant, in the modeled word (CVC).

The treatment session need not concentrate on word intelligibility as its only goal. When the child is able to produce monosyllabic or bisyllabic words with substitutions more typical of the child with developmental errors (in-class errors), the clinician can introduce traditional programming on selected phonemes or even use a distinctive feature approach.

In conclusion, the child with multiple articulation errors poses a special problem for the clinician. The child is typically very difficult to understand by almost everyone except certain members of the family. Unless the child's remarks are intelligible, they will not be reacted to appropriately by strangers and friends of the family. This reinforcement is vitally important if children are to attempt conversation with people in their environment. Often, the severely involved child refuses to attempt speech because of bad experiences in social exchanges.

Typically, there are so many phonemes in error that merely selecting one phoneme or feature seems futile when what the child needs is to be understood immediately by others. The procedures discussed in this chapter suggest that when the goal is intelligibility of utterances, a child with multiple articulation errors will come to use his or her speech in a functionally useful way.

**REFERENCES**

Compton, A. 1970. Generative studies of children's phonological disorders. J. Speech Hearing Disord. 35:315–339.

Hodson, B. 1978. A preliminary hierarchical model for phonological remediation. Lang. Speech Hear. Serv. Schools 9:236–240.

Hodson, B. 1980. The Assessment of Phonological Processes. The Interstate Printer and Publishers, Danville, IL.

Ingram, D. 1976. Phonological Disability in Children. Elsevier, New York.

Menyuk, P. 1971. The Acquisition and Development of Language. Prentice Hall, Englewood Cliffs, NJ.

Rieke, J. A., Lynch, L. L., and Soltman, S. F. 1977. Teaching Strategies for Language Development. Grune & Stratton, New York.

Weiss, C. 1978. Weiss Comprehensive Articulation Test. Teaching Resources Corporation, Boston.

CHAPTER 5

# Facilitating Phonological Development in Children with Severe Speech Disorders

*Barbara Williams Hodson*

> *Children with unintelligible speech require special attention and special techniques. Hodson uses a phonological process analysis to develop a plan of intervention for these children.*

1.  Why does Hodson suggest the use of a phonological process approach to classify children's articulation errors? How does she implement this classification system to develop a methodology for the remediation of articulation errors? In your answer to this last question, define and describe Hodson's use of the term targeting.

2.  What are the phonological processes most common in the speech of unintelligible children according to Hodson? What do you think these phonological processes represent?

3.  In each cycle, Hodson focuses on several different phonological processes. Do you agree with this approach, or do you think phonemes for only one phonological process should be targeted during each cycle?

4.  Hodson recommends the use of a number of traditional articulation training procedures to teach phonological patterns. What are these procedures?

5.  What procedures does Hodson recommend for probing? How is this information used to plan subsequent sessions?

6.  What rationale does Hodson provide for teaching /s/ in clusters before /s/ in singletons?

A KINDERGARTEN YOUNGSTER ENTERS THE SPEECH-LANGUAGE ROOM and says, /dɪ ɪ dʌ naɪ wɪ do wum/. Where does intervention begin? How much remediation time will be required before comments such as "This is a nice little room," will be readily understood? Will this child be "ready" to succeed in phonics, spelling, and reading activities? As a profession, our success rate for children with mild to moderate artic-ulation disorders has been excellent, but what has been our "batting average" with perhaps the most challenging speech client, the unin-telligible child?

Our observations and reports from clinicians and parents indicate that unintelligible children typically attend speech classes an average of 5 years targeting one phoneme at a time. Reportedly, the children eventually become intelligible, but not before they have experienced a considerable amount of academic underachievement and a great deal of frustration. In addition, the total number of hours typically expended for articulation programming for unintelligible children has been some-what difficult to justify.

A method that radically expedited intelligibility gains is summa-rized in this chapter. The maximum time that was required for a child to become intelligible using this facilitative phonological approach on a once-a-week basis was 18 months. The method evolved over a period of 6 years while providing individualized remediation services to over 100 children with severe speech disorders (Hodson, 1981, 1982; Hodson and Paden, 1983).

## CLIENTS

The children who participated in the Phonology Remediation Program were between 3 and 8 years of age when they enrolled in the clinic. They were referred by relatives, pediatricians, and speech-language pathologists. All were experiencing difficulty communicating verbally. Intelligible children were excluded from the Phonology Program.

In most instances, there were no "identifiable" significant etio-logical factors at the time of their diagnostic evaluations. Many had histories of otitis media, however, and in some instances, myringotomy surgery had been performed and pressure-equalizing tubes had been inserted. Four of the children had repaired cleft palates, and three had submucous clefts. One child had been diagnosed by Mayo Clinic as having "severe developmental apraxia." Three children had educa-tional placements in classes for the mentally retarded. Some of the children evidenced neurological "soft signs," such as poor balance and coordination, but none was severely involved, and most appeared to be within normal limits developmentally.

Most of the preschool children had not received prior articulation intervention programming. However, the 6-, 7-, and 8-year-old children had all been enrolled previously in public school speech classes for from 1 to 5 years.

Case history information indicated that these unintelligible children typically produced few consonants before their third year. Diagnostic reports revealed that at the time of the onset of their respective remediation programs, their consonant repertoires typically consisted of some of the following singletons: /p, b, t, d, m, n, w/.

## PHONOLOGICAL EVALUATION

The Assessment of Phonological Processes (Hodson, 1980) was used to examine the phonological performance of each child. This instrument involves having the children spontaneously name common objects, body parts, and simple concepts. Administration of the diagnostic form (55 items) requires 15–20 minutes, and the screening form (20 items) requires less than 5 minutes. Each child in the Phonology Remediation Program was assessed individually.

Percentage-of-occurrence scores were derived for the 10 major phonological processes by dividing the actual number of occurrences by the possible number of occurrences. Those processes that were utilized less than 40% typically did not require intervention. Those that occurred more than 40% were examined to determine which ones should be targeted.

## BASIC PHONOLOGICAL TERMS

A number of terms are used to describe phonological elements. *Consonant clusters* refer to consonants that are contiguous within a syllable, such as /sp/ and /ts/, as in the word spots. Consonant *singletons* occur next to a vowel or syllabic liquid and are not part of a consonant cluster (e.g., pot). *Prevocalic consonants* precede vowels or "vocalic" liquids within a syllable, and *postvocalic* consonants follow these elements. For example, /h/ is prevocalic and /t/ is postvocalic, in the words "hat" and "hurt." *Sonorants* are vowel-like and typically voiced. Vowels, liquids /l, r, ɚ/, glides /w, j/, and nasals /m, n, ŋ/ are sonorants. *Obstruents* are noise-like and nonsonorant. They include stops /p, b, t, d, k, g/, fricatives /f, v, θ, ð, s, z, ʃ, ʒ, h/, and affricates /tʃ, dʒ/. *Strident* consonants are those which occur when a forceful air stream is directed against the upper teeth. These include the sibilants

/s, z, ʃ, ʒ, tʃ, ʤ/, and also /f, v/. Frontal lisps are also strident. The tongue is protruded, but stridency is maintained. A frontal lisp differs from the less frequent /θ/ for /s/ substitution, because /θ/ is nonstrident.

The sound errors of unintelligible children typically fall into several classes or categories. These categories are called phonological processes to denote changes that affect classes of sounds. *Cluster reduction* refers to the omission of one or more elements in a consonant cluster (e.g., string → /tɪŋ/, /trɪŋ/, or /srɪŋ/). *Stridency deletion* refers to the loss of stridency, either via the total omission of the strident target (e.g., soap → /oup/; hats → /hæt/) or by substituting a nonstrident sound (e.g., soap → /toup/, /houp/, or boup/). *Stopping* refers to substitution of a stop consonant (p, b, t, d, k, g/ for "nonstop" consonants /f, v, θ, ð, s, z, ʃ, ʒ, h, m, n, l, r, w, j/ (e.g., nose → /douz/). *Gliding* refers to substitution of a glide /w, j/ for another phoneme (e.g., red → /wɛd/; soap → /woup/). *Vowelization* involves replacing a syllabic or postvocalic liquid with a "true" vowel (e.g., chair → /tʃɛu/; table → /teɪ bo/). *Liquid deviations* refer to the loss of the quality of /l, r, ɚ/ either by omission or by substitution. The most common phonological processes affecting liquids are gliding, stopping, and vowelization. *Fronting* refers to any forward place of articulation change. *Fronting of velars* involves the substitution of alveolars, particularly /t, d, n/, or labials, particularly /p, b, m/, for velars /k, g, ŋ/. *Backing* involves substitution of velars /k, g, ŋ/ or glottals /h, ʔ/ for other phonemes. *Glottal replacement* refers to the production of a glottal stop in place of another sound (e.g., hat → / hæʔ/). *Assimilation* serves to make the altered phoneme more like the one influencing it (e.g., spoon → /fpun/). Assimilations can occur even if phonemes are not contiguous (e.g., spoon → / spum/).

Several terms explain the procedures of remediation. The term *phonological pattern* is used to denote the converse of the term phonological process. A phonological pattern refers to the correct phonological usage of phonemes. For example, cluster reduction is a phonological process, but the correct usage of clusters is a phonological pattern. The term *target* refers to the phonological elements that are being taught. *Target phonemes* (e.g., /k/) are elements of target patterns (e.g., velars) and are not always equivalent to the phonemes of the word. For example, the target for /r/ in rock might initially be /ɝ/. Teaching or facilitating emergence of a phonological pattern is referred to as *targeting*. *Cycle* refers to the time period during which a group of phonological patterns is targeted. The first presentation of a series of patterns is referred to as cycle I, the second as cycle II, and so on. Most phonological patterns are *recycled* one or more times. Patterns which are beginning to emerge in a child's spontaneous utterances are not recycled. Each cycle becomes increasingly more difficult for the child as more difficult phoneme combinations are added.

## UNINTELLIGIBLE CHILDREN'S COMMON PHONOLOGICAL PROCESS

All of the highly unintelligible children who were evaluated, evidenced varying degrees of difficulty when attempting to produce liquids, stridents, and consonant clusters (Hodson and Paden, 1981). The older children, who had already received considerable articulation training, typically produced word-initial singletons /f/, /s/, and /l/, although /s/ productions were frequently distorted. It was observed that /s/ clusters were particularly lacking in the speech samples of the older children as well as the younger children. Whereas the younger children regularly omitted the strident phoneme (e.g., spoon → /pun/), the older children typically produced a word initial strident sound, but omitted the second element of the cluster (e.g., spoon → /sun/ or /fun/).

Deletion of the stop element by the older children may be more a reflection of prior articulation training than of normal development. Traditionally, children with severe speech disorders are taught to say singleton prevocalic /s/ first, even though they may exhibit a natural tendency for producing /s/ clusters. It has been observed that the children who say /tænd/ for both "sand" and "stand" usually begin producing /s/ by saying /s:tænd/ when targeting a word such as "sand." Because an articulation training goal for the older children most likely had been to teach correct prevocalic singleton /s/ rather than an /s/ per se, the unintelligible child may have been taught not to produce /s/ clusters at a time when consonant cluster productions may have actually been more facile.

Although over 40 phonological processes were observed in speech samples of these unintelligible children, it was neither necessary nor appropriate to target every process. In fact, the only phonological processes which all of these unintelligible children needed to remediate were stridency deletion, cluster reduction, and liquid deviations.

It was observed also that our clients demonstrated individual preferences for certain other phonological processes. We found that there were four additional, rather common processes which needed to be targeted by a substantial number of unintelligible children: singleton consonant deletion, particularly postvocalic obstruents (e.g., hat → /hæ/); velar fronting (e.g., gun → /dʌn/); backing (e.g., tub →/kʌg/); and syllable reduction (e.g., basket → /bæ/).

Not every child needed to remediate these latter processes, of course, and individual children needed to develop additional, less common phonological patterns. In addition, there were several rather frequently occurring processes that rarely required intervention: assimilation (e.g., gun → /nʌn/); prevocalic voicing (e.g., tub → /dʌb/); glottal replacement (e.g., hat → /hæʔ/); and stopping (e.g., leaf → /dip/). It was observed that as the children's phonological systems developed, the number of occurrences of these latter processes declined even though they were not targeted directly (Hodson and Paden, 1983).

## REMEDIATION

### Facilitating Emergence of Phonological Patterns via Cycles

The traditional practice of teaching each phoneme to a designated criterion level is incredibly time consuming for the child with unintelligible speech. We have found that an alternative method, which involves systematically targeting all of the major phonological processes in successive time periods of 2 to 3 months, results in rapid overall intelligibility gains. Each of these time periods is referred to as a *cycle*. During each cycle, phoneme targets are presented for each of the major patterns. For example, if a child has five major processes, and if 2 to 4 weeks are to be spent on representative phoneme targets of each of the major patterns, a cycle might be as short as 10 weeks or as long as 20 weeks.

A restriction was imposed on the length of the cycles in our Phonology Program in that they had to coincide with the university calendar. During the regular academic year, each cycle was approximately 12 weeks long. Summer cycles averaged 6 weeks in length. The children participated once a week for 60 to 90 minutes.

Although several phonological patterns were presented during each cycle, only one phonological pattern was facilitated at a time. Furthermore, we did not remain with a pattern or a phoneme until a predetermined criterion level was reached. Rather our goal was to start the emergence of each major phonological pattern in order to develop the child's entire phonological system. Thus we were interested in facilitating the emergence of a number of phonological patterns, rather than in perfecting phoneme segments. The number of sessions devoted to each phonological pattern varied. Generally a minimum of two phoneme targets was provided for each pattern per cycle. Also, rarely were more than 4 or 5 weeks spent on any element of a phonological pattern during any given cycle.

Typically, the easier target phoneme(s) for each target pattern were presented during the first cycle, with increasingly more difficult phoneme combinations and groupings being presented during ensuing cycles. Reassessment occurred between cycles to ascertain which phonological patterns, if any, were beginning to emerge in spontaneous speech. Very little carryover is expected during the first cycle. If an adequate foundation is laid, however, extensive progress occurs during the next few cycles. Each succeeding cycle becomes increasingly more complex. More difficult phoneme combinations are incorporated, and previously presented phoneme targets for a given phonological pattern are grouped together.

**Remediation Sessions**

Each remediation session begins and ends with a few minutes of auditory bombardment, amplified slightly through an auditory training unit. The child listens to the clinician read approximately 15 words which incorporate the session's target phoneme(s). For example, for the phonological process velar fronting, the phoneme target may be the voiceless prevocalic velar /k/, in words, such as "come, coke, cat," and so on. The clinician reads to the child who listens attentively while engaged in a quiet manipulative activity. The child does not repeat the "auditory bombardment" words, and, therefore, these words do not have to be chosen with special care.

A second set of two to five words are selected which meet the following criteria: 1) are representative of the week's target pattern; 2) can be pictured or be presented as an object; 3) include neither consonants nor vowels that may produce unwanted assimilation effects (particularly during the first cycle); and 4) can be elicited without struggle, although tactual cues and auditory and visual stimuli are often incorporated during early production practice activities. Words such as "cow" and "car" meet these criteria and are illustrative of those used to introduce prevocalic voiceless velars during Cycle I. Words such as "cat" and "can" are deemed to be poor preliminary choices for production practice words during the first presentation because they contain alveolar consonants, which typically produce regressive alveolar assimilation. It is usually difficult at first for a child who exhibits velar fronting not to say /tæt/ for "cat." Thus, when teaching velars, words containing alveolars should be reserved until later cycles when the child has developed some facility in producing velars.

This second word list is used to develop a set of stimuli which serves to elicit spontaneous verbal responses. Objects are utilized for children whose general level of functioning is below the age of 3. Index cards (5 × 8 inches) are used for children who are ready for two-dimensional stimuli. The "nonreaders" and older children who are poor readers draw pictures of their target words after first saying them, and the clinicians write the names of the pictures under them so that adults are able to identify the pictures. Because older children with severe speech disorders typically are poor readers, pictures are used frequently for these older children. Whenever possible, reading activities are incorporated into later cycles.

The objects and picture cards are used to elicit spontaneous productions of the target words in a variety of child oriented activities, such as bowling, fishing, and so on. The child or clinician names a picture, saying the phonological pattern's target phoneme(s) correctly before taking a turn. The clinician provides as many tactual, verbal, or auditory cues as are necessary to ensure success. For example, a clinician might provide tactual cues, such as touching the child's throat when eliciting /k/ to indicate "backness." Sometimes a verbal assist is utilized, for example, asking the child, "Is it tar or car?" In some instances, it is necessary to break a word apart stressing the vowel (e.g., /kə̣ ɑːɚ/) in order to eradicate the /t/. Cues are gradually reduced as the session progresses and as the child gains facility with a sound.

Initially, the child need not necessarily produce the whole word correctly. It is essential, however, that the child correctly produce the actual target phoneme(s) for the particular phonological pattern being facilitated. As defined above, the target phonemes are not necessarily equivalent to the phonemes of the word. Rather, they are pattern elements that are being targeted. Because it has been observed that these children do not gain anything by practicing target phonemes incorrectly, it has been deemed preferable to teach correct production of a limited number of targets in words, rather than to allow error productions to occur. If the child cannot say the targets even with cues, the clinician should reconsider the choice of targets.

At the conclusion of the production practice activities, probes are used to determine which phoneme(s) to target during the next session. The assessment is made by having the child imitate the clinician's productions of potential target words. Although general phonological patterns have already been identified by means of the phonological evaluation, the actual progression week by week depends upon each child's individual abilities. For example, initial /s/ clusters are more stimulable for some children, whereas others have less difficulty with final /s/ clusters. Furthermore, some cluster combinations can be elicited more readily than others. For example, when probing for an /s/ cluster target, the clinician asks the child to repeat words such as "star," "spoon," "snake," "smoke," "boats," and "mops." The combination that is the easiest to elicit is selected as the target for the next session.

As indicated above, auditory bombardment is repeated at the end of each clinical session. The week's "listening list" of words is then given to parents and/or to school personnel with the instruction to provide auditory bombardment of the week's phoneme target(s) on a daily basis between clinic sessions. In addition, the children take their picture cards with them so that the target words may be practiced once a day. When the targets represent the same phonological pattern, the children may take the cards home for several weeks. Thus, if the preceding week's target was also initial /s/-clusters, the child takes both sets of cards home. If the child targeted velars last week, and initial /s/ clusters this week, however, the clinician withholds the velar pictures until the next cycle. The child brings the picture cards back to the clinic each time and names them for the clinician before the new lesson begins. If the same phonological pattern is targeted during the new lesson as during the preceding session, the cards from the prior session are also used in some of the production practice activities.

### Targets for Profoundly Unintelligible Children

The least intelligible children are the ones who omit entire classes of sounds. A few produce no obstruents, either prevocalically or post-vocalically (e.g., bed → /ɛ/ or /wɛ/), and a very small number produce no sonorants (e.g., run → /ʌ/).

Children who produce no glides may spend a week targeting initial /w/. Children who omit word-final nasals usually target final /m/ for one week and final /n/ for the next. The children who produce some sonorants, but no obstruents, typically target final /p/ one week, followed by a week of final /t/ or final /k/, whichever is more stimulable. We have found that stimulating final voiceless stops for a couple of weeks helps a child become aware that many words have endings. Typically the child begins spontaneously to produce some final consonants a few months later.

Children who are able to produce V<u>C</u> or <u>C</u>V but not <u>C</u>V<u>C</u> (consonant-vowel-consonant) syllables profit from targeting words such as "pipe," "pop," and "pup" for a week. The goal is not to produce perfect consonants or words, but rather to teach the child to produce word endings and word beginnings in the same word.

Speech samples of some profoundly unintelligible children are restricted to monosyllables and occasional bisyllabic utterances. These children profit from targeting "syllableness" for a couple of weeks. Equal stress compound words such as "cowboy" and "baseball" are presented for one week, followed by combinations such as "cowboy hat" and "baseball bat" the next week. The goal here is to produce the appropriate number of syllables, rather than to produce specific phonemes or perfect words.

Children who demonstrate the ability to produce some multisyllabic combinations and some singleton obstruents, although not necessarily the correct ones, are ready to begin developing other aspects of their phonological systems. Typically, children do not need to "recycle" singleton "consonantness" nor "syllableness."

## Targets for Children with Severely Unintelligible Speech

Children with severely unintelligible speech also evidence some omissions, particularly in consonant clusters, but their omissions are not as extensive as for the profoundly unintelligible children. Severely unintelligible children profit from targeting classes of sounds which are deficient.

Many of the children in our Phonology Program experienced difficulty producing velars, particularly in the prevocalic position. Some children were unable to produce velars even in isolation during the first cycle. In such instances, velars were stimulated auditorily and tactually, but were not presented in production practice words until a later cycle. In general, we found that word-final /k/ was easier to elicit than prevocalic /k/.

A small number of children evidenced backing. They readily produced /k, g, ŋ, h/, but experienced difficulty producing alveolars. For these children, it was usually necessary to target final /t/ followed by initial /t/ for a couple of weeks for two or three cycles.

No two children evidenced exactly the same phonological system and no two children followed exactly the same cyclic progressions. Every one of these unintelligible children, however, needed to target stridents, liquids, and consonant clusters to some extent.

A major component of this remediation approach involves teaching /s/ clusters. We have found that it is effective to teach unintelligible children who substitute stops for stridents to produce /s/ or the stridency feature in an /s/ cluster (e.g., star, spoon) before teaching prevocalic /s/ (e.g., sun). The reason is that children often insert /t/, as in /s:tʌn/ for "sun" during their first attempts to acquire /s/ clusters. At first, more time and effort are often required to teach singletons than clusters because attention must be given to the elimination of the stop consonant while teaching the production of /s/. Also, it has been found that less time is required later to teach singleton /s/.

For some children, word-final clusters that contain a stop and an /s/ (e.g., /ts/) are the easiest initial targets for eliciting stridency. Usually, the concept of plurals is incorporated when targeting final /s/ clusters, and in some instances, third person singular present tense verbs (e.g., "eats") and some possessives (e.g., "Pat's") are taught.

The younger children in our phonology program demonstrated excellent ability to generalize to all /s/ clusters. The older children, however, usually had to target virtually every type of /s/ cluster at some time, including medial (e.g., "mi_ster") and three-consonant clusters (e.g., "straw").

One phrase which was usually incorporated by the third cycle to facilitate generalization of stridency was, "It's a _____." In the first week of this cycle, children labeled items whose names contain no strident phonemes (e.g., "It's a door"), and in the second week they used this carrier phrase when naming their /s/ cluster pictures (e.g., "It's a spoon"). The "It's a" phrase was used only to facilitate stridency.

In the first year of the Phonology Program liquids were not targeted until all other phonological patterns had begun to emerge. Subsequently, it was discovered that an extraordinary amount of time and effort was required at the end of the Phonology Program to teach liquids, particularly /r/. We then began introducing liquids during the first cycle and observed that the early introduction of liquids resulted in increased facility in their production and faster transition into spontaneous speech.

The primary goals for teaching liquids during cycle I were to develop auditory and kinesthetic awareness, and to reduce the gliding process by eliminating the intruding /w/ or /j/. Also, when teaching prevocalic /r/, it proved useful to break the sounds of each word apart and to prolong the vowel following the liquid. Thus, the model for "rock" during cycle I was /ɝɑɑk/ rather than /ɝːɑk/. Premature attempts at blending /r/ and a vowel have consistently resulted in the child's saying /ɝwɑk/.

## CASE EXAMPLES

Child A entered the Phonology Program at age 6. His speech was characterized by cluster reduction, stridency deletion, and liquid deviations. He did not delete singleton consonants, and he produced classes of sounds other than stridents and liquids appropriately. His conversational utterances were judged to be 10% to 15% intelligible.

During cycle I, Child A targeted the following (one per session): word-initial /sp/, /st/, /sk/, /sm/, /sn/; word-final /ts/, /ps/, /ks/; and word-initial /l/, /r/. The second cycle he targeted /sp/, /st/, and /sk/ during one session, followed by /sm/ and /sn/ the next. The third session he targeted final /ps, ts, ks/. The fourth session of cycle II, Child A used "It's a" phrases (e.g., "It's a table") to name words that did not contain /s/. During the fifth session of cycle II, he named /s/ cluster pictures using "It's a" phrases (e.g., "It's a star"). In the sixth session, he targeted prevocalic /f/, and in the seventh session he targeted prevocalic /s/. Liquids were presented again during the last three sessions of cycle

II: prevocalic /l/ in the eighth session, followed by prevocalic /kl/ and /gl/ clusters in the ninth session, and prevocalic /r/ in the tenth session. During cycle II, more difficult target words were added to those that had been used in cycle I.

During his third and last cycle, Child A targeted /sp, st, sk, sm, sn/ all in the first session. The second session he targeted /ps, ts, ks/, again. In the third session, he named his initial /s/ cluster pictures using the "It's a" carrier phrase. The remaining sessions were spent targeting more difficult consonant cluster combinations including final and medial /s/ clusters (e.g., "mask" and "mister"). Conversational speech samples at the end of cycle III and the results of post-testing indicated that stridents, liquids, and consonant clusters were emerging in A's spontaneous utterances.

Child B entered the Phonology Program at age 4 producing neither prevocalic nor postvocalic obstruents. His utterances consisted mainly of monosyllables, which included occasional prevocalic nasal productions and the glide /w/. He was judged to be completely unintelligible. Gesturing was his means of communication.

Final /p/ was targeted during the first session, final /k/ in the second, and final /t/ in the third session. In the fourth session, Child B targeted "syllableness" in spondee words, and during the fifth session another word was presented with each spondee word (e.g., "cowboy hat"). In the sixth session, Child B targeted C̲V̲C̲ (i.e., initial and final consonants of CVC syllables). The target words were "pipe," "pup," and "pop." He targeted final /ts/ during the seventh session of his first cycle. Initial /sp/ was presented the following week. His next easiest /s/ cluster, which was /sm/, was taught during the ninth week. Word-final /ɚ/ was "stimulated" during the tenth week. By the end of cycle I, Child B was saying some final consonants, and he was using two and three words together in spontaneous utterances.

Child B targeted velars during the first two sessions of cycle II, final /k/ in the first session, and initial /g/ in the second session. Plurals were targeted during the third session with the model being /s/ rather than /z/. Thus for the target word "boys," the model was /bɔɪs/ rather than /bɔɪz/. Children with severe speech disorders typically say /bɔɪd/ for "boys" when the final /z/ model is presented. Furthermore, because normally developing young children rarely produce voiced final obstruents (Hodson and Paden, 1981), it was deemed inappropriate to teach voiced final consonants. It did not seem appropriate to ask our unintelligible clients to produce more "correct" sounds than their more intelligible peers use. Furthermore, we observed that as their phonological systems developed, the children sorted out the voicing contrasts.

Cycle III involved "retargeting" velars, /s/ clusters, singleton stridents, and liquids. Increasingly, more difficult target words were added during cycles IV and V, with the emphasis placed on velars, liquids, stridents, and especially consonant clusters. By the end of cycle V, Child B (at age 5½ years) was using velars and stridents fairly consistently in spontaneous utterances. Also at that time, liquids and consonant clusters were emerging in his speech.

These are examples of cycles utilized for two unintelligible children. Each child's cyclic progression was individualized. No two children in the Phonology Remediation Program followed exactly the same sequence. Reassessment occurred between cycles to ascertain which patterns were emerging and which needed to be recycled. Child A was essentially intelligible after three cycles (12 months) and Child B after five cycles (18 months). Their speech was not 100% perfect when they were dismissed, but both boys continued to develop their phonological systems on their own. Reevaluation, which occurred approximately 6 months after dismissal, demonstrated that spontaneous speech performances of both boys were continuing to improve. Furthermore, neither boy required additional articulation programming, although Child B received some training in syntax in his public school.

## DISCUSSION

The remediation approach which is described in this chapter is facilitative and integrative in nature and is based on developmental phonology principles. According to this approach, the primary intervention goal is to increase intelligibility by facilitating development of each child's phonological system. A major consideration has been the concept of facilitating emergence of phonological patterns in contrast to the tradition of perfecting phoneme segments. Many university training programs advocate reliance on singleton phoneme acquisition norms and on behavioristic programs to provide guidelines pertaining to the selection of which sounds to train and when to train them. Many speech-language pathology graduates report that when they have unintelligible children in their caseloads, they typically choose an "early" singleton phoneme (e.g., /f/), and teach it in word-initial, word-final, and word-medial positions (and occasionally in clusters) until a designated criterion has been reached (e.g., 90%). Thus, a semester or two may be spent on each and every phoneme. Such programming seems to be appropriate for a child who misarticulates only a few phonemes (e.g., the child who substitutes /f/ for /θ/ and/or has a frontal lisp), but it has been found to be incredibly time consuming for children who miss more consonants than they produce.

The first step in planning remediation programs for unintelligible children involved analyzing their phonological systems. Each child's spontaneous utterances elicited via administration of The Assessment of Phonological Processes (Hodson, 1980) then were recorded and then were analyzed for the presence of phonological processes. Every one of the unintelligible children in the Phonology Program needed to target stridents, consonant clusters, and liquids. There were many children, of course, who needed to target more basic phonological patterns first (e.g., final consonants). Each child's remediation program was *individualized*. By identifying and starting at the *optimal* place in each individual's phonological system, we were able to provide situations whereby even the most unintelligible children could experience immediate and tangible success.

No two children followed exactly the same sequence. Cycles were utilized that varied in length from 6 to 14 weeks. A week or more within each cycle was spent on each major phonological process. Reassessment occurred between cycles, and those phonological patterns that had not yet begun to emerge were recycled. The cycles became progressively more demanding. Target words that contained increasingly more difficult combinations of phonemes and consonant clusters were added during later cycles.

Auditory bombardment utilizing an auditory training unit that was set at a low level was incorporated twice in *every* session to develop auditory *awareness* of the targets and to improve listening skills. Production practice was used to increase facility in producing the respective targets and to develop kinesthetic awareness of a new way of producing the targets.

Semantic differences between a child's particular production for a pattern and the adult's production were explained to the child when appropriate, and occasionally a picture of a "foil" word was incorporated (e.g., "top" along with the /st/ cluster words which included "stop"). However, routine use of minimal pairs for production practice activities was usually too difficult for our clients during their early sessions.

This Phonology Remediation Program was designed for unintelligible children. It is neither necessary nor realistic to use this approach for the child who has a mild articulation disorder. Children who began participating in our Phonology Program at 3 or 4 years of age was essentially intelligible and was able to experience success in reading, phonics, and spelling activities in school, except in instances where there were other complications such as learning disabilities. The children who began their Phonology Programs at second or third grade had already experienced considerable academic failure and frustration.

The longest time required for any of these unintelligible children in the Phonology Program to become intelligible was 18 months. Although most did not exhibit "perfect" speech at the time of their dismissals, all were judged to be intelligible. Furthermore, their phonological systems continued to develop after dismissal. Reevaluations indicated that progress continued even for those who did not receive additional intervention in their schools.

Although the Phonology Remediation Program was created and refined in a university clinic, it has been adapted successfully for use in public schools and in hospitals. The approach appears to be serving rather efficiently the needs of a low incidence population of highly unintelligible children. Posttest measures (Hodson, 1980; Hodson and Paden, 1983) indicate that the program is accountable. The approach is still evolving. Efforts continue to be directed toward improving and refining evaluation and remediation procedures, so that unintelligible children can be served even more expeditiously in the future.

**REFERENCES**

Hodson, B. 1980. The Assessment of Phonological Processes. Interstate, Danville, IL.

Hodson, B. 1981. Evaluation and remediation of phonological disorders. Communicative Disorders: An Audio Journal for Continuing Education. Grune & Stratton, New York.

Hodson, B. 1982. Remediation of speech patterns associated with low levels of phonological performance. In: M. Crary (ed.), Phonological Intervention: Concepts and Procedures. College-Hill Press, San Diego, CA.

Hodson, B., and Paden, E. 1981. Phonological processes which characterize unintelligible and intelligible speech in early childhood. J. Speech Hear. Disord. 46:369–373.

Hodson, B., and Paden, E. 1983. Targeting Intelligible Speech: A Phonological Approach to Remediation. College-Hill Press, San Diego, CA.

# CHAPTER 6

# Correcting Multiple Misarticulations

*Donald Mowrer*

*Mowrer provides a rationale for the diagnosis and treatment of the articulation errors of Clifford, a young child for whom most of the consonant sounds were in error. Of interest are the detailed treatment strategies indicated by Mowrer and the utilization of these teaching strategies.*

1. *A phonologic process approach was used by Mowrer to analyze Clifford's articulation patterns. What were the major patterns that characterized Clifford's articulatory deviations? Was the phonological process analysis the basis for Mowrer's goals for treatment?*

2. *What was Mowrer's reasoning for selecting some of the fricatives as the first sounds to teach to Clifford? Do you agree with this strategy? Mowrer's treatment approach involved motor practice. What is your evaluation of this approach in view of the fact that a phonological process analysis was used to categorize the articulation errors?*

3. *In view of Clifford's success, do you think that parents can be trained to work with their children as the primary clinical instructor under the guidance of a speechlanguage pathologist? If yes, under what circumstances would you recommend the utilization of parents in this way?*

I WILL DESCRIBE THE STRATEGY used to change the phonological system of a 5-year-old child, Clifford, who misarticulated or omitted most of the English consonant sounds. At the time of testing, his hearing was normal. No organic factors were identified that could account for his articulation problem. Clifford is one of many children whose problem would be considered a "functional" articulation problem.

## TELEPHONE USED TO PROVIDE SERVICES

Clifford resided in a rural area 100 miles from an area where he could obtain formal articulation training, therefore, the telephone was used to monitor speech treatment. Although using the telephone to provide instructional services is not a new idea, it is not a common approach. Whether or not a phone is used to deliver services is a secondary issue. My intention is to show that the teaching strategy described here can be applied to a large number of children who demonstrate similar types of articulation problems.

## DESCRIPTION OF THE PROBLEM

Clifford attended kindergarten in a rural community. His parents, concerned about his slow speech development, arranged for a speech evaluation at a university speech and hearing clinic.

### Testing Procedure

The Goldman-Fristoe Test of Articulation (Goldman and Fristoe, 1972) was used to assess Clifford's articulation. Clifford's responses to the Sounds-in-Words Subtest are shown in Table 1. Also indicated in Table 1 are explanations for the diacritical markings used to code Clifford's speech.

One way to understand Clifford's phonological system is to superimpose his system on the adult system. Consonants can be classified in terms of place of articulation and manner of production. Manner of production (stops, fricatives, and affricatives) will be considered first.

*Analysis of Stop, Fricative, and Affricative Sounds*  Each of Clifford's articulation responses to the test words of the Goldman-Fristoe Test was compared with the adult model. The purpose was to determine how the two systems differed. The sounds /b/ and /d/ are often used as substitutions for /k, g, v, ð, tʃ, dʒ/. Clifford produced /t/ and /p/ without aspiration, consequently these two consonants sounded like /d/ and /b/, respectively. The only fricative Clifford produced was /f/, which occasionally was substituted for /ʃ/.

Table 1.   Clifford's responses to test words of the Sounds-in-Words Subtest of the Goldman-Fristoe Test of Articulation (1972)[a]

| Test word | Clifford's response | Test word | Clifford's response |
|---|---|---|---|
| house | [aʊ] | this | [dɪ] |
| telephone | ['tɛləfon] | carrot | ['tɛw't] |
| cup | ['tʌp] | orange | [ɔn] |
| gun | [dʌn] | bathtub | [bæf'tɔb] |
| knife | [naɪf] | bath | [bæ] |
| window | [fɪndo] | thumb | [dʌm] |
| wagon | [fædən] | finger | [fində] |
| chicken | ['tɪʔn̩] | ring | [fɪŋ] |
| zipper | [ipə] | jumping | [dʌmpɪn] |
| scissors | [idə] | pajamas | [pədæmə] |
| duck | [dʌʔ] | plane | [pen] |
| yellow | [io] | blue | [bu] |
| vacuum | [bæʔum] | brush | [bʌ] |
| matches | [mæʔə] | drum | [dʌm] |
| lamp | [læmp] | flag | [fæg] |
| shovel | [fʌbə] | Santa Claus | [æntə 'tɔ] |
| car | ['ta:] | Christmas tree | ['tɪmʔ 'ti] |
| rabbit | [fæbɪt] | squirrel | ['tɛə] |
| fishing | [fɪʔn̩] | sleeping | [ipən] |
| church | ['tʌʔ] | bed | [bɛd] |
| feather | [fɛʊ] | stove | ['to] |
| pencils | ['pɛnɔ] | | |

[a] ['], unaspirated; [ ̩], syllabic consonant.

***Analysis of Liquids and Glides***   The second area of concern was Clifford's use of liquids and glides. The /l/ was produced correctly inconsistently in the initial and medial positions, and consistently in the final word position and in clusters. The /f/ was substituted for the consonantal /r/ in the initial position. In the final position, the post-vocalic /r/ variants were substituted by a /w/, the lengthening of a single vowel, a vowel addition, or deleted. The /r/ in blends was omitted. The /f/ was also substituted for initial /w/.

The substitution of /f/ for glides and liquids is not commonly found in the speech of young children. Sound substitutions within the obstruent group or within the liquid and glide group are frequent, but substitutions for sounds between groups does not generally occur. We would expect substitutions like /f/ for /s/, /t/ for /k/, and /s/ for /ʃ/, but not /t/ for /r/, /f/ for /r/, or /k/ for /l/. Although Clifford's substitution of /f/ for /r/ and /w/ is unusual, the other substitutions and omissions noted in Clifford's speech are those often produced by young children.

***Analysis of Nasals***   The nasals were generally not in error. However, /n/ was sometimes substituted for /ŋ/ when the velar consonant following the nasal was fronted as, for example, [fində] for /fɪŋgɚ/. Note that /ŋ/ in the word *ring* is correct.

## Analysis of Clifford's Phonological System

According to Ingram (1976), children pass through three sound simplification processes from about the ages of 1 through 4 years. They are referred to here as *syllable structure, assimilation,* and *substitution.* It is interesting to compare Clifford's system with each of these processes.

### Syllable Structure

1. *Omission of final consonants*   Although Clifford often omits final consonants, the few consonants present in his repertoire also occurred in final position slots, as evidenced by the use of final consonants in the words *cup, gun, lamp, rabbit,* and *knife.* If Clifford possessed fricatives, there is a good chance he would have used them in final position. Consequently, I did not feel that omission of final consonants constituted a major problem for Clifford.
2. *Reduplication*   Clifford does not reduplicate syllables.
3. *Cluster reduction*   A problem exists with respect to Clifford's use of clusters. He usually omits the second consonant in the cluster, often a liquid or glide, and omits the first consonant if it is a fricative. He appears to be in the second stage of cluster reduction according to Ingram's (1976) scheme of cluster learning. Ingram states that the first stage is omission of both clusters. The second stage is omission of the second cluster, and the third stage involves a substitution of one sound in the cluster.
4. *Omission of unstressed syllable*   There was no evidence of this phonological process. Syllable structure, for the most part, does not appear to be a problem for Clifford.

### Assimilation

1. *Vowel assimilation*   There appears to be no evidence of vowel assimilation.
2. *Vowels affecting voicing*   The omission of aspiration for /p/ and /t/ was probably responsible for their sounding voiced.
3. *Consonant assimilation*   There was no clear evidence of consonant assimilation in Clifford's substitution pattern.

**Substitution**   Substitutions comprised the bulk of Clifford's articulation problem. Each of the six areas in this classification is discussed with regard to his misarticulations.

1. *Stopping*   The use of stops for fricatives and affricatives was frequent as illustrated by ['tʌʔ] for "church" and [dɪ] for "this." On

the other hand, fricatives were often omitted as in the case of [idə] for "scissors" and [bʌ] for "brush." In other instances, /f/ was used correctly and, as noted above, was substituted for /w/ and /r/. The process of stopping was present, but not always consistently used.

2.  *Fronting*  Fronting was present in many instances as when [b] and [d] were used in place of velars /k/ and /g/. A tendency toward fronting also was evidenced by a ['t] for /tʃ/ as in ['tʌʔ] for "church," and an [f] for /ʃ/ in [fʌbə] for "shovel."

3.  *Use of alveolar nasal for velar nasal*  This substitution may have occurred because the nasal assimilated the place of articulation of neighboring front stops produced by the child, as in [fɪndə] for "finger." When a front stop was not present, /ŋ/ was produced as in [fɪŋ] for "ring." However, for the *-ing* suffix [n] was used.

4.  *Liquid replacement*  Sometimes the /l/ was used correctly except in clusters and in the final position where it was omitted. The consonantal [r] was replaced by [f] in the initial position ([fæbɪt] for rabbit), and by /w/ in the medial position (['tɛw't] for carrot).

5.  *Syllabic [ɝ] and [ɚ] replacement*  The [ɝ] and [ɚ] were replaced by a [w], a lengthened vowel, or were deleted. This substitution was consistent, and is typical of the misarticulations of young children in the lower elementary grades.

6.  *Omission*  Clifford omitted many consonant sounds. Sounds frequently omitted were the alveolars, dentals, palatals, and fricatives (except /f/), and the glottal fricative (/h/).


## DEVELOPING GOALS FOR TREATMENT

The phonological analysis of Clifford's articulation indicated five areas as targets for treatment. Each target involves the addition of sounds.

1.  *Fricatives must be added.*  The addition of frication will enable him to produce eight sounds, namely /s, z, θ, ð, v, ʃ, ʒ, h/, all of which he does not produce. This addition will contribute most to increasing his intelligibility.

2.  *Affricates /tʃ, dʒ/ must be added.*  These sounds should be taught after the fricatives are learned.

3.  *Velar stops /k, g/ must be added, even though [g] appears in "flag."*  The velar nasal /ŋ/ is present, and probably will be used more often as the velar stops are acquired.

4.  *Consonantal [r] and vocalic [ɝ] and [ɚ] must be added.*  Each of these sounds may require different teaching strategies. Possibly mastery of one may facilitate the learning of the others.

5. *Cluster addition*   One member of each of the consonant clusters
   must be added to complete cluster development.

These five goals for the treatment program were, for the most part,
ordered sequentially. The addition of fricatives was the first step in
training. We believed that the use of these sounds would contribute
greatly to Clifford's intelligibility. For example, consider the sentence
"He sat on the bush." Clifford would say this sentence as follows: [i
æt ɔn dʌ bʌ]. Obviously, this statement is unintelligible without the
presence of /h, s, θ, ʃ/. These fricatives were absent in all required
contexts in 31 of the 43 test words shown in Table 1. According to
Weiss et al. (1980, p. 55), the fricatives /s, z, ð, h, v/ occur 14.4% of
the time in English, whereas [r, ɝ, ɚ] occur 8.3%, and /k, g/ occur only
4.7% of the time. By establishing the single feature of frication and
adding voicing, the number of sounds Clifford can utilize will be increased; and the resultant increase in intelligibility will produce the
greatest change in his speech.

A second reason why the teaching should begin with fricatives is
that most fricatives are easy to evoke using simple verbal and visual
cues. We had Clifford stick out his tongue and blow over the top of it
to produce /θ/ or a close approximation of it. Even though the airstream
initially was produced laterally, Clifford gained experience with the
fricative feature. Frication can also be evoked by asking Clifford to
close his teeth, push his tongue up against the teeth, and blow. A
sibilant type feature can be produced in this way. By providing additional cues regarding tongue, teeth, and lip placement fricative production can be shaped through a series of successive approximations.
I have found that several fricative sounds can be evoked within 10 to
15 minutes during the first session; but affricatives and liquids cannot
be evoked as easily. I recommend addition of frication as the first goal
chiefly because this feature holds the greatest potential for rapid gains
in intelligibility, and because they are easy to produce.

The second goal was the teaching of /k, g/. The sounds were to
be introduced early during the treatment sessions after /s/ and /θ/ (as
well as their voiced cognates) were used correctly in words. Because
Clifford could produce stops (including the glottal stop), it was believed
that learning to use /k/ and /g/ could be acquired easily.

Once Clifford correctly produced words in phrases and used the
/θ, h, s, v, z/ consistently, /ʃ, ʒ/ were introduced. When these sounds
were used correctly in words, the third goal was to teach /tʃ, dʒ/ because the stops (/t/ and /d/) and fricatives (/ʃ/ and /ʒ/) that make up
these affricatives had been acquired.

The fourth goal was to teach the vocalic [ɝ, ɚ], and the consonantal [r] in this order. I have found these sounds are among the more

difficult to evoke, in part, because a visual model of tongue position is difficult to provide. Another reason that /r/ sounds are difficult to evoke is because positive transfer of the relevant articulatory features is not usually possible. For example, learning /s, z/ can facilitate the learning of /ʃ, ʒ/ because both pairs of sounds share many common features. On the other hand, the features of [r, ɝ, ɚ] are sufficiently different from those of other sounds to preclude transfer.

The last goal was to improve cluster production. All sounds of a cluster should be available as singles before consonant blending is taught. The teaching of clusters can be ordered in terms of ease of production. One logical starting point is with the fricative-sonorant combinations, namely /sm, sn, sl/. The reason fricative-sonorants are introduced first is because both sounds of this cluster are continuous sounds and the clinician can prolong the sounds when they are taught. The fricative-stops /sp, st, sk/ were taught next, and then the stop-liquids /bl, tr, kl, dr, gr, gl/ were introduced.

### EXECUTION OF THE TREATMENT PLAN

One factor that complicated deliver of the treatment plan was that Clifford lived in a remote rural area and he was unable to attend regular clinical sessions. The use of the telephone to provide instructions placed obvious constraints upon the treatment program, so Clifford's mother was asked to carry out much of the treatment in the home. Thus, the distance factor did not influence adversely the selection or execution of clinical goals. Calls were placed with a WATS line at least three times each week, including holiday periods.

### Motivation

A token economy system was used as the motivational technique. Accordingly, Clifford's mother was instructed to provide Clifford with a token after each correct response. Clifford exchanged the tokens for toys. The definition of a correct response for each objective was clearly explained.

### Teaching Fricative Production

The first goal was to teach Clifford production of several sounds containing frication. The first sound selected for training was /s/, which was taught using the S-PACK (Mowrer et al., 1974), a commercially available instructional program. This sound was selected over /θ/ as the first sound because: 1) intensity is greater; 2) the S-PACK, designed to teach correct /s/ production, has proven to be a highly successful program; and 3) the written instructions and follow-up program of the S-PACK could be used effectively by Clifford's mother.

The S-PACK program consists of a step-by-step hierarchy of production tasks beginning with [s] in isolation, followed by [s] in nonsense syllables, in words containing [s], in phrases containing [s], and finally, in words in simulated conversational speech situations. Often it was difficult for the clinician to discriminate between correct and incorrect [s] productions over the telephone. Nevertheless, Clifford's attempts to produce frication could be detected. Any success at producing frication during [s] production was rewarded. His mother, who was provided with an S-PACK program, was able to monitor correct [s] productions, and often was asked to verify to the clinician whether an [s] attempt was correct or not. When Clifford completed the first three parts of the S-PACK, his mother was asked to continue the training on a daily basis for 3 consecutive weeks with the S-PACK program.

A program similar to the S-PACK, designed to correct the [θ] and [ð], was later sent to Clifford's mother. This program was introduced as the S-PACK was being presented. The same training sequence was used to teach these two sounds. Training began with production in isolation and proceeded to practice in conversational speech situations. After the third week of training, Clifford began using [s, z, θ, ð] occasionally in conversational speech.

### Teaching Velars

The /k/ was introduced when it was observed that Clifford spontaneously said /k/ correctly in the word *think*. This occurrence of /k/ was fortunate and caused us to deviate from our original plan. Although originally we decided to introduce /k/ after several fricatives had been acquired, the spontaneous occurrence of /k/ suggested that this sound be taught simultaneously with the fricatives.

The /k/ was imbedded in carrier phrases as the final sound in the word *make,* and followed by a variety of other sounds. Here are some examples:

> make a book
> make a soap
> make a boy
> make a sun
> make a zoo
> make a thumb
> make some money
> make some food
> make the bell

These phrases were selected to provide practice in coarticulation sequences using /k/ as a releaser of schwa or to precede the consonants /s/ or /ð/. These phrases were said without a pause between words, and spoken in a rhythmical fashion with primary stress on the first and last words. When /k/ was produced correctly at least 95% of the time, it was taught in other contexts as a releaser and arrester of syllables.

At this time, the voiced cognate /g/ was introduced in phrases. Examples are as follows:

> I'm a goat
> bug a boo
> it's a gun
> he can go
> there's a girl
> it's a girl

The /h/ was introduced next in a manner different from the /s/ and /θ/. After training was underway, it was observed that sounds sharing features with /s/ and /θ/ were relatively easy to evoke. Therefore, there was no necessity to teach /h/ in isolation. Syllable sequences, such as [hʌm, hʌm, hʌm, ho, ho, ho], and [hʌm, ho, hʌm, ho], words (*him, ham, hope, hat, hand,* and *hit*), phrases containing /h/, and sentences were modeled for Clifford. At this time he repeated these models accurately.

In all sessions sound production practice was limited to about 8 minutes and was followed by a brief period or practice in conversation. Clifford's articulation errors during conversation were noted and phrases containing these errors were used subsequently as practice items. For example, Clifford said [ai ad ə æmbəgə] (I had a hamburger) in conversation. A series of phrases emphasizing /h/ was used for practice during the remainder of that session, and during the following session. Examples of practice items for the /h/ phrases were:

> I had a hamburger
> I had a coat
> I had a soup
> I had a goat
> I had a thumb
> I had a home
> I had a hat

The /z/, /ð/, and /g/ were introduced in the intervocalic position because assimilation of voicing of the surrounding vowels usually facilitates the production of voiced fricatives. Examples of phrases in which /z/, /ð/, and /g/ were introduced are:

> he's a man (/z/)
> either you (/ð/)
> he goes home (/g/)

Certain phrases were selected to maximize contrast in place and manner of production. Place features were contrasted by using phrases

that required rapid successive movements from the front (f) of the
mouth to the back (b), as illustrated in the following examples:

It's a bug body
     f  b  f

There's a tug boat
      f  b  f

It's a flag pole
    f  b  f

He makes buildings
   f b   f   f  b

Grandpa comes home
 b     f  b  f

Manner contrasts are illustrated by the following examples (s =
stop, c = continuant, and n = nasal):

like some tar
  s   c  n   s

cook for me
    s c   n

give him pepper
 s c    n s

there's papa
     c s

After 20 sessions of practice, Clifford produced fricatives /s, z, θ,
ʃ, v, ʒ, h/ and velars /k, g/ correctly. When conversing with his mother
he produced them correctly most of the time. Also his speech was
intelligible to strangers, although before treatment only about 10% of
his speech was intelligible.

### Introduction of [ɝ], [ɚ], and [r]

After the fricatives and velar stops were used correctly in connected
speech, [ɝ] was introduced. Instructions were given to Clifford's
mother regarding tongue placement for [ɝ]. Clifford was told to curl
his tongue tip up and back and produce [ɝ]. He produced a close approximation of [ɝ] during his first few attempts. With repeated practice
and encouragement from his mother, Clifford was able to produce [ɝ]
correctly with consistency in isolation. Then [ɝ] was practiced initially
in the word *her*. Later phrases were introduced as follows:

her coat
her comb
her gun
her gas
her cold
her soap
her thumb

Early in training, words were used in which velar stops immediately followed [ɝ] because they are regarded as a facilitating context for [ɝ]. In the following session two-syllable words were used in order to provide opportunity to practice [ɚ]. These words were *mother, father, sister, heater, bumper, feather,* and *either.* Finally, [r] was practiced in contexts in which it is preceded by vowels, as in the following phrases:

> see the arm
> the barn is big
> his car is nice
> far away

Clifford practiced phrases that assisted him in acquiring coarticulation skills. Conversational speech involves rapidly coarticulated speech sounds, and unless these movement patterns are practiced, correct articulation in conversational speech cannot be acquired. Ideally, phrases should be selected from those used in daily conversational speech, although most of the phrases used early in treatment were constructed to take advantage of coarticulatory contexts and assimilation.

Also, the consonantal [r] was taught in phrases by pairing it with the vocalic [ɚ] in phrase types such as the following:

> mother    read
>  [ɚ]      [r]

> fire     rope
> [ɚ]      [r]

The rationale for placing [r] next to [ɚ] was to transfer the retroflex articulation from [ɚ] to [r]. The next step was to whisper the first word in the sequence and to voice the second word in order to emphasize the second word. Finally, the first word in the phrase was omitted, whereas the second word was spoken aloud.

## Introduction of Affricatives

Words were selected containing /tʃ/ in final position like *match, catch, batch,* and *latch,* and placed in phrases as follows:

> catch a man
> catch a boy
> catch a girl
> patch a book
> catch a door
> pitch a ball

The reason /tʃ/ was practiced in word-final position was because it appears more often in this position in conversational speech. Also note that a vowel always followed /tʃ/ to foster prolongation of /ʃ/. In this way, the release of /ʃ/ can be slowed to facilitate /tʃ/ production. In effect, Clifford was encouraged to say *catch a man* in the following manner: [kɛt ʃ:ə: mæn].

## Introduction of Consonant Clusters

The final phase of instruction involved the teaching of initial clusters, namely /sm, sn, sk, st, sp, sl/, followed by initial stop clusters /kl, bl, gr, kr, pl, gl/. The /s/ was prolonged when modeled to help Clifford identify the following vowel. For example, *snake* was modeled as [s:n ek], *sky* was modeled as [s:k aɪ], and so on. After successful repetition of 30 models which contained a lengthened [s], Clifford repeated words spoken at a normal speaking rate until his accuracy reached 90%. Finally, stop + liquid and stop + glide consonants were presented. When Clifford experienced difficulty with a particular cluster, a vowel was inserted between the two consonants (epenthesis) to accentuate the two consonants. The strategy was to prolong sounds and exaggerate them so Clifford would be able to perceive movement patterns at the slowed rate. The consonants were spoken at a more rapid rate in following steps until, finally, the vowel was eliminated.

## EVALUATION OF PROGRESS

Clifford was seen at the speech clinic by the author three times during the 4-month treatment period. During each visit the Goldman-Fristoe Test of Articulation (Goldman and Fristoe, 1972) was administered. The scores from these tests provide a detailed account of changes in his phonological processes during the treatment period. The first test was administered 1 month after onset of treatment, followed by a second test given 2 months after onset of treatment. Little change was noticed on the picture naming or story naming tasks. His ability to imitate sounds in isolation and in nonsense syllables showed marked improvement in both tests. It was not until the third test was given after 4 months of treatment that significant changes in articulation were noted on the picture naming and story telling tasks. Fricatives and velars were almost always correct. The sounds [ɝ], [ɚ], and [r] were correct 50% of the time, and the affricatives were distorted. At that time Clifford's speech was regarded as intelligible and treatment was terminated.

Five months later, Clifford was enrolled in the first grade. A school speech pathologist, unaware that Clifford had received speech training, noted a few articulation errors but did not enroll him for treatment. Eight months later, when Clifford completed the first grade, there was no trace of the original articulation problem.

Several factors contributed to Clifford's rapid success in learning new articulation skills. First, there was no evidence of a neurologic or motor problem. Second, at the time treatment was initiated his hearing acuity was within normal limits. Third, he was a cooperative child, well motivated to follow instructions and engage in speech activities. Finally, his mother created a favorable learning environment and followed through with assigned activities.

## REFERENCES

Goldman, R., and Fristoe, M. 1972. Goldman-Fristoe Test of Articulation. American Guidance Service, Circle Pines, MN.

Ingram, R. 1976. Phonological Disability in Children. Elsevier, New York.

Mowrer, D., Baker, R., and Schutz, R. S-programmed articulation control kit. Ideas Publishing Co., Tempe, 1974.

CHAPTER 7

# Articulation Training Based on Coarticulation

*Elizabeth Prather and Patricia Whaley*

*A model for articulation instruction that includes coarticulation drill and conversational experience is presented by Prather and Whaley. They provide guidelines for each stage of instruction, and procedures for the assessment of progress.*

1. *Do you agree with Prather and Whaley's premise that only accurate productions should be practiced and that these be transferred immediately to linguistic material?*
2. *Describe Prather and Whaley's baseline approach which is used to assess articulatory performance. Is spontaneous speech part of this process? Do you agree with these procedures?*
3. *What are the four guidelines that are proposed for deciding on the order in which sounds are to be treated? Are there any others that you would include? Which principle do you regard as the most important one?*
4. *Distinguish between the following three training procedures: coarticulation drill, parallel transfer, and probe testing. How are these procedures used to effect automaticity in speech production?*
5. *How do Prather and Whaley assess successful transfer in carryover? What are their recommendations when successful transfer does not take place?*

ARTICULATION IS A COMPLEX SUBPROCESS of speech production, and speech production is only one manifestation of language. Articulation errors can result from many physiological and phonological variables and combinations. No one treatment approach is effective for everyone. The articulation training procedures we are presenting are designed to change motor production patterns and are greatly influenced by McDonald's (1964a, 1980) sensori-motor approach to articulation testing and treatment. We recommend these procedures be used for clients who have established faulty, automatic articulation patterns for one or more phonemes.

We have used the program successfully with children and adults who have disordered articulation related to hearing loss, dysarthria, and ideopathic functional etiologies. These procedures are especially appropriate for clients who need to increase the number of phonetic contexts they can articulate correctly and those who need to transfer correct articulation from a deliberate, consciously controlled level to an automatic level with normal rate of articulation.

Key components to our approach to articulation treatment are that the client drill only successful (accurate) productions and that the drill material be transferred immediately to meaningful linguistic use. The final goal of correctly articulated speech is accomplished via five levels of testing and training: 1) baseline diagnosis; 2) coarticulation drills; 3) parallel transfer; 4) probe testing; and 5) generalization to social conversation. The following sections describe the procedures we use at each level of the treatment regimen.

## BASELINE DIAGNOSIS

The purpose of a baseline diagnosis is to describe the client's articulatory movements and the resulting acoustic patterns. Articulatory movements and acoustic accuracy vary with phonetic contexts (coarticulatory effects) and with speakers. Thus, to obtain a representative sample of the client's articulation, it is necessary to observe and to listen to a variety of phonetic contexts.

We typically start by determining which phonemes a client misarticulates. We use a combination of the McDonald Screening Deep Test for Articulation (McDonald, 1964b) and conversational speech to obtain a sample of most English phonemes in a small number of phonetic contexts. During these initial screening procedures the clinician may transcribe errors phonetically or simply judge productions as correct or incorrect. This first step is completed when the clinician can list the phonemes that are frequently misarticulated and those that are usually accurate.

The major portion of the baseline diagnosis is spent sampling incorrectly articulated phonemes in a wide variety of phonetic contexts. We rely on the McDonald Deep Test of Articulation (McDonald, 1964b) and spontaneous conversational speech samples for the necessary observations. The McDonald Deep Test (picture or sentence form) samples the client's productions of any phoneme as it is preceded or followed by most other consonants and vowels. Almost always the tested phoneme will be produced correctly in one or more contexts. Kneler (1980), for example, reported that her severely hearing-impaired teenage client correctly articulated /tʃ/ when it was followed by /p, b, r, æ, and ʌ/, and when /tʃ/ was preceded by a wide variety of consonants and vowels. In all other contexts he produced a sound similar to /ʃ/.

Although we would expect the target articulatory movements to be most significantly affected by the immediately preceding and following movements (sounds), Daniloff and Moll (1968) demonstrated that coarticulation effects may extend across several phoneme units and even syllables. That is, a target movement and the resulting sounds may be altered by several of the preceding or following sounds.

A second process that accounts for normal variance in articulation is undershoot. According to Harris (1978), *undershoot* refers to articulatory movements that are interrupted before they are completed. Thus, movement toward a target area begins, but the articulatory movement is stopped or the direction of the movement is changed before the target is reached. Undershoot is most likely to occur during the production of unstressed syllables or during rapid speech.

The bi-syllable McDonald Deep Test does not allow us to evaluate all of the effects of undershoot or the coarticulation effects described by Daniloff and Moll. We therefore urge observation of the client's productions of target phonemes during spontaneous conversational speech. These "deep test" spontaneous speech samples may be obtained by asking clients to talk about, describe, tell stories about, or explain specific topics. The topics may be selected to evoke many productions of the target phonemes. Kneler (1980), who wanted her client to produce /tʃ/, asked him to tell stories about "Witches on Halloween" and "Mr. Chicken Goes to Church."

If no accurate productions have been heard during the formal testing or during the spontaneous speech sample, we recommend that imitation procedures be used. The clinician may first try word combinations and phrases that are linguistically meaningful. Only if the client still fails would nonsense syllable combinations be used. The purpose of the imitation procedure is to discover phonetic contexts the client can produce accurately at least 90% of the time.

For clients who have multiple phonemes in error, specific target articulations need to be selected. We suggest clinicians consider the following factors before deciding on the order in which the client will learn correct articulation of the error phonemes:

1.  It is necessary to find at least one context in which a phoneme is articulated accurately and automatically.
2.  Articulatory feature generalization can be expected. If most alveolar consonants are produced with the tongue forward, generalization from one or two target phonemes should occur to all or at least several of the other affected phonemes. For example: Jane, age 20, came to our clinic to improve her articulation for a radio/television broadcasting major. Baseline diagnosis revealed that she used a forward tongue placement (her tongue touched the back of her upper teeth) for /t, d, n, l, tʃ, dʒ/. In addition her tongue tip approached her teeth for /s, z, ʃ, ʒ, r/. We selected /tʃ/ and /s/ as the initial phoneme targets, and during treatment she correctly changed the forward tongue movement for these two phonemes as well as the other involved phonemes.
3.  The number of contexts in which the client uses a target phoneme in error should also be considered. Phonemes that are produced correctly more often than not would have a lower priority than those which are usually erred.
4.  Certainly the effect of the incorrect articulation on the client's speech intelligibility is an extremely important consideration. Given a choice, always select targets that will affect a real change for the client. Such a guideline would eliminate /θ/ and /ð/ as early targets because these two phonemes contribute little to speech intelligibility.

## COARTICULATION DRILL, PARALLEL TRANSFER, AND PROBE TESTING

### Training Stimuli

Early training sessions consist of coarticulation drill, parallel transfer, and probe testing. The stimuli used at these three levels are similar but represent successive steps to the goal of correctly articulated conversational speech. The practice items used during coarticulation drill are the phonetic contexts the client articulated correctly during baseline

Coarticulation Drills: Ten repetitions per stimulus; entire drill is repeated once. The client practices phonetic contexts that were articulated correctly at the 90% level during baseline diagnosis or probe testing.

Methods of Presentation: Imitation, reading, or picture naming.

Coarticulation Drill Example Stimuli:
1. cheesestore
2. bookstore
3. shoestore
4. kite string
5. dance tonight
6. was tired
7. his turn
8. this tree
9. like sodas
10. likes it
11. leaks air
12. likes cheese
13. walks home
14. bakes it
15. hates it
16. can't see
17. don't see
18. iced tea
19. ice cream
20. his dog
21. his daughter
22. this dog
23. house dog
24. mouse trap
25. basket

Figure 1.   Coarticulation drill procedures and examples of training stimuli.

diagnosis, and parallel transfer exercises consist of these same contexts used meaningfully. For example, if an item in coarticulation drill was cheesestore, a parallel transfer question could be, "Where do you buy cheese?" The client would answer, "Well, at the cheese store," and parallel transfer would be accomplished. Other examples are presented in Figures 1 and 2. Note in both figures that /s/ and /z/ are drilled in the same session when the voicing contrast is correct.

Probe tests consist of unpracticed phonetic contexts, new stimulus items representing previously drilled phonetic contexts, or previously erred phonetic contexts (Figure 3). We create probe tests so we can prepare drill stimuli for the next training session. The clinician may probe with entirely new contexts or may pattern probes from the pre-

---

*Parallel Transfer*: One response per stimulus; repeat entire list once.

*Example Stimuli*:

| Clinician: | Client: |
|---|---|
| 1. Where do you buy cheese? | At a cheese store |
| 2. Where do you buy books? | At a bookstore |
| 3. Where do you buy shoes? | At a shoestore |
| 4. How do you hold a kite? | With a kite string |
| 5. What will you do tonight? | I'll dance tonight |
| 6. Was he rested? | He was tired |
| 7. Was it her turn? | No, his turn |
| 8. Did you climb that tree? | No, this tree |
| 9. Do you like malts? | No, I like sodas |
| 10. Does he like it? | Yes, he likes it |
| 11. Does it hold air? | No, it leaks air |
| 12. Does he like cheese? | Yes, he likes cheese |
| 13. Does he run home? | No, he walks home |
| 14. Does she boil it? | No, she bakes it |
| 15. Does she like spinach? | No, she hates it |
| 16. Can you see it? | I can't see it |
| 17. Do you see it? | I don't see it |
| 18. Do you like hot tea? | I like iced tea |
| 19. Is that yogurt? | It's ice cream |
| 20. Is that her dog? | It's his dog |
| 21. Is that his son? | No, his daughter |
| 22. Do you mean this cat? | No, this dog |
| 23. Is it a wild dog? | No, a house dog |
| 24. Is it a bear trap? | It's a mouse trap |
| 25. Is that a box? | No, a basket |

Figure 2.   Parallel transfer procedures and examples of training stimuli.

viously practiced material. For example, previous success on "can't sing" may suggest probe test items like "don't sing, won't sing, or can't sing." When a client articulates a probe item at least 90% correctly, the probe becomes an item in the next coarticulation drill.

Methods of presenting the training stimuli will vary with clients' needs and interests. When clients are able to articulate correctly the training items without a model, we use pictures or a written presentation. Imitation can be used during drill and probe testing as long as the clinician and the client use normal prosody and voice. Imitation is never used during parallel transfer or spontaneous conversation. Typically, the clinician can evoke meaningful use of a context (parallel transfer) by asking short questions, and spontaneous conversations can be established with pictures or questions.

Probe Testing: Client repeats each item 10 times to test for 90% accuracy; if error is made on two trials before 10 repetitions, terminate the item. Failed items can be used for probe testing at a later time. Passed items are added to drill list for the next training session.

Probe Test Example Stimuli:
1. cheese sandwich
2. plays ball
3. rosebush
4. on Tuesday
5. on Wednesday
6. guess who
7. Miss Baldwin (client's teacher)
8. less time
9. fix it.
10. bus stop

Figure 3.   Procedures for probe testing and examples of test stimuli.

## Training Procedures

Essential aspects of training are the use of automatically produced speech and daily practice schedules. All responses from probe testing through drill and conversational speech should be produced on an automatic level with normal prosody, voice, timing, and correct articulation. Even the slightest pause or juncture before the target phoneme is not acceptable. Clients are not directed to think about articulation placement or movement. Remember, the training stimuli are those phonetic contexts the clients can articulate correctly; therefore, practice on an automatic level is easily accomplished.

Ling (1976), who developed a speech production program for deaf children, also recognized the importance of practicing speech production on an automatic level. He stated that " . . . extensive conscious control [of speech production] is incompatible with our quest for the automaticity necessary for fluent serial ordering and coarticulation in speech. . . ." We have all talked to the client who produces slow, deliberate, correct articulation but does not "take the time" to use correct articulation outside of treatment. If the client never learns conscious control, the client will not have to unlearn conscious control. Morley and Fox (1969) also indicated the necessity for the development of automatic sequences, or neurophysiological patterns, because "voluntary conscious control would be impossible at the required speed and complexity" for conversational speech.

Daily practice of correct articulation is an absolute necessity. Ideally, a client will practice 3 to 4 minutes three to five times each day in addition to regularly scheduled clinical sessions. These recommendations are based on hypotheses relative to the function of short-term memory, rehearsal, and long-term memory processes. Klatzky (1975) hypothesized that short-term memory and long-term memory are separate memory processes and that rehearsal or practice renews information in short-term memory so that it is tranferred to long-term memory. Klatzky reported evidence that the more a behavior is practiced, the more likely it is that the rules for the behavior will become a part of long-term memory. Simply stated, the more we practice, the more quickly we learn. Thus, we suggest the client practice only correct articulation (90%) to learn the new rules and that he practice several times each day.

The amount of practice each client can tolerate may vary from session to session and certainly will vary among all clients. A minimum amount of practice within a training session and a minimum number of practice sessions seems necessary, however, to ensure continuous acquisition of correct articulation.

Courtright and Courtright (1976) suggested a single repetition of an item does not effect a change in long-term memory. A client must repeat the item often enough to pass through the limits of short-term memory (echoic memory) to involve the long-term memory processes. For children, we assume short-term memory limits to be four to five digits or syllables, and for adults, the limit increases to six or eight. Thus, we recommend that clients repeat each coarticulation drill/probe test item at least five times without interruption. Younger clients, 2 or 3 years old, may be able to repeat only three times following a model. Ideally, 10 repetitions are suggested to ensure exceeding short-term memory limits, and to facilitate data collection for the clinician.

When clients can maintain correct articulation with or without a model across an unlimited number of repetitions, Kneler's (1980) program may serve as a guide for determining the number of rehearsals per stimulus item and the amount of practice per training session. Kneler asked her client to repeat each stimulus 10 times during articulation drill and probe testing. Kneler's coarticulation drills were comprised of 25 stimulus items with a variable number of phonetic contexts and the probe tests were comprised of 10 stimulus items also with a variable number of different phonetic contexts. Parallel transfer was comprised of 25 items. The coarticulation drill and parallel transfer exercises were presented twice during each training session. Thus, her client produced 500 coarticulation drills and 50 parallel transfer exercises during each session. The probe testing included 100 productions (10 stimuli, each repeated 10 times). As treatment progressed, she decreased the drill time and increased the parallel transfer time.

The number of practice sessions each week will depend upon the clinician's schedule and the availability of monitors (peers, siblings, parents, spouse) who can conduct short practice sessions with clients. Both clients and monitors are usually willing to commit themselves to three to five practice sessions daily because each session is limited to around 3 minutes. It is important, however, that they understand the necessity for practicing only accurate productions using normal prosody, voice, and timing. We have effected this program using various treatment schedules ranging from daily clinic sessions down to only one per week. As the number of clinic sessions is reduced, however, the load carried by the client and monitor increases. In situations where no monitor is available, we strongly recommend daily clinic sessions.

**GENERALIZATIONS TO SOCIAL CONVERSATION**

At the end of each training session, we can probe the client's ability to articulate correctly in spontaneous conversation. We capitalize on the client's correct articulation to elicit the speech sample. For example, if the client has been successfully articulating contexts that contain the word *cheese* we might ask the client to tell how to make a cheese sandwich. Older clients could compare various types of cheeses or tell about a favorite cheese recipe. The client can continue speaking until the accuracy rate for the target phoneme drops below 90%. If the client misarticulates the phoneme, we add items that represent the incorrectly articulated phonetic context to the probe test of the next session.

The final stage of treatment is continuous/spontaneous speech. Topics of discussion are selected to capitalize on the client's interests and correct articulation. The clients speak continuously until they have articulated the target phoneme in at least 30 instances. Spontaneous speech practice should be discontinued, however, if clients do not use the target phoneme correctly 90% of the time. It is essential that spontaneous speech practice occur outside of the clinical session and we recommend that clients practice for a few minutes several times each day.

**SUMMARY**

To summarize, during coarticulation drill and parallel transfer, clients practice correctly articulated phonetic contexts and immediately use these contexts meaningfully. The following is a review of the clinical procedures from baseline diagnosis through spontaneous speech.

1. *Baseline diagnosis*   Determine correctly articulated phonetic contexts, methods of presenting contexts, and the number of times the client can repeat practice items.
2. *Coarticulation drill (Figure 1)*   Present 10 to 25 practice items one at a time to the client who repeats the item correctly from five to ten times in close succession. The client must produce the item correctly at least 90% of the time. If the accuracy drops below the 90% level, the client is instructed to stop repeating the item. The incorrectly articulated drill items will be used as probe test items during later sessions.
3. *Parallel transfer (Figure 2)*   Begin parallel transfer when the client has successfully drilled meaningful word strings that can be used to answer short questions or identify pictures or objects. Questions about the coarticulation drill items seem preferable because the client is required to think about which among the drill stimuli can be used appropriately. The client attends to the linguistic meaning of the response rather than the articulatory movements. Clients may respond using two word phrases or complete sentences. We recommend the clients use complete sentences when they are capable.
4. *Probe test (Figure 3)*   Test 10–25 new stimulus items each session. Items articulated correctly (90% or better) are included in coarticulation drills for the next session. Probe test items produced incorrectly (below 90%) are dropped for several sessions but are retested at a later time.
5. *Spontaneous conversation*   Select topics of conversation that are interesting to the client and will result in the client using the target phoneme at least 30 times. The client must use correct articulation (90% or better). Spontaneous speech practice three or four times daily is recommended until the client articulates the target phoneme correctly during all speech.

**REFERENCES**

Courtright, J. A., and Courtright, I. C. 1976. Imitative modeling as a theoretical base for instructing language disordered children. J. Speech Hear. Res. 19:655–663.
Daniloff, R. G., and Moll, K. L. 1968. Coarticulation of lip rounding. J. Speech Hear. Res. 11:707–721.
Harris, K. S. 1978. Physiological aspects of articulatory behavior. Status Reports on Speech Research. Haskins Laboratories, New Haven, CT.
Klatzky, R. L. 1975. Human Memory: Structures and Processes. W. H. Freeman and Company, San Francisco.

Kneler, S. 1980. An articulation training program using a real time spectrographic display with a severely hearing impaired adolescent. Unpublished master's thesis, Arizona State University, Tempe.

Ling, D. 1976. Speech and the Hearing-Impaired Child: Theory and Practice. The Alexander Graham Bell Association for the Deaf, Washington, D.C.

McDonald, E. T., 1964a. Articulation Testing and Treatment: A Sensory-Motor Approach. Stanwix House, Pittsburgh.

McDonald, E. T. 1964b. A Deep Test of Articulation. Stanwix House, Pittsburgh.

McDonald, E. T. 1980. Disorders of articulation. In: R. J. Van Hattum (ed.), An Introduction to Communication Disorders. Macmillan Publishing Co., New York.

Morley, M. E., and Fox, J. 1969. Disorders of articulation: Theory and therapy. Br. J. Disord. Commun. 4:151–165.

# CHAPTER 8

# The Case for Individual Variation in the Management of Children with Articulation Disorders

*John E. Bernthal and Nicholas W. Bankson*

*Bernthal and Bankson show how general principles of phonological development can be applied to the growth patterns of individual children. They discuss the clinical implications of a model of training based on individual acquisition patterns and contrast this approach with a developmental model based on the acquisition of discrete sound segments.*

1. *What are some reasons for the variability in articulation patterns observed in the early words of children?*
2. *What do the authors mean by the term* sound preference? *Is this term operationally different from the term* sound substitution? *What are some possible reasons why children emphasize some sounds over others?*
3. *Bernthal and Bankson distinguish between mastery and customary production. What is the difference between these two terms as they apply to articulation performance? What principles of phonological development can be used to explain differences in articulation performance across age levels for an individual child?*
4. *What objections do Bernthal and Bankson have to a model of articulation training based on the developmental norms of individual sounds? In this regard, how do they address this issue of individual differences? Are their suggestions for training based on phonological principles or neuromotor development? Do you agree with their suggestions?*

THE STUDY OF LANGUAGE ACQUISITION in children typically has focused on commonalities in children's language patterns. Investigators have looked for a universal order of acquisition and universal operations, rather than examining individual differences and variations that occur during this period. In the study of phonological development, the primary emphasis has been on the acquisition of individual segments, including the universal order of sound acquisition, commonality in mastery of individual sounds, acquisition of sound contrast, and the identification of phonological processes that occur across children and languages. Individual variation in these and other aspects of phonological acquisition, for the most part, has been ignored. There is obvious value in the search for general trends, similarity in patterns of development, and universal operations. However, the study of individual variation during speech sound acquisition is also of interest to the speech clinician. Because the clinical process requires attention to individual variation, knowledge of individual patterns of development may be more critical in the evaluation and management of a child with an articulation disorder than common trends and universal orders.

Until recently, only a minor role has been given to individual cognitive abilities that may contribute to the development of a child's phonological system. Earlier, investigators emphasized innate and environmental constraints in studying the acquisition of similar patterns of phonological acquisition. They did not generally consider individual variations. Individual variation during phonological acquisition should be expected because it is not likely that all children would derive identical phonological systems during the developmental period. We know that certain children evidence unique phonological patterns during the speech sound development period. In fact, one could argue that many children are identified by speech clinicians as disordered or deviant in articulation by virtue of the individuality seen in their phonological development. Recognition of phonological variation may lead to an increased understanding of children's phonological systems, which in turn may influence the use of remediation strategies. The intent of this chapter is not to argue against the presence of commonalities during phonological acquisition, but rather to point out that superimposed on the commonality is a great deal of individuality and to suggest how individual variation may influence clinical procedures.

## VARIATIONS OBSERVED DURING
## THE PHONOLOGICAL ACQUISITION PERIOD

A number of investigators has suggested that the period during which the first 50 words are acquired differs significantly from the pre-word stage before it, and the two-word utterance stage after it, and view the first 50 words as a separate period in phonological acquisition (Ingram, 1976; Schwartz and Prelock, 1982). Schwartz and Prelock (1982) have suggested that the limited vocabulary size is not the critical aspect of this stage, but rather a "cluster of linguistic and cognitive behaviors" which separates the first 50 words from later phonological behavior. During this period, there is variation among children in their phonological productions, variability within a child in the production of a given word, and variability in the productions of individual segments across words. In other words, the child may not maintain a stable representation of the underlying adult form of specific lexical items and thus will not have consistent productions of either individual lexical items or individual sound segments.

One aspect of the variation seen in phonological patterns that has been studied is the individual segments utilized by children during the development of early words. Leonard et al. (1980) studied productions of speech sounds in 10 young children (age range 1 year, 4 months, to 1 year, 10 months). Specifically, they observed word-initial consonant productions. They reported that no subject's set of phone classes was identical to that of any other subject. Certain phones were produced by all subjects and certain adult targets were attempted by all subjects. For example, all subjects exhibited word-initial [m], [b], and [d] in their repertoires, and nine subjects used word-initial [kʰ]. Six subjects used word-initial [g] and word-initial [w] appropriately, and five used word-initial [n]. Five subjects used word-initial [h], but two subjects deleted initial [h]. At least two subjects used word initial [tʃ], [f], and [dʒ], although these phones are not typically seen in the speech of very young children. Certain voiced consonants were preferred to their voiceless cognates as four subjects substituted [b] for [p] and five substituted [d] for [t]. On the other hand, no subject produced [θ], [ð], [l], [z], or [r]. Leonard et al. (1980) summarized by stating that some phones are reflected in the early speech of most children, other phones tend to be used by only a small percentage of children, and still other phones may not be reflected in the early speech of any child. This statement would suggest that, although individual differences are seen across children in their use of early sounds, these variations are within certain limits.

Schwartz and Prelock (1982) speculated that some variability is the result of the child's unstable representations of the target words. An alternative explanation would be that such segments only reflect the lexical items the child chooses. A third explanation might be that the sounds seen in the child's lexicon are the result of the child's sound preferences and avoidances. These latter two topics are discussed in more detail later in this chapter. Ideally, we need diary studies from sizeable groups of children which would trace initial or early emergence of phones to customary production, to sound mastery, and to consistent production of those phones in continuous speech.

Ferguson (1976) has pointed out that a child may frequently regress in some of his or her phonological productions, and he compares such variation to extensions and overgeneralizations found in other aspects of language development. In other words, during phonological acquisition, the child discovers patterns by testing and revising hypotheses. He also noted that when a child is at the stage of first word productions, utterances may fluctuate considerably. For example, he reported that the following types of fluctuations may occur at this stage: the final consonant may be present or absent, the voiced and voiceless cognates are used alternately, low central or mid-front vowels may be used interchangeably, and stop or spirant consonants are used interchangeably. Furthermore, Ferguson (1976) suggested that some variant pronunciations which are different from the adult target are "natural" in that they reflect the kind of processes found in historical sound change and second language learning, whereas other variation may reflect the child's perceptual and production skills and strategies. This process of "regularization" in phonological development has also been used as a basis for a cognitive model of phonological acquisition (Macken and Ferguson, 1981).

Klein (1981) has identified two production strategies for the production of adult polysyllabic words in four children aged 20–24 months toward the end of this first 50-word period. She found that two of the children used a "syllable-maintaining" strategy, whereas the other two used a "syllable reducing" strategy when attempting to produce polysyllabic words. Although such strategies reveal more regularity than is typically seen in children earlier in this period, it does demonstrate different strategies across children.

One way the children use a syllable maintaining strategy is by producing polysyllabic words in which the syllables are reduplicated. Syllable reduplication is apparently an easy way to produce polysyllabic words because the sounds of the syllable do not need differentiation. Such strategies represent the types of phonological patterns typically seen in normal children from 20–40 months when children's sound productions tend to be regular, presumably because they reflect a more consistent use of phonological processes.

## SOUND PREFERENCES

It has been suggested that some children have a preference for certain phonetic segments and avoid other segments during the phonological acquisition period (Ingram, 1976). Sound preferences are reported by both normally developing children and those with phonological disability (Weiner, 1981). Weiner defines sound preference as the replacement of a group of sounds with similar feature(s) from the same sound class, by one or two similar sounds. Fokes (1982) has proposed that "the cautious child may produce only what he is able, or wishes, to attempt . . . although the child may have extensive concepts, he may refuse to pronounce a word that is not consistent with his system" (p. 18). In other words, the child who uses preferred forms may be less venturesome than the child who freely mispronounces forms that are not yet acquired. It is important to point out that the concept of "sound preferences" based on performance criteria is a reasonable possibility. An investigation related to this issue was the second study reported in the Leonard et al. (1980) paper, in which they observed variations in the production of speech sounds in a pair of identical twins. These subjects were 19 months of age during the initial visit and were seen at weekly intervals, with some deviations in this schedule. The linguistic environment for these twins was assumed to be similar because their mother was the principal caretaker for both. The phone classes of these two subjects showed considerable variation and were "no more similar" than those of any two of the 10 children discussed earlier. Each twin produced bilabial nasals, alveolar stops, and velar stops as their first consonants, but /θ/, /ð/, and /l/ or /r/ were not observed in either of the child's first 50 words. However, by the eleventh visit, which was approximately 14 weeks after the first visit, there were individual differences in the production of fricatives. One twin was producing [s] while the second produced [f], [z], and [n], all of which were absent in the production of the first subject. These findings again demonstrated the presence of sound variation across children and the possibility of sound preference and avoidance, because the linguistic input for both twins was presumed to be equivalent. It is possible that some lexical items may have been more significant to one child than to the other child, and thus, could reflect the different acquisitional strategies used by the two children.

The differences between the twins found in the Leonard et al. (1980) study are in contrast to findings from most other studies of twins. An explanation for the differences may be the fact that these twins were examined during the early period of linguistic development when individual differences in phonological characteristics are common. Such differences in output between twins raised in the same linguistic environment suggest the cognitive factor of individual differences in phonological acquisition. Most previous studies of identical twins studied older children and reported similar sound production in both members of the pair.

One explanation for the differences in the data for the younger twins and those at the two utterance stages and older is that at the earliest stages each child is experimenting, that is, categorizing and discovering patterns by testing and revising hypotheses (Macken and Ferguson, 1981). This experimenting and hypothesis testing may result in a number of individual differences and is reflected in the data reported by Leonard et al. (1980). The similar speech pattern reported for older twins may be the influence of the child's experience with language as well as the child's cognitive ability and physiological capabilities. The language interactional experiences between older twins may be a critical influence in this later stage of phonological development and thus account for more similar phonological patterns as the children's phonology becomes increasingly stabilized.

## SOUND PREFERENCE IN CHILDREN
## WITH PHONOLOGICAL DISABILITIES

Ingram (1976) and Weiner (1981) have both presented data from children with phonological disorders that seem to indicate sound preferences in this population. Ingram pointed out that several children with phonological disorders showed a preference for fricatives and a tendency to use a fricative or affricate in place of other sounds. He also noted that several children demonstrated a nasal preference. Weiner (1981) reported that sound preference was a common attribute in 8 of 14 children ranging in age from 3 years, 5 months to 5 years, 10 months, all with unintelligible speech. A child was considered to have a sound preference if one or two similar sounds replaced an entire sound class more than 70% of the time. The number of preferred sounds seen in the speech of these eight children ranged from one to four and varied from child to child. For example, one child replaced initial voiceless fricatives and affricates with [θ], and voiced fricatives, liquids, and glides with [ð]. A second child used four palatal sibilants for several sound classes. Preferred sounds were substituted most frequently for fricatives.

If a child uses one or two preferred sounds in his or her productive phonology, the probability for the occurrence of homonyms increases. A homonym is defined in this context as two or more different adult words produced by a child in the same phonetic form. For example, a child we recently observed substituted [h] for all fricatives and all voiceless stops. Because the fricatives and many of the stops were collapsed into a single sound, the number of contrasts was reduced and a relatively large number of homonyms was present in his speech. For example, [hæ] was used for *hat, pat, sat,* and *cat.*

Farwell (1976) postulated that children select and produce certain words because of specific segments that make up the words. She observed a very young child who produced /s/, /ʃ/, /tʃ/, /dʒ/ and thus produced words like *ice, eyes, shoes, keys, cheese,* and *juice,* whereas a second child of a similar age avoided almost all adult words which contained fricatives or affricates for several months. Both children presumably heard many plural nouns and other forms containing fricatives and yet their word patterns were different—one frequently produced fricative sounds, whereas the other produced few words which contained fricatives. An alternative notion has also been advanced as an explanation for the different segments that different children use during the early stages of phonological acquisition. Ferguson and Farwell (1975) and Leonard et al. (1980) have noted that the sounds children use may vary as a result of lexical choice.

These authors have hypothesized that initially children learn words, not sounds or phonemic contrasts, and that early acquired phonemic oppositions in children's speech serve to differentiate words. Leonard et al. (1980) stated that they found little evidence that children established contrasts on the basis of individual phonemic segments, but rather the subjects studied by these authors were more concerned with establishing contrasts between words. It would follow, then, that the lexical items the child uses will determine which phonetic forms are produced. Leonard et al. also pointed out that even though subjects were able to produce a sound in a lexical item on one occasion, there was considerable phonetic variation in the subsequent productions of the item. Variability seen in a child's production of the same word would be expected because the words are not "strictly phonemically principled." In other words, because phonemic contrasts may not have been fully developed, the child's productions are not restricted by a set of phonemic contrasts or a limited group of allophones. From this perspective, development of phonetic forms is secondary to the production of lexical items.

Moskowitz (1980) also proposed that early words have a communicative basis. She regards the first 50 as phonological idioms or independent units. These idioms are acquired outside the phonological system, even though some may be similar to adult pronunciation, a position held also by Fokes (1982).

As we stated earlier, it is likely that some children limit their active lexicon to words which can be produced fairly accurately. Others prefer to build vocabulary more rapidly, pronouncing many of the words inaccurately and without much evident phonological organization. Because phonological and lexical factors interact during the process of speech acquisition, it is difficult to determine whether the lexical items a child chooses determines the segments and the syllable structure that a child uses or if, conversely, sound preference, syllable shapes, and prosodic factors determine the lexical items a child uses.

## CUSTOMARY PRODUCTION AND MASTERY

Although phonological variability decreases about the time the child begins to produce two-word utterances, variability in segmental production remains. During this period, however, children's productions become much more regular, the child is described as using phonological processes and is given credit for the acquisition of specific sound segments and stable underlying forms. The child tends to simplify certain adult forms with processes such as final consonant deletion, stopping of fricatives, and cluster reduction. Early in this period there may be a loss of accuracy of previously correct forms because of overgeneralization. In addition, selectivity (sound preference and avoidance) is seen, especially in children with disordered phonology. Because most of what we know about segmental development during this time is based on classical studies of speech sound development, we will review such investigations and discuss articulation variability that has been identified through such efforts.

Classical studies of speech sound development (Poole, 1934; Templin, 1957; Wellman et al., 1931) provide developmental norms that are based on cross-sectional data from relatively large groups of children and indicate the age levels at which specific speech sounds are produced with a high degree of accuracy. These norms identify the upper age limits of sound productions and reflect the mean ages at which either 75% (Templin), 90% (Wellman et al.), or 100% (Poole) of the children in a particular sample correctly produce speech sounds in word-initial, word-final, and sometimes word-"medial" positions. As Winitz (1969) has pointed out, however, such developmental norms represent points at which some level of mastery has been achieved but do not indicate earlier successive points in a learning sequence.

It may even be that just because a sound appears late in the child's production, it doesn't necessarily mean that it was learned late. When such norms are considered to represent universal expectations of speech sound development, the following considerations are overlooked: 1) the large amount of individual variability in the ages at which individual children produce specific speech sounds; 2) the order in which speech sounds are produced by an individual; and 3) the gradual and fluctuating process including regressions with which a sound may be acquired.

Sander (1972), in his reanalysis of Templin's (1957) data, emphasized the fact that acquisition of speech sound production is gradual and variable. He pointed out that criteria traditionally associated with norms for the age of mastery of sound production are both arbitrary and stringent. He suggested that a more realistic perspective of speech sound acquisition may be gained by considering sound development as it moves from a point of customary production (correct articulation in two of the three word positions) to mastery (correct articulation in all three word positions). One could even argue that from a clinical perspective, sounds that are consistently produced correctly in even a single word position have been acquired.

Sander's (1972) reanalysis, in combination with phonological acquisition data in children aged 24 to 48 months reported by Prather et al. (1975), indicate that when customary production and sound mastery are considered as a range on a temporal continuum of sound acquisition, the process of speech sound development appears to be gradual and reflects variability seen among children and among sound segments. For example, 50% of children produced /s/ in two positions by 2 years, whereas it was not until 8 years that 90% of children produced the sound in three word positions. On the other hand, customary production of the /k/ occurred by 2 years, whereas mastery was achieved at 4 years. Although such data do not deal with the time period required for a particular child to move from customary production to sound mastery for an individual sound, they seem to indicate that some youngsters remain in the process of either acquiring or refining their productive control of certain sounds, such as /s/, for several years. For other phonemes, such as /k/, the acquisition period is shorter. It should also be pointed out that some children may master a sound before the age group associated with customary production, yet others may begin to produce a sound later than the age associated with sound mastery. Children may vary greatly in the amount of time they need to move from initial production to mastery of different sounds. Viewing sound development across a temporal continuum enhances our appreciation for the fact that, although there are general patterns of sound development within a range of possibilities, there is no precise sequence for speech sound acquisition that occurs across all children. Rather, children develop sounds in varying orders and at different times with the amount of phonetic variation differing for specific phones and different contexts.

Using a group of 12 kindergarten children with defective /s/ production, Stephens and Daniloff (1980) studied longitudinal acquisition of correct /s/ productions. None of the subjects received clinical instruction during the period of the study. Improvement in /s/ productions was based on a sample of sentences that was repeated at eight intervals across a school year. They reported that the children varied in their developmental patterns. Three subjects made orderly progress, two made rapid and then slow progress, and the remainder experienced periodic regression in their overall progress. These data support the observation that fluctuations in speech sound productions are found not only in young children, but also in older children (age 5) who are refining particular phonological productions.

## CLINICAL IMPLICATIONS

That a range of variability exists in speech sound acquisition for children between 24 and 60 months is helpful in case selection and in choice of target behaviors. A traditional procedure in determining need for intervention has been to relate a client's phone productions to his or her chronological age in comparison with mastery norms. The target behaviors selected for treatment of the client have often been based on the same comparison.

We suggest that the clinician may be better advised to allow the factors of intelligibility and error patterns as well as syllable shapes to have greater importance in the selection of cases and target behaviors than developmental norms for segments. A clinician may give priority in case selection to young children with intelligibility problems and may select relatively late developing contrasts as target behaviors because a particular process is operating on such sounds. For example, if a child substitutes stops for fricatives, we would suggest that the clinician seek to establish the stop/fricative distinction without preconceived notions about which fricative is typically observed early in the child's production repertoire. This suggestion implies the use of a multiphonemic approach in which any member of a target sound class would be acceptable for initial instruction. For example, to begin training with /s/, for a child who substitutes stops for fricatives, is predicated on the assumption that he or she will learn /s/ before /z/, /ʃ/, /ʒ/, /f/, /v/, /θ/, /ð/, a probabilistic prediction at best.

In the single sound approach to management, the assumption is that the clinician can predict which fricative(s) will be acquired first by the child. We do not recommend this approach, but rather agree with the notion of cycles as proposed by Hodson (1982) in which phonemes which reflect a phonological pattern are focused on for a cycle and then presented again at a later time. We also have had success with this approach.

One way to examine the variability of production in a specific sound is through phonetic contextual testing using, for example, the Deep Test of Articulation (McDonald, 1964), the Sound Production Task (Shelton et al., 1967) or some other measure that allows for an in-depth assessment of a sound in a number of different phonetic contexts. These procedures for testing might provide the clinician with an overall indication of the development of a specific sound. One might speculate that the greater the number of contexts in which the sound is produced correctly, the greater the level of phonetic proficiency. One might further speculate that as the consistency of correct productions increases, the probability is greater that the sound will be acquired without remediation or that more rapid progress will be made when remediation is given. The tests identified above, however, only deal with the potential facilitory effect of segmental phonetic context. The effect of syllable shape and suprasegmental variations should also be examined.

In those cases where a child exhibits a single sound preference, that is, the single sound is substituted for an entire class of sounds, a management strategy might be to contrast the preferred sound with individual members of the sound class that is collapsed into the preferred sound. For example, if [h] is substituted for fricatives and affricates, intervention might focus on contrasting [h] and [s], [h] and [tʃ], and so on. Thus, the goal may be to establish contrasts between a preferred sound and individual sounds which are not seen in the child's productive repertoire.

It is interesting to speculate whether an increase in the child's productive lexicon will result in an increase in the number of sound segments and the regularity of their use in a child's productions. If a child's impoverished sound system is reflective of a restricted number of lexical items in his or her repertoire, then remediation should focus on the introduction of additional lexical items, rather than teaching segments. The additional words will likely require the use of additional phones, which may then result in the use of simplification processes to cope with the increase in phones. Initially, simplification processes may produce phonetic forms which are less like adult forms than some of the earlier productions. The results may be, however, that the child will become phonologically "tuned in," and the constraints and influence of the selected items on the child's productive phonology will decrease.

As pointed out above, it is difficult and sometimes impossible to determine the relationship between sound preferences and lexical items. What may appear to be a sound preference in some children may be the result of a particular lexical repertoire. On the other hand, a child may have a sound preference which is reflected in a restricted lexicon. Regardless of which may be the case, remediation should take the form of contrasting lexical items.

In summary, we suggest that clinicians sample an individual's phonology with enough depth and breadth that individual patterns and variability can be discovered. It is suggested that the target behaviors selected for remediation, and the instructional methodologies should vary from traditional approaches because of this knowledge. Such information will hopefully lead to a treatment program designed to help the client move toward the adult standard in a more efficient manner than an approach in which segments are taught in a similar manner and protocol, regardless of the client's error patterns.

## REFERENCES

Farwell, C. G. 1976. Some ways to learn about fricatives. Paper read at the 8th Child Language Research Forum, Stanford University. April, Stanford, CA.

Ferguson, C. 1976. Learning to pronounce: The earliest stages of phonological development in the child. Papers Rep. Child Lang. Devel. 11:1–27.

Ferguson, C., and Farwell, C. 1975. Words and sounds in early language acquisition: English initial consonants in the first 50 words. Language 51:419–439.

Fokes, J. 1982. Problems confronting the theorist and practitioner in child phonology. In: M. Crary (ed.), Phonological Intervention, Concepts and Procedures. College Hill Press, San Diego, CA.

Hodson, B. W. 1982. Remediation of speech patterns associated with low levels of phonological performance. In: M. Crary (ed.), Phonological Intervention, Concepts and Procedures. College Hill Press, San Diego, CA.

Ingram, D. 1976. Phonological Disability in Children. American Elsevier, New York.

Klein, H. B. 1981. Strategies for the pronunciation of early polysyllabic lexical items. J. Speech Hear. Res 24:389–405.

Leonard, L., Newhoff, M., and Mesalam, L. 1980. Individual differences in early child phonology. Appl. Psycholinguistics 1:7–30.

MacDonald, F. I. 1964. Screening Deep Test of Articulation. Stanwix House, Pittsburgh.

Macken, M. A., and Ferguson, C. A. 1981. Phonological universals in language acquisition. In: H. Winitz (ed.), Native Language and Foreign Language Acquisition, Volume 379, Annals of the New York Academy of Sciences, New York.

Moskowitz, B. A. 1980. Idioms in phonology acquisition and phonological change. J. Phonetics 8:69–83.

Poole, E. 1934. Genetic development of articulation of consonant sounds in speech. Elementary Engl. Rev. 11:159–161.

Prather, E. D., Hedrick, D., and Kern, C. 1975. Articulation development in children aged two to four years. J. Speech Hear. Res. 40:179–191.

Sander, E. K. 1972. When are speech sounds learned? J. Speech Hear. Disord. 37:55–63.

Schwartz, R., and Prelock, P. 1982. Cognition and phonology. In: J. Panagos (ed.), Children's Phonological Disorders in Language Contexts, Seminars in Speech, Language, and Hearing, Vol. 3. Thieme-Stratton, New York.

Shelton, R. L., Elbert, M., and Arndt, W. B. 1967. A task for evaluation of articulation change: II. Comparison of task scores during baseline and lesson series testing. J. Speech Hear. Res. 10:578–585.

Stephens, M. I., and Daniloff, R. 1980. Spontaneous self-improvement among /s/ misarticulating kindergarteners. Paper read at the 1980 Annual Convention of the American Speech-Language-Hearing Association, Detroit.

Templin, M. 1957. Certain language skills in children, their development and inter-relationship. Institute of Child Welfare, Monograph Series, No. 26. University of Minnesota Press, Minneapolis, MN.

Weiner, F. F. 1981. Systematic sound preference as a characteristic of phonological disability. J. Speech Hear. Disord. 46:281–286.

Wellman, B. L., Case, I.M., Mengert, I.G., and Bradbury, D. E. 1931. Speech sounds of young children. University of Iowa Studies in Child Welfare, 5, No. 2. University of Iowa, Iowa City.

Winitz, H. 1969. Articulatory Acquisition and Behavior. Prentice-Hall, Englewood Cliffs, NJ.

## CHAPTER 9

# Generalization in Articulation Training

*Barbara K. Rockman and Mary Elbert*

*Factors which contribute to the generalization of articulation responses are carefully considered by Rockman and Elbert. They enumerate conditions that facilitate generalization, and also discuss areas that require further study.*

1. *Distinguish between contextual and situational generalization in the treatment of articulation disorders. Which type of generalization traditionally has been identified with carryover?*
2. *Distinguish between across phoneme generalization and within phoneme generalization. Which term best describes word position generalization? According to Rockman and Elbert's summary, is word position an important consideration in the generalization of articulation responses? Furthermore, what is the influence of the use of syllables in articulation training on articulation generalization?*
3. *What are some considerations in the teaching of articulation when training is based on phonological processes? How can generalization be used to show the psychological validity of phonological processes?*
4. *Summarize your impressions of the type of probes that can be used to assess generalization? What factors should be considered when making a probe list?*
5. *How is articulation generalization facilitated? Can you think of several conditions that might serve as facilitators that were not considered by Rockman and Elbert?*

GENERALIZATION HAS BEEN DEFINED by Stokes and Baer (p. 350, 1977) as follows:

> The occurrence of relevant behavior under different non-training conditions (i.e., across subjects, settings, people, behaviors, and/or time) without the scheduling of the same events in those conditions as had been scheduled in the training conditions. Thus, generalization may be claimed when no extratraining manipulations are needed for extratraining changes.

In speech pathology, generalization, as defined above, has traditionally been called "carryover" and has referred to the process by which a client begins to use behaviors learned in the clinical setting in other settings. This kind of generalization has been called *situational* or *extraclinic generalization*. In addition, however, speech-language pathologists are interested in the generalization processes that occur during a client's acquisition of new behavior. This type of generalization has been called *intratherapy* or *contextual generalization*, and concerns how a new behavior is acquired and incorporated into the phonological system of the client from isolated sound production to words, to various word positions, to utterances of varying length. It is with this latter type of generalization that this chapter is concerned.

The expectation that generalization will occur is implicit in the work we perform as speech-language pathologists. To believe otherwise implies the necessity of training each target sound in every possible word and context in which it occurs. No one expects training or learning to follow this course. Rather, we assume that at some point, generalization of information learned in one context or situation will occur in similar untrained contexts and situations.

Both the research literature and our clinical experience have demonstrated adequately that when subjects or clients are provided with training, generalization usually occurs. There is less agreement concerning how or why it occurs, and it is this question that continues to plague both experimental investigators and clinical practitioners. What accounts for generalization? Why do some subjects generalize so readily and others so poorly? Given the importance of generalization to changing articulatory/phonological behavior, what do we know about it?

Much of what we know about generalization in articulation training has emerged only recently from a handful of training studies done within the past 15 years. Principles we now accept as givens have been empirically demonstrated only within this period of time, for example, the assumption that training on a specific phoneme will result in similar changes in its voiced or unvoiced cognate. These studies have explored a variety of factors in an attempt to discover variables which may contribute to or account for generalization. We, as clinician-researchers, have come to view the assessment of generalization as an important and regular aspect of our clinical work. We would like to persuade the clinician that it is both possible and desirable to include generalization procedures routinely in clinical practice. It is our belief that by evaluating generalization routinely during clinical training, we afford ourselves a window into the client's changing articulation/phonological system and into the effectiveness of our own procedures as well.

It is our purpose in this paper to present for clinicians a number of procedures extracted from the research literature in articulation generalization which may be applied clinically to measure and facilitate generalization. First, we will provide an overview of the research on generalization in articulation training studies and discuss clinical implications. Second, we will describe procedures for measuring generalization in clinical situations. Third, we will suggest ways in which generalization may be facilitated.

**OVERVIEW OF RESEARCH FINDINGS AND CLINICAL IMPLICATIONS**

McReynolds (1981) provides an excellent review of the experimental work in articulation generalization. In this section, we shall highlight only a few of the most relevant findings and relate these to clinical problems. McReynolds acknowledges the difficulty in extracting broad general principles from these studies because of differences in research design, type of subjects, and type of training provided.

McReynolds notes that generalization has been investigated on at least two levels:

(1) linguistic context generalization—these studies have been concerned with generalization of behaviors learned in a specific linguistic unit (isolated sound, syllable, word, word-position) to other, more advanced linguistic contexts (words, other word positions, sentences, spontaneous utterances).
(2) situational generalization—these studies are concerned with generalizing behaviors learned in the clinical situation to other environments or to individuals other than the clinician.

In this chapter we are concerned with the first level of generalization.

**Generalization across Phonemes**

*Research Findings*    The role of similarity among phonetic features in effecting phoneme generalization was initially demonstrated by Winitz and Bellerose (1963). One of the first well-documented examples of across phoneme generalization in articulation training was provided by Elbert et al. (1967). When children were trained on /s/, improvement occurred on untrained /s/ contexts, but not on the control phoneme /r/. Improvement was also noted, however, on the second control phoneme, /z/, on which no training had been provided. Here was clear-cut evidence that learning one phoneme could result in changes in another, closely related behavior. The authors accounted for the generalization on the basis of the phonetic similarity of the phonemes involved. The work of McReynolds and Bennett (1972) and of Costello and Onstine (1976) extended this concept of phonetic similarity by investigating the role of distinctive features in phoneme generalization.

In these studies, the experimental approach was to address a specific feature that occurred in several of the sounds on which the subject erred and which could have accounted for each of the errors. Training was provided on this feature for one preselected phoneme, and its generalization was monitored for other phonemes which contained this feature. For example, the feature value of [ + strident] was determined to be in error for one subject for whom the production of the class of strident phonemes, namely /f/, /v/, /s/, /z/, and /tʃ/, was in error. The procedure was to train [ + strident] through the phoneme /f/ and to determine generalization of [ + strident] for the strident phonemes. McReynolds (1981) notes that the findings of these studies indicate that some degree of *across phoneme generalization* for phonemes that share distinctive features is an anticipated outcome of training.

*Clinical Implications*   Let us consider a client whose errors include all fricatives and the velar stops /k/ and /g/. The clinician must decide where to begin training. A strategy of teaching based on across phoneme generalization is to train frication initially because the majority of sounds in error share this distinctive feature. Thus, in this instance, one might argue that training that begins with fricatives, rather than velars, is more efficient because, through the process of generalization, improvement in a greater number of phonemes is potentially possible.

## Generalization within Phonemes

*Across Position Research*   In another group of studies the effect of the position of the target sound in the training item (word-initial, -medial, or -final) on the generalization measure (Elbert and McReynolds, 1975, 1978; McReynolds, 1972; Powell and McReynolds, 1969) has been an issue of concern. In these studies, investigators were interested in within phoneme generalization, across word positions. At issue was whether training a phoneme in a particular position is more likely to result in generalization than training in some other position or combination of positions. The results have been somewhat mixed, but suggest that, in general, the position in which a target sound is trained is not a key factor in generalization. In most studies, the procedure was to begin training in the initial position, and then to progress to final and then to medial training. One exception to this sequence was the Elbert and McReynolds (1975) investigation in which the children were trained on varying positions and contexts of /r/. In these studies, for the most part, there was generalization to all word positions. McReynolds (1972) noted, however, that as additional positions are trained, greater generalization occurs across positions.

In similar studies, position generalization was not confirmed for retarded children (McLean, 1970; Raymore and McLean, 1972) nor for children of normal intelligence with severely restricted phonetic inventories (Rockman and Elbert, 1982). In this latter study, training was provided sequentially in nonsense syllables and monosyllabic words containing the target sounds /s/ and /k/ in final position, for example, /ik/ and "peek," /us/ and "moose." Generalization was tested not only in final position but also in initial position and in two-word–medial contexts. These children generalized the target phoneme to untrained words in the final position, but showed little or no generalization across positions. No doubt individual differences among subjects may have accounted for the lack of consistency among studies on word position.

*Clinical Implications*    Traditionally, training in articulation begins with the teaching of single sounds in the initial word position, with the second stage on final position, and the final stage on medial position. Clusters or blends are relegated to a separate stage of training. As reviewed above, the results of several studies indicate that this sequence is not particularly important, and they suggest a different approach. One procedure is to train a sound in all three positions simultaneously to provide the client with additional contexts to broaden his or her insight into the nature of the sound that is being taught. Perhaps this procedure will provide for rapid generalization across word positions. Clinicians who feel that training should begin with one position only may not be taking full advantage of generalization across word positions.

*Across Contexts*    Still other studies have been concerned with the generalization of a phoneme across various linguistic levels or contexts. That is, given training on one linguistic level, for example, nonsense syllables or words, what type of broader generalization may be expected? In exploring these questions, investigators have looked at the role of both the training items and the measures or tasks used to evaluate generalization.

Most of the experimental studies have used nonsense syllables for training the target sound and then tested generalization of that sound in words or longer utterances (Costello and Onstine, 1976; Elbert and McReynolds, 1975, 1978; Elbert et al., 1967; McReynolds, 1972; McReynolds and Bennett, 1972; Powell and McReynolds, 1969; Wright et al., 1969). McReynolds (1972) also examined the effects of training a sound in isolation on generalization to spontaneously produced single words. She found no generalization during training in isolation and reported that generalization did not begin to occur until training was provided in the initial position of a nonsense syllable. In all of the studies cited above, subjects typically showed generalization to untrained items at other linguistic levels, although to varying degrees. Whereas the value of using nonsense items in acquisition training is well established (Winitz, 1969, 1975), the relative value, for generalization purposes, of training a target sound in nonsense syllables versus other contexts is still unclear.

Of interest in other studies are the types of tasks used to evaluate generalization. Some studies have included only imitative generalization measures, whereas others have looked at both imitative and spontaneous tasks. Imitative tasks have included lists of words or other units (Costello and Onstine, 1976; Elbert and McReynolds, 1975, 1978; Elbert et al., 1967). One procedure commonly used is the Sound Production Task (SPT), described by Elbert et al. in 1967. SPTs are 30-item imitative tasks that sample the production of a sound in isolation, nonsense syllables, words, and phrases in a variety of phonetic contexts. Spontaneous tasks have included naming pictures (Costello and Onstine, 1976; Elbert and McReynolds, 1978; McReynolds, 1972; McReynolds and Bennett, 1972), reading, and spontaneous talking (Wright et al., 1967).

In general, studies that have looked at both imitative and spontaneous single word or short utterance responses have found that generalization occurs to both response modes about equally. When we examine generalization in relatively long spontaneous utterances, the evidence is less clear. After training on /s/ in isolation, syllables, sentences, and connected conversational speech, Wright et al. (1969) compared generalization on imitated Sound Production Tasks (single words and short phrases/sentences) with that in longer spontaneous utterances in reading and spontaneous talking. Subjects did consistently better on the imitative than on the spontaneous tasks. Even when subjects could consistently produce 90% of the imitated probe items, little correct use of the trained phoneme was seen in reading or conversation. Diedrich and Bangert (1980), on the other hand, report that in older school-aged children there was comparable generalization on imitative SPTs and spontaneous talking tasks. Research that points to the most effective strategy for facilitating generalization to spontaneous, longer utterances is still needed.

A somewhat different question pertains to the effect of phonetic context on generalization. Elbert and McReynolds (1978), explored the effect of phonetic contexts on generalization of /s/. Training was provided in the context of nonsense syllables using the neutral vowel /ʌ/. Generalization probes were designed to examine the effects of a variety of phonetic contexts, such as high and low vowels and front and back consonants and vowels, on the production of /s/. The effects of syllable shape, such as CV (consonant-vowel) VC, CCV, CVCC, on generalization were also examined. There was no evidence that any particular context was more facilitating for generalization than another, particularly when training was provided in this neutral context. Rather, children generalized across many different contexts.

Still another question pertains to the effect of grammatical context on generalization. As noted earlier, Rockman and Elbert (1982) provided training sequentially in nonsense syllables and monosyllabic words containing the target sounds /s/ and /k/ in final position, for example, /us/ and "moose"; /ik/ and "peek." Generalization was tested in final and initial position and in two-word–medial contexts. In one medial context, the target sound was contained in a single morpheme, for example, echo, pickle. In the other, the target sound was contained in a two-morpheme word, for example, baking, walking. This latter group consisted of words similar to those used in training, for example, hook, peek, to which another morpheme (grammatical inflection -ing, -er, -y) was added. The investigators hypothesized that greater generalization would occur for the two-morpheme medial position because the target sound had been learned in the final position of morphemes. They predicted that when an inflection was added to similar morphemes, placing the target sound in medial position, subjects would maintain correct production of the target in this medial context, and thus, generalization in medial position for the two-morpheme words would be greater than single morpheme medial contexts. This prediction was not confirmed, as there was no difference in generalization to either of the medial contexts. In fact, little generalization was shown to any position other than final position on which training had been provided. Had generalization occurred for the two-morpheme words and not for the single morpheme contexts, it might be inferred that underlying morphological and phonological structure influences articulatory generalization. The results of this study seem to suggest, however, that articulatory generalization is largely constrained by phonetic factors.

*Clinical Implications*   The research findings indicate that children generalize to untrained linguistic contexts when trained on nonsense syllables. In clinical practice, however, clinicians have to weigh the advantages and disadvantages of training on presumably abstract forms such as nonsense syllables versus real words. A distinction also must be drawn between training for acquisition or learning of a new sound and training for maximal generalization of that sound. Real words, which are more concrete and presumably meaningful to children, may well present a degree of difficulty in training for acquisition as a result of interference from prior learning (Winitz, 1969, 1975). Using real words in training for generalization, however, would seem to have some advantage in that they stand a greater chance of occurring in the environment and being reinforced than do nonsense syllables. Finally, these studies indicate that it is important to sample a wide variety of linguistic levels both imitatively and spontaneously, especially for relatively long sentences, to obtain a true picture of an individual's generalization pattern.

### Generalization Based on Phonological Processes

Recently a procedure called the *phonological process approach* has been applied to the treatment of children's sound errors (Hodson, 1981; Ingram, 1976; Weiner, 1981). This approach is largely directed to the generalization process through the use of preestablished phonological categories. Some common phonological processes are: *final consonant deletion*, in which children produce CVC syllables as CV; *velar assimilation*, in which alveolar consonants become velars, for example /gɔg/ for dog; and *fronting*, in which palatal velar consonants are replaced by alveolars, for example /tʌp/ for cup.

   In the phonological process approach, articulation errors are described according to phonological categories or processes, and furthermore, the articulation errors that are accounted for by a process are treated collectively. In some cases, generalization based on a phonological process analysis falls into the category of *across phoneme* generalization, because the phonemes are governed by the same phoneme class, as for example, the process of "stopping" which affects fricatives and converts them to stops. In other cases, generalization based on a phonological process analysis occurs *across phoneme classes*. For example, the processes of final consonant deletion and cluster reduction involve members of several sound classes; both stops and fricatives, among others, may be deleted by these processes. The correction of stopping for a given fricative, with demonstrable generalization to other fricatives which were substituted by stops, may be accounted for on the basis of across phoneme generalization. Similarly, the correction of final sounds from different phoneme classes may be accounted for by generalization that occurs across phoneme classes. If the omission of final consonants is governed by rule or process, irrespective of sound class, elimination of the process for a member of one sound class should result in or allow for the production of final consonants in all classes.

Results of the few studies on the effectiveness of approaching sound errors through phonological processes have been mixed. Weiner (1981) reported a significant reduction of final consonant deletion across phoneme classes after training using a contrast or minimal pair procedure. In his procedure two words are contrasted: one is the result of the child not producing a final consonant and the other is a different word formed by adding a final consonant, for example, bow-boat, ray-race. It should be noted that, in this task, Weiner accepted the production of any final consonant as a correct response and interpreted any final consonant as evidence that the process of final consonant deletion had been suppressed or eliminated. He also reported that subjects produced a high percentage of correct responses as a result of the training. Other studies have not shown similar across class results (Elbert and McReynolds, 1980; McReynolds and Elbert, 1981). Subjects with errors characterized as final consonant deletions received training on several examplars of either final stops or final fricatives. Subjects generalized to other sounds within the same phoneme class, but not across phoneme classes. This approach to remediation raises the question of whether linguistic categories (such as phoneme classes or other phonological classes, such as word position) can always be assumed to be psychologically real categories. Lack of generalization across classes might argue for psychological or conceptual distinctiveness for specific linguistic categories. Broad generalization across classes could be viewed as evidence to the contrary. LaRiviere et al. (1974), using a categorization task, explored the conceptual reality for adults of selected distinctive features. Results were mixed, with nasal, strident, and vocalic features showing conceptual reality, whereas continuant and voice features did not.

*Clinical Implications*     There is no clear interpretation regarding the use of phonological processes for articulation training. Although Ingram (1976) states that phonological processes should be the target of treatment, at the same time he expresses reservations regarding the generalization hypothesis, noting that the data thus far have not been entirely convincing. He concludes that it may be "safer to attack a process by training on all the affected segments." If this is the case, the advantage of approaching sound errors based on phonological processes is unclear. At this stage, clinicians can best maintain careful records and examine generalization based on phonological processes for themselves.

In this brief overview, we have examined the kinds of generalization questions that have been raised in the research literature. We have suggested that clinicians can use generalization measures to address clinical questions of their own and to determine the effects and effectiveness of many of their procedures. In the following paragraphs, we present procedures that are typically used in research to assess generalization and which also lend themselves to clinical use.

## MEASURING GENERALIZATION

### Basic Considerations

Generalization is measured through the use of *probes*. A generalization probe can take many forms. It may be a list of words that clients imitate, a set of pictures that they name, a sample of their reading for a specified length of time, or a timed sample of their use of spontaneous speech. A probe consists primarily of behavior not directly trained and is administered at regularly scheduled intervals throughout the course of training. A subset of the probe list is often selected for training. In this way, it is possible to monitor generalization of trained as well as untrained items.

It is important to differentiate between the type of probe used in programmed instruction and that used to measure generalization. In programmed instruction, at the conclusion of each phase of a program, it is common practice to "probe" the next level of difficulty. As an illustration, when a client reaches criterion on the imitation of training words, the clinician would probe the client's ability to perform at the next level, which is to name or produce spontaneously those same words without a model. In this way, the clinician can determine whether any change has occurred on the basis of prior training and whether it is necessary to provide training on this step at all. This type of probe, then, is different from administration to administration, because it is always directed to the next level of difficulty within a program. The generalization probe, on the other hand, remains the same from administration to administration.

Generalization measures are designed to examine changes in untrained behaviors over time. In speech-language pathology, we have traditionally adopted a before and after framework for measuring change, and frequently have not looked at related untrained behavior or generalization. The before measure or pretest has typically consisted of an articulation test. These tests, if scored as directed using a sub-

Table 1.    Example of a 30-item /k/ generalization probe

| Initial | Medial | Final | Clusters | |
| | | | Initial | Final |
| --- | --- | --- | --- | --- |
| /k-/ | /-k-/ | /-k/ | cloud (/kl/) | desk (/sk/) |
| can | racoon | book | cream (/kr/) | milk (/lk/) |
| key | pickle | chalk | queen (/kw/) | |
| car | knocking | knock | | |
| comb | rocker | duck | | |
| kite | echo | sidewalk | | |
| cup | pocket | take | | |
| castle | bacon | stick | | |
| captain | | | | |

stitution, omission, or distortion category system, provide only one example of each phoneme in each word position. Because many children show highly variable articulation performance, often word specific errors, this type of testing does not provide an adequate initial measure or pretest of behavior.

When a more formal pretest is used, it typically consists of the specific behavior the clinician intends to train. Thus, if a child is being trained on /r/, the pretest might consist of 10 /r/ words on which the child initially obtains a score of zero. Training is then provided on /r/ in these words and at the final stages of training the child is able to produce all of these words correctly. There really is no need for a posttest assessment, because the child has been trained to produce these words correctly. It should be easy to see, then, that there has been no measure of generalization here. There has been no attempt to measure behavior other than that specifically trained nor to evaluate change between the beginning and end of training. If an articulation test is administered again at the end of training, and the articulation test words are not those that were trained, then a very brief and minimal look at generalization is possible.

The use of a well-designed probe list before and during training provides a clear view of the child's learning on words other than the specific training words. What is needed is a particular list or selection of words that samples the distribution of a given phoneme in the same variety of contexts that it enjoys in the language. For example, if the clinician intends to train /k/, it is important to include occurrences of /k/ clusters on the proble list as well as singleton /k/. It is important to try to evaluate /k/ in words containing both lesser and greater phonetic complexity in order to explore fully the child's generalization and control over /k/ production, as indicated in Table 1. The items in Table 1 are shown before randomization to illustrate the framework by which items were selected. To keep the number of items at 30, not all /k/ clusters are represented on the probe list.

## Baseline Measures

In order to talk about the generalization of behavior, a clinician must demonstrate how that behavior operated or occurred before the introduction of treatment. Unless the clinician has good documentation of behavior at the outset, it is difficult to demonstrate convincingly that change has occurred. This documentation takes the form of baseline measurements. The baseline may be thought of as a pretest, although a baseline is frequently taken over more than one session to document the stability of a behavior. For example, the same probe might be administered three times before the initiation of training. This same probe is administered throughout training to measure change. The client's baseline performance serves as a control measure before the administration of treatment. Any changes that might be noted on later administrations of the same measure (probes) are interpreted as reflecting the effect of training.

Before making an assessment of generalization, clinicians should be clear about the kinds of generalization they wish to explore. Also, before beginning articulation training, they should anticipate what the outcomes may be and should be prepared to probe these behaviors. In addition, they should determine which aspects of generalization are to be examined and what changes are to be identified, so as to plan and devise appropriate measures.

## Constructing a Probe List

Although we have discussed a variety of forms a probe may take, a probe list provides the most direct and rapid measure of generalization. What are some of the factors to be taken into consideration when constructing a probe list?

*Number of Items*   The probe list must be sufficiently long to sample various contexts of the phoneme of interest. At the same time, it must be of reasonable length to be tolerated by clients over frequent administrations and to fit into training sessions without being disruptive. Probe lists containing between 30 and 40 items seem to meet these conditions.

*Within the Child's Understanding*   Needless to say, unless the words are within the child's knowledge, they are essentially nonsense words. They also pose problems in repetition tasks. We recommend that probes be words that children are likely to know.

### Phonetic Composition

*General Complexity*  It may be that the greater the phonetic complexity present in a word in addition to the target phoneme, the greater the likelihood of error on the target. For a child with errors on all fricatives and affricates, probe words for /s/ that contain other fricatives and affricates may be more difficult than words not containing these sounds. The issue here is whether a child with this particular error pattern is any more likely to produce /s/ correctly in probe words like *bus* or *house*, which contain no other fricatives or affricates, than in words like *juice* or *face*, in which the initial consonant is also in error for the child. Although this is an issue that lends itself to empirical study, it has not been examined, to our knowledge, and we present it here as a factor for consideration in selecting probe words.

Similarly, it has been our experience and the suggestion of others that, for some children, the presence of /l/ in a probe word for /r/ will cause difficulty in the production of /r/ (McNutt and Keenan, 1970; but see also Shriner and Daniloff, 1971). The explanation for these interfering factors is not always clear. In the case of /r/ and /l/, it has been our experience that although children have no errors involving /l/, its presence in an /r/ word may result in confusion over which liquid to produce.

*Use of Error Sound*  Another factor thought to affect production of a newly learned target sound adversely is proximity of the error substitution sound in the stimulus item (McNutt and Keenan, 1970). Shriner and Daniloff (1971), in a discussion limited to the possible negative effect of /w/ on /r/ in the phrase *one red ball*, argue that there is no basis for this position in coarticulation in that the distance between the error sound /w/ and the target sound /r/ is such that coarticulatory effects would not apply. Winitz (1975), acknowledging that his rationale is psychological rather than physiological, has suggested that during acquisition training, clinicians avoid phrases and sentences in which a sound similar to the error substitution is adjacent to or near the position occupied by the error sound.

To illustrate this point, let us take the case of a child learning to produce /k/, for which /t/ is substituted. For this child, the inclusion of probe words like *kite* or *tick* on the probe list may cause confusion between the child's target sound and the error substitution. Words of this type also may add to difficulty of production because of the potential for assimilation, either progressive or regressive. Therefore, although it may be desirable to include some of these items on probe lists to assess the child's mastery of the target sound, clinicians should recognize that words of this type may be more difficult than words not containing the error sound.

*Multiple Instances of Target Phoneme*   Probe words that contain the target phoneme in more than one position may present additional difficulty and are also subject to assimilation problems. Thus, the use of the word *scissors* to assess production of medial or intervocalic /z/ is confounded by several factors, such as another /z/ sound in final position that is part of the consonant cluster /rz/, further adding complexity, and another fricative in the initial position. For these reasons, production of medial /z/ in *scissors* seems more difficult than in a word such as *busy* or *daisy*. Although it may be desirable to include words like *six* on an /s/ probe test or *cake* on a /k/ probe test, for example, the increased difficulty posed by their presence should be recognized.

*Syllable Shape*   This factor is related to phonetic complexity. It is important to be aware of the syllabic configuration of the words included on the probe list. It is desirable to have both monosyllabic and polysyllabic words represented while remembering that polysyllabic words will generally be phonetically more complex. Words should represent CV, VC, and CVC configurations as well as more complex shapes, such as CCVC, CVCC, or CVCVC.

*Position of Target Phoneme*   Probe lists should sample phonemes in all word positions and in as many naturally occurring contexts as feasible. These generally include word-initial, -medial, and -final positions and consonant clusters in all word positions. For example, in the /k/ probe list (Table 1), /k/ is sampled in a variety of clusters and word positions and in nonsense syllables.

*Vowel Representation*   Care should be taken to see that the target sound is sampled with a variety of adjacent vowels, representing different vowel heights and front to back positions.

The construction of the probe list, seen from this perspective, should provide the clinician with a good professional exercise in examining and evaluating the factors noted above. We view the making of the probe list as a healthy challenge, not unlike a good crossword puzzle.

### Administering Generalization Probes

*Frequency*   One of the major decisions in probing for generalization concerns the scheduling of the probes. How often should probes be administered? In some of the research studies cited earlier, probes were administered at each training session. In others, they were administered on a criterion based schedule, that is, as the client achieved specific levels of success on the training tasks.

There are advantages and disadvantages to both schedules. Daily probes, those taken at each training session, provide an in-depth and detailed look at articulation change. On the other hand, they require more time both in and out of the clinical session, time in session for administration, and time outside for scoring and analysis.

Probes administered on a criterion based schedule enable clinicians to examine the effects of specific steps within the training sequence. The clinician cannot always conclude that a change in articulation on the probe test from one administration to the next is the result of the training that occurred in that interval. The results of training in each phase in all likelihood are cumulative. This type of probe schedule, however, provides some insight into the number of steps and amount of training necessary for a given client before generalization begins to occur.

The frequency of probe testing is less important than a commitment to use probes to test for generalization. We recommend that clinicians experiment with a variety of probe test schedules, such as every session, every third session, weekly, at the conclusion of specific training phases, until they are able to establish a basis for the frequency at which probes are to be used.

*Reinforcement/Feedback*    Probes are traditionally treated as tests, that is, no specific reinforcement or feedback is provided for correct or incorrect responses. The clinician may provide general verbal reinforcement for good attention or behavior during the probe, or tangible reinforcement may be provided at the conclusion of the entire probe for the same general behaviors, but no distinction is made on probe items between correct and incorrect responses. The clinician simply records the client's responses; there is no evaluation.

*Mode of Administration*    Probe lists are generally administered in an imitative mode. The same questions that apply to any imitative task are often asked with regard to imitative probes. Aren't imitated responses easier to produce correctly? Does imitation really test generalization? Don't clients simply learn the probe list responses? Our experience has been that the client's implicit insight into the articulation behavior under consideration seems to be the primary factor determining correct performance on the probe list. Clients typically do not begin producing probe list responses correctly until they have developed some rudimentary insight into the relationship between the sound they are being taught to acquire and the sound or sounds that are tested on the probe list. It may help to bear in mind that often, in research studies, the subjects are not told that the probe list is in any way related to the sound training part of the experiment. No feedback or shaping of responses is provided. Thus, this type of administration is viewed as valid in measuring the child's developing tacit awareness and control of specific phoneme production.

Many researchers and clinicians elect to present probe lists on tape to avoid subtle and potentially biasing variations in stress and duration on target sounds. By using a taped presentation, the clinician ensures that changes on the probe are not the result of unintentional cuing during stimulus presentation. If taping is not practical, the clinician should be aware of the tendency to emphasize target sounds and try to minimize these differences.

Whether the probe is presented via tape or live voice, we recommend that the order of the words on the probe be varied from administration to administration. When using a taped presentation, at least two forms of the list should be prepared. In this way, the client does not come to expect a specific order of the probe words.

It may be important to examine the differences between an imitative and a spontaneous probe administered within the same time frame. The spontaneous probe may be presented by using a set of pictures to represent the items on the imitative probe list. The client who is able spontaneously to produce the target phoneme in words is demonstrating a level of phonological awareness and articulatory control in advance of the imitative response. Again, clinicians must decide what is practical for them in the clinical setting. If a spontaneous probe is desired, a baseline measure of spontaneous production should be obtained before training.

Similarly, as mentioned earlier, probes may take many forms: reading the same passage at regular intervals and tabulating the number of correct versus incorrect responses on the target phoneme, describing a set of pictures or providing a narrative on a given topic, with the same tally of correct versus incorrect productions. The only requirement concerning the mode of administration is that it must be constant from baseline to final testing in order to provide a valid measure of generalization over time.

In this section we have discussed many procedures for evaluating generalization in the clinical population. In the final section of this paper, we turn our attention to the issue of active facilitation of generalization.

## FACILITATING GENERALIZATION

The studies on generalization reported above are not intended to describe how to facilitate generalization. Instead, their purpose was to observe generalization patterns as they naturally occurred. In an article discussing the technology of generalization, Stokes and Baer (1977) refer to these kinds of studies under the category of "train and hope," implying that nothing had been done directly to promote generalization.

There is little research, beyond the observational, which directly addresses the question of facilitation of articulation generalization. With this information on articulatory generalization, however, we can speculate about variables that may be important in promoting generalization (Stokes and Baer, 1977).

## Variables

*Extensive Practice*    It is important to recognize that many of the subjects in training studies showed generalization. How did this happen? Let us first look at the level of training that is provided. All of the research programs involved a high level of learning; that is, practice was provided until the subjects could correctly produce the training items consistently over a large number of trials. Because articulatory behavior is, at least in part, a motor skill, this extensive practice to the point of automatic production may ensure that the production aspect is readily available to the person. Learning studies indicate that in situations in which one learns successive tasks of the same class, transfer is greater when extensive practice occurs on the early tasks in the series (Ellis, 1972). It seems unlikely that any substantial generalization would occur before the error sound or sounds can be produced with some ease and automaticity. The opportunity to practice the correct response extensively appears to be a critical factor, although it is recognized that the amount of training required before generalization occurs will vary from child to child. Some children begin to generalize very early in training, whereas others require more extensive training and practice.

*Type and Number of Exemplars*    A second factor that is related to generalization concerns the type and number of exemplars of sounds taught. To facilitate generalization to probe lists, should we train a sound in one position in several exemplars or train several exemplars with the sound in different positions? Is it more productive to train a few exemplars that represent greater diversity or many exemplars with limited diversity? In the learning literature, the importance of practice under varied task conditions for producing transfer is emphasized (Ellis, 1972). This notion is illustrated nicely by Ellis (1972), who notes that one's understanding of a topic can be improved not so much by repeated rereading of the same text, but by reading another text on the same subject matter. The importance of varied context and examples is stressed. Stokes and Baer (1977) also emphasize that there must be sufficient diversity among examplars trained to reflect the dimensions of the desired generalization.

In articulation training studies, questions concerning the type or form of exemplar to be used in training have focused largely on positions of the target sound in the training item (McReynolds, 1972; Powell and McReynolds, 1969; Rockman and Elbert, 1982). Winitz (1975) illustrates the type of paradigm that would be necessary to examine the actual effects of training position on transfer to other positions and concludes that this issue has not been settled with regard to generalization learning. Given the information we have thus far, it would seem that once sound acquisition has been established in a limited context, generalization to probe lists would be facilitated by training words in all positions simultaneously.

Another question related to the choice of exemplar concerns whether to train a phoneme as a single entity or use contrasting examplars. For example, for the child who substitutes /t/ for /k/, one strategy would be to train sequentially words containing /k/, for example, key, cap, cone, back, book, sack, whereas another strategy would be to train two exemplars at a time, contrasting the error and target sounds, for example, key-tea, cap-tap, and so on. This type of contrast training has often been called the minimal pair strategy and may be used to train both phonetic and phonological errors (Elbert et al., 1980). Both of these strategies have been used in articulation research and generalization has been shown to occur with each procedure.

*Probe List*   When the child is trained on only a few items but tested on a longer, highly diverse list (probe), we may be arranging a situation that is optimum for generalization. By training a few exemplars to a high automatic level at which the child can produce the response with ease, we are assuring that the motor skill is established and available for use. At this point, when the probe list is presented the child may begin to observe the similarity between the training items and the many other possible uses of a particular sound and reach the needed insight which is the basis of generalization. The probe list itself may serve as a powerful facilitation device. It may be essential to differentiate between training a lengthy, diverse set of words and probing the same list. Too many training examples may inadvertently promote a type of rote learning which may interfere with the more cognitive processes which are important to generalization. The child may view the task more as "list learning" than "system learning." Thus, the probe list may serve as more than a measurement device. It is possible that it may provide a valuable opportunity to the learner to make observations, form hypotheses about the sound system, and begin actively to make changes in his or her own system.

*Programming Steps and Reinforcement*   Generalization may be enhanced through the use of specific programming steps. Both a change in the type of response and the reinforcement schedule may lead the child to assume more responsibility for his or her own productions and make the response more readily available for correct usage. In research studies, subjects usually begin with extremely low baseline scores, which indicates that the target behavior is either entirely absent or infrequent. The target behavior is established through shaping procedures and imitation of the researcher's models. When the response is produced correctly consistently, procedures are changed to require a spontaneous response. The spontaneous response calls for retrieval of the correct production from memory because the auditory model is no longer available. Reinforcement is an important component of the training procedure because a behavioral approach is used most often in generalization studies. At first, reinforcement is continuous until the response is stable; then a variable reinforcement schedule is introduced. Variable reinforcement schedules are known to result in behavior that is more resistant to extinction and, in the case of the misarticulating child, may help to stabilize the target response.

As the training sequence progresses from imitated responses with continuous reinforcement to spontaneous responses on a variable schedule of reinforcement, the child is presented with increasingly difficult tasks that require increasing control of the response. Although the effects of variable reinforcement schedules on articulation generalization have not been investigated directly, it is possible that they contribute to generalization. Thus, the clinician may wish to explore varying reinforcement schedules throughout training.

## CONCLUSION

In this chapter we derive from research literature strategies for measuring and facilitating generalization in the clinical setting. We encourage clinicians to play an active part in the ongoing development of the technology of generalization by using the procedures we describe, as well as their own, in the training situation. Clinicians have frequent opportunities to evaluate their procedures and to examine an individual child's learning using the generalization procedures described. By adopting a generalization orientation to clinical practice, the clinician can actively participate in the research process, answering questions and generating new hypotheses for the future.

## REFERENCES

Costello, J., and Onstine, J. M. 1976. The modification of multiple articulation errors based on distinctive feature theory. J. Speech Hear. Disord. 41:199–215.

150    Rockman and Elbert

Diedrich, W., and Bangert, J. 1980. Articulation Learning. College Hill Press, Houston.
Elbert, M., and McReynolds, L. V. 1975. Transfer of /r/ across contexts. J. Speech Hear. Disord. 40:380–387.
Elbert, M., and McReynolds, L. V. 1978. An experimental analysis of misarticulating children's generalization. J. Speech Hear. Res. 21:136–150.
Elbert, M., and McReynolds, L. V. 1980. The generalization hypothesis: Final consonant deletion. Unpublished investigation. Bloomington, IN.
Elbert, M., Rockman, B., and Saltzman, D. 1980. Contrasts: The Use of Minimal Pairs in Articulation Training. Exceptional Resources, Austin, TX.
Elbert, M., Shelton, R. L., and Arndt, W. B. 1967. A task for evaluation of articulation change. I. Development of methodology. J. Speech Hear. Res. 10:281–289.
Ellis, H. C. 1972. Fundamentals of Human Learning and Cognition. Wm. C. Brown Co., Dubuque, IA.
Hodson, B. 1981. Phonological processes which characterize unintelligible and intelligible speech in early childhood. J. Speech Hear. Disord. 46:369–373.
Ingram, D. 1976. Phonological Disability in Children. Edward Arnold Ltd., London.
LaRiviere, C., Winitz, H., Reeds, J., and Herriman, E. 1974. The conceptual reality of selected distinctive features. J. Speech Hear. Res. 17:122–133.
McLean, J. E. 1970. Extending stimulus control of phoneme articulation by operant techniques. ASHA Monogr. No. 14, Washington.
McNutt, J. C., and Keenan, R. A. 1970. Comment on "The relationship between articulatory deficits and syntax in speech defective children." J. Speech Hear. Res. 13:666–667.
McReynolds, L. V. 1972. Articulation generalization during articulation training. Lang. Speech 15:149–155.
McReynolds, L. V. 1981. Generalization in articulation training. Anal. Intervention Devel. Disabil. 1:245–258.
McReynolds, L. V., and Bennett, S. 1972. Distinctive feature generalization in articulation training. J. Speech Hear. Disord. 37:462–470.
McReynolds, L., and Elbert, M. 1981. Generalization of correct articulation in clusters. Appl. Psycholinguistics 2:119–132.
Powell, J., and McReynolds, L. 1969. A procedure for testing position generalization from articulation training. J. Speech Hear. Res. 12:629–645.
Raymore, D., and McLean, J. E. 1972. A clinical program of carry-over of articulation therapy with retarded children. In: J. E. McLean, D. E. Yoder, and R. L. Schiefelbusch (eds.), Language Intervention with the Retarded. University Park Press, Baltimore.
Rockman, B., and Elbert, M. 1982. An experimental investigation of individual differences and generalization in articulation training. Unpublished Manuscript. Bloomington. IN.
Shriner, T. H., and Daniloff, R. G. 1971. Reply to "Comments on the relationship between articulatory deficits and syntax in speech defective children." J. Speech Hear. Res. 14:442–444.
Stokes, T. F., and Baer, D. M. 1977. An implicit technology of generalization. J. Appl. Behav. Anal. 10:349–367.
Weiner, F. 1981. Treatment of phonological disability using the method of meaningful minimal contrast: Two case studies. J. Speech Hear. Disord. 46:97–103.

Winitz, H. 1969. Articulatory Acquisition and Behavior. Appleton-Century-Crofts, New York.

Winitz, H. 1975. From Syllable to Conversation. University Park Press, Baltimore.

Winitz, H., and Bellerose, B. 1963. Phoneme-sound generalization as a function of phoneme similarity and verbal unit of test and training stimuli. J. Speech Hear. Res. 6:379–392.

Wright, V., Shelton, R., and Arndt, W. B. 1969. A task for evaluation of articulation change. III. Imitative task scores compared with scores for more spontaneous tasks. J. Speech Hear. Res. 12:875–884.

# CHAPTER 10

# Correcting Misarticulations by Use of Semantic Conflict

*Edwin A. Leach*

*Leach describes a procedure for treating the articulation er-*
*rors of children which he calls the* Semantic Conflict Approach. *He provides the rationale for this approach and its*
*implementation.*

1. *What does Leach mean by the Semantic Conflict Ap-*
   *proach? What is Leach's rationale for this approach?*
2. *What is the primary clinical goal of the Semantic Conflict*
   *Approach? What is the clinical procedure that Leach*
   *recommends for implementation of this goal? At what*
   *point in articulation training would you recommend*
   *using this approach? If this approach is successful, do*
   *you think it will provide for carryover?*

ANYONE WHO HAS STUDIED A CHILD'S DEVELOPMENT of communication cannot help but be impressed by the fact that it begins very early and progresses rapidly. Soon after birth, healthy infants communicate general body conditions of comfort, discomfort, and contentment, show early forms of socialization, and exhibit responsiveness to speech. At the time the first word is uttered, most parents can cite an extensive list of communicative behaviors used by their young infant. Slightly later, when speech continues to be limited to single word elements, parents can interpret a variety of utterance meanings for unfamiliar listeners (Nelson, 1973). Imperfect as this early communication may be by adult standards, the normal child is a relatively successful communicator.

There are a number of factors that contribue to the young child's success in communication. First, virtually all of the meaning intended by young children is limited to the content of the immediate environment in which the communication occurs. An abundance of cues, in the form of clothing, toys, books, food items, and actions, often makes the adult's interpretation of the communication fairly accurate. Also, the children's focus of attention, indicated by head position and eye gaze, will often provide helpful cues.

Second, the repetition of daily experiences, such as bathing, dressing, and eating and the locations in which the child is placed (bedroom, kitchen, grocery store, etc.) restricts the content variety for communication. With a small number of possible interpretations, the odds favor the adult when interpreting a child's communicative intent.

Third, in the early years during which children are acquiring basic syntactic and phonological skills, their audience is limited in number and variety. A high percentage of a child's listeners are immediate family members, and perhaps a few family friends. At times, children appear to resist the addition of new listeners. When children of 2 or 3 years of age are placed in the company of other children their own age, the typical outcome is one of minimal interaction, verbal or otherwise. This restricted audience to whom most communication is directed means simply that children usually have an audience that is familiar with their communication patterns. Family listeners, who have a significant communication history with the child, will have a much better chance of correctly interpreting communicative intents than will unfamiliar listeners. Older siblings are especially adaptable to young children's speech and often function as "interpreters" when unfamiliar listeners are present. These interpreters further guarantee successful communication.

Finally, the early imperfect speech of children does not always result in confusion about an intended word. For example, when we examine the alternative words produced by children who substitute /p/ for /f/ initially, some interesting characteristics may be noted. Of those 90 words common in the vocabulary of children which contain /f/ as the initial sound (see Table 1), only 41 (45%) of the derivative productions are actual English words; the remaining 49 (55%) are non-English productions (American College Dictionary). Of the 41 actual words, about one-third are unlikely to be spoken by 5- or 6-year-old children (*pace, pact, pang, par, parse, pawn, peer/pier, peat, pelt, pew, pyre, pox, pun, pone*). Of the 27 words that are conceivably within the vocabulary of young children, nine words form a different part of speech when /p/ is substituted for /f/: (fail-verb/pail-noun, pale-adjective; fat-adjective/pat-verb; field-noun/peeled-verb; file-noun/pile-verb; fill-verb/pill-noun; fir-noun, fur-noun/purr-verb; foot-noun/put-verb; for-preposition, four-noun/pour-verb, poor-adjective; full-adjective/pull-verb). Only 18 words of the original 90 /f/-initial words (20%) may be a source of confusion to the listener when /p/ is substituted for /f/.

This low percentage suggests that for a child who misarticulates p/f, only a small number of words beginning with /f/ is potentially a source of confusion for the listener. Although success in communication does not appear to be impaired greatly by p/f substitutions, this circumstance might not necessarily hold for all sound contrasts. The /r/, however, which is a frequent misarticulation, seldom contrasts with /w/, a common substitution for /r/. For those few pairs of words for which /r/ and /w/ contrast, the words of the pair are usually different grammatical parts of speech. For example, *rag* is a noun and *wag* is a verb, *rest* is a verb and *west* is a noun or an adjective, and in many instances, /r/-/w/ minimal word pairs from the same grammatical class, do not contrast in the context of a sentence. For example the verbs *rent* and *went* are unlikely to be confused in the context of a sentence were the /r/ to be substituted by /w/.

It is my contention that the lack of listener confusion or the low frequency of its occurrence is a significant factor in the continuation of some children's misarticulation patterns, especially when only one or two sounds are involved. The basis for this contention is stated as follows: 1) most listeners with whom a young child communicates are seldom confused about the child's communicative intents; 2) communication is successful in spite of a child's articulatory errors; and 3) there is little motivation on the part of children to correct their misarticulations until they come into contact with new listeners who may respond negatively to their speech. Perhaps for this reason,

Table 1.   Most common /f/ words for initial position and /p-f/ substitution derivatives

| | Word | p-f derivative | | Word | p-f derivative |
|---|---|---|---|---|---|
| 1. | Face | Pace | 46. | Fern | |
| 2. | Fact | Pact | 47. | Fetch | |
| 3. | Factory | | 48. | Fever | |
| 4. | Fad | Pad | 49. | Few | Pew |
| 5. | Fade | Paid | 50. | Fib | |
| 6. | Fairy, Ferry | | 51. | Fiddle | Piddle |
| 7. | Fag | | 52. | Field | Peeled |
| 8. | Fail | Pail, Pale | 53. | Five | |
| 9. | Faint | Paint | 54. | Fight | |
| 10. | Fair | Pair, Pear, Pare | 55. | File | Pile |
| 11. | Fall | | 56. | Fill | Pill |
| 12. | Faith | | 57. | Film | |
| 13. | Fake | | 58. | Fin | Pin |
| 14. | False | | 59. | Find | Pined |
| 15. | Fame | | 60. | Finish | |
| 16. | Family | | 61. | Fine | Pine |
| 17. | Famous | | 62. | Finger | |
| 18. | Fan | Pan | 63. | Fir, Fur | Purr |
| 19. | Fancy | | 64. | Fire | Pyre |
| 20. | Fang | Pang | 65. | First | |
| 21. | Far | Par | 66. | Fish | |
| 22. | Farce | Parse | 67. | Fist | |
| 23. | Farewell | | 68. | Fit | Pit |
| 24. | Farm | | 69. | Fix | Picks |
| 25. | Farther | | 70. | Foe | |
| 26. | Fast | Past | 71. | Fog | |
| 27. | Fasten | | 72. | Fold | |
| 28. | Fat | Pat | 73. | Folk | Poke |
| 29. | Fate | | 74. | Follow | |
| 30. | Father | | 75. | Food | |
| 31. | Fault | | 76. | Fool | Pool |
| 32. | Favor | | 77. | Foot | Put |
| 33. | Fawn | Pawn | 78. | Four, Fore, For | Pour, Poor |
| 34. | Fear | Peer, Pier | 79. | Force | |
| 35. | Feast | | 80. | Forget | |
| 36. | Feet, Feat | Peet, Peat | 81. | Fork | Pork |
| 37. | Feather | | 82. | Forest | |
| 38. | Fee | Pea | 83. | Found | Pound |
| 39. | Feed | | 84. | Fox | Pox |
| 40. | Feel | Peel | 85. | Fuel | |
| 41. | Fellow | | 86. | Full | Pull |
| 42. | Felt | Pelt | 87. | Fun | Pun |
| 43. | Female | | 88. | Furniture | |
| 44. | Fence | | 89. | Future | |
| 45. | Fell | | 90. | Phone | Pone |

speech-language clinicians often recommend that it is advantageous for children with articulation errors to be enrolled in preschool.

The remedial approach considered here takes into account the premises presented above with regard to the relationship between articulation errors and communicative intent. We recommend this approach for children during the formative years of speech development, 3 to 6 years of age, when a consistent pattern of misarticulation is observed. As we will see, this approach involves systematic presentation of instances of semantic conflict as a way to indicate to children that they have not communicated properly. Care must be exercised when using this approach because it may represent an abrupt change in the way listeners react to the child's speech. Also, this approach should be practiced by as many individuals as possible in the child's environment, so that a high degree of response consistency is achieved.

## A SEMANTIC CONFLICT APPROACH

The beginning point for this approach, like other approaches, is to test thoroughly the child's articulation pattern. Here, the speech clinician may make use of any articulation testing form which provides a clear profile of phonetic errors by word position. Next, a single phonetic element is chosen for remedial work based on the following factors: 1) the sound exhibits a significant influence on the child's intelligibility; and 2) the sound is consistently misarticulated. Typically, initial-word position substitutions are targeted for treatment first. Beyond these considerations, the rationale for the selection of the training sound is not a major factor in this approach.

As the next step, the clinician should develop a list of words used by the child in which the training sound appears. At this point, the clinician should become familiar with as many words as possible used by the child in which the training sound occurs. For example, if the child substitutes p/f in the initial position, the clinician should record all /f/-initial words used by the child.

From this list of words, the clinician will choose one or more subsets of 6 to 10 words, each based upon the following criteria: 1) they are easily picturable; and 2) they occur relatively often in the child's daily conversational speech. A group of 6 to 10 words is convenient for remedial training, but the number may be larger or smaller if desired.

Next, two pictures are selected or drawn to represent each of the /f/ words chosen for remedial training. One of the two pictures will represent the intended word *farm*, and the other, the unintended misarticulated word, *parm*. For the intended word, *farm*, a picture of a farm is used; for the unintended misarticulated word, *parm*, a nonsense picture is drawn. These pairs of pictures are chosen for each of the training words selected.

For example, if *farm, fan, finger,* and *food* are among the /f/-initial training words chosen, a nonsense drawing is made for each of the three non-English words which results when /p/ is substituted for /f/ in addition to the picture for each intended word. Nonsense drawings would be made for *parm, pinger,* and *pood* in addition to the pictures for the intended words, *farm, finger,* and *food*. The /p-f/ substitution for *fan* produces an actual English word, *pan*; therefore a picture of a pan would be used among the nonsense drawings, and a picture of a fan among the intended words.

In this manner, the clinician chooses two sets of pictures: one set portrays the words which the child intends (e.g., *farm, fan, finger,* and *food*); the other set portrays the p/f substitution word equivalents (e.g., *parm, pan, pinger,* and *pood*). Care must be exercised by the clinician to be sure the nonsense drawings are used to represent only the same misarticulated word. For example, the nonsense drawing for *parm* must be used only with the appearance of this utterance and not with any other utterance. The drawings must not be mixed up because semantic conflict is the basis for this remedial approach.

The central goal is to establish separate semantic identities for each intended word and its corresponding unintended utterance. The clinician chooses several words and their corresponding picture pairs and then names each pair for the child: "Here is a *farm* and here is a *parm*"; "Here is a *finger* and here is a *pinger*"; etc. "Now, you name them and I will point to them as you name them." A variation is to reverse roles and have the child name and point to each pair or for the child to point to the pictures as the clinician names each of them. Also, the clinician can tape record each item in random order and present the recording to the child for correct identification of each picture. Similarly, the child's pronunciation of each item may be tape recorded for later presentation in which the child identifies the pictures from his or her own speech. This approach may be adapted easily for use with small groups because no special combination of children grouped by type of articulatory error is necessary.

The semantic conflict approach advocated here promotes awareness on the part of the child between the pronunciation of the intended picture (e.g., *farm*) and the alternative picture (e.g., *parm*). This approach is not to be regarded as a replacement for the traditional procedures of phonetic placement and discrimination. Instead, it is one way to help a child realize that an articulatory error is being committed. The clinician should develop this approach in the spirit of a positive, helpful attitude and stand ready to assist children as they try to understand the confusion between alternate word pairs. This approach is viewed as a strong motivator toward articulatory improvement.

The semantic conflict approach is founded on the principle that the basic unit for remediation in misarticulation training is the word. Fractionalizing approaches that dissect words into sound units for remediation are often exceedingly abstract to children, especially young children, and may not be clearly understood. These procedures should be used also by parents and other family members. It is important for children to gain a sense of awareness about their error patterns from their parents or others in addition to the speech clinician to bring about a change in articulatory patterns.

## REFERENCES

Nelson, K. 1973. Structure and strategy in learning to talk Monogr. Soc. Res. Child Devel. 38:1–2.

CHAPTER 11

# Expanding the Clinic Cubicle Through the Use of Media

*Susan J. Shanks*

*In this chapter, Shanks provides guidelines and procedures for the use of media to teach carryover skills to children with articulation errors. Her techniques are illustrated with the presentation of several case studies.*

1. *Carryover traditionally has been relegated to the terminal state of articulation training. Shanks presents a different position. What is her position?*
2. *Describe the several potential advantages that the use of media has in creating an environment for the social development of articulation.*
3. *Summarize some of the technical procedures that are used when children work with media for the purpose of acquiring carryover skills. Can you think of additional procedures or techniques you might want to try?*
4. *What are some general guidelines for media planning?*

CONTRIBUTORS TO *For Clinicians by Clinicians* address significant issues in the intervention process with positive changes in articulation and language as a universal goal. The numerous and varied management procedures in use are represented in this work, which is typical of most texts presenting more than one mode of intervention. The titles of the chapters emphasize concern for all age groups and diversified etiologies.

## CARRYOVER

Each contributor, a speech-language pathologist, has as his or her final goal, whether describing how to remediate misarticulations or build language form and content, the use or carryover of new communication skills in all environments. All speech-language clinicians consider carryover or habituation as an important component in their treatment hierarchy. Unfortunately, the carryover of newly learned sounds and symbols has often been viewed as a final step in the intervention process. An exception to this trend is seen when a pragmatic approach to intervention is emphasized. *Pragmatics* as used by the speech-language pathologist refers to the interactive functions of language in context including the use of language and the reasons why people speak. The pragmatics movement of the mid-1970s has stimulated important questions about the utilization of highly structured intervention sessions (Prutting, 1979).

Clinicians who adhere to a highly structured format usually do so because they are planning their sessions in conformance with behavior modification principles. The use of target sounds and sentences that are presented as stimuli or models to be imitated is usually a final step in the behavior modification treatment structure.

Early integration of newly learned communication segments into conversation is the core of the pragmatic thrust. The use of media as a method of strengthening this carryover process is the focus of this chapter. The approach will be of special interest to those persons who, like myself, have through necessity had to supervise students in a clinic cubicle and have searched for ways to expand its four walls.

### Carryover in the Treatment Hierarchy

During the preparation of this chapter, I began to review the evolution of our profession to determine what has kept us in the clinic cubicle and why carryover now is viewed often as a separate and final stage of the learning process in many treatment programs. The early clinicians who were mainly from schools of psychology did not delineate separate carryover procedures. To them, the goal of teaching was to improve interpersonal communication in the clinic. In an early text, Backus and Beasley (1951), pioneers in group communication-oriented speech and language training, presented this viewpoint. They strongly recommended that the incidental learning of sounds, sentences, and other linguistic units should be integrated into social interactions. In this way, they believed, the focus of training was on the whole child rather than on parts of communication.

As professionals in our field began to emulate other sciences, they formulated a part-to-whole approach to treatment. Soon analytical methodology in the remediation of speech and language problems became the mode. Young and Hawk (1938), who were instrumental in the development of a physical approach to intervention, formulated a motokinesthetic method to teach the production of individual speech sounds. Their target population had neurogenic speech disorders, and, therefore, they did not expect carryover until very late in the treatment process.

As we became recognized more and more for our value in helping people communicate, the pendulum swung more and more toward highly structured methodologies carried out within the clinic cubicle. Social interaction was not emphasized until late in the training sequence when carryover techniques were introduced.

In 1966, Engel and his associates became concerned about the lack of carryover that resulted from speech and language training. They offered suggestions on how to help children use their newly learned speech outside of the clinic cubicle. Many articulation texts refer to Engel et al. (1966) as a source of carryover ideas. Some authors dedicate a chapter of their book to this component of training (Bosley, 1981; Winitz, 1975). Others include recommendations for carryover in a chapter on management approaches. The terms *carryover, transfer, generalization, habituation,* and *maintenance* are used interchangeably in many texts and articles to describe the incorporation of newly learned behaviors during communication outside of the clinic (Bernthal and Bankson, 1981; Weiss et al., 1980). Weiss et al. (1980) differentiate transfer or generalization from maintenance or habituation, but they state that the stages often overlap. In this chapter, all of these terms refer to the carryover process.

Clinicians strive for carryover in different ways. In some instances, prescribed, structured clinical procedures are performed by parents, caregivers, and peers, first in the clinic, and then in other settings, such as at home or at school (Schiefelbusch, 1978). Essentially, this approach entails moving the cubicle to another site. Other clinicians encourage the use of sounds and language units in conversation during treatment. Later, these same elements are practiced in running speech with a variety of individuals in other settings (Gerber, 1973; Guess et al., 1978).

Many clinicians speculate that behavior modification as a method of treatment has been a key factor in keeping clinicians from using early carryover activities. Recognizing this fact, Gray and Ryan (1973), at the beginning of each behavior modification training session, used a show and tell period as a form of carryover. I observed their program in 1971 and 1972 and noted that the carryover activity was so structured that there was little similarity between their programmed carryover training and the interpersonal communication that takes place in the home.

The above review has provided a reference for my three-fold bias regarding carryover: 1) carryover should be incorporated early in training for articulation and language disorders; 2) the child should use new verbal units in simulated "natural" communication situations in the clinic; and 3) significant others who care for the child should be told about the problems in and benefits of obtaining early carryover.

## INCORPORATION OF MEDIA IN CLINICAL PLANNING

Two students whom I supervised in clinic practicum searched for media in order to incorporate this three-fold approach of mine into a workable carryover plan. Professor Karen Jensen and her students in the California State University, Fresno, Education of the Deaf training program who were learning to use media with deaf children provided the incentive for this thrust.

Media is defined by Webster (1959) as "that through which anything is conveyed or carried on, an intermediate means or channel . . ." (p. 1528). Educators of the deaf use media to integrate natural communication into the classroom learning experience. They use overhead transparencies, filmstrips, 35mm slides, and 8mm movies or videotapes made of the children on field trips. Their use of materials is limited only by their imagination and money. Although media presentations may be costly, there are ways to obtain media materials if the worth of their use can be demonstrated.

During previous semesters, my student clinicians used language masters, tape recorders, and the usual assortments of puppets, sequencing cards, and kits found in the speech-language clinic. The clinicians next began to study the materials found in our media center (Anna Michelson Memorial Instructional Media Center for the Deaf) for methods to encourage carryover. According to Kemp (1968), the first step in planning a media presentation is to search the closets of the audiovisual materials center for anything that would hold the child's attention. One group of transparencies produced by Robert Newby[1] met this criterion. Questions asked about these transparencies were: How can they be used to teach carryover of target sounds? Can the words illustrated by the transparencies be incorporated into a natural conversation? Can objectives be prepared that include peers and parents in the use of the transparencies in carryover activities?

Clinician 1 found multimedia fascinating and decided to use several media to incorporate teaching machine concepts (Holland and Mathews, 1968) into her treatment with an unintelligible, uncontrollable child. My clinical impressions of her success are found in Case Study 1, which follows.

Clinician 2, a novice, decided to employ transparencies in her work with two children. One child had been extremely negative in treatment the previous semester and the other, although easily motivated, did not initiate any communication in the cubicle. Case studies 2 and 3 describe the way Clinician 2 developed her media sessions.

## MEDIA IN SPEECH-LANGUAGE PATHOLOGY

Before turning to the case studies, the reader should know that we did not consider ourselves pioneers in the use of media for speech and language training (Bangs, 1968; Withrow and Nygren, 1976). Media have been used successfully in aphasia treatment by Wepman and Morency (1963), who described how film strips stimulated adults with aphasia to talk more, and by Keenan (1975), who utilized media to develop treatment programs for brain-damaged patients.

## PREPLANNING

Several aspects of the treatment program became apparent as the student clinicians began to plan their use of media for carryover activities. Their role as interventionist changed from primary sender of communication to include receiving messages. Traditionally, the clinician has initiated most communicative interchange by modeling or asking questions. Media are useful in reversing this role. The clinicians found the child became the leader in communicating ideas. Presentation of media enabled the child to view and hear the stimuli before communication began. Familiarity with the topic to be discussed encouraged the child to assume the role of sender more easily. The students also discovered that characteristically treatment had been restricted to the

[1]Newby Visualanguage, Inc., Box 121, Eagleville, PA 19408.

here and now of the clinic cubicle. They, like many clinicians, lacked knowledge of the children's past, present, and future experiences, which is necessary in structuring natural communicative interaction.

How could they use media to obtain information about the child's experiences that would enable them to interact naturally with each child? Words and/or topics had to be selected with full understanding of the child's background if they were to have communicative value (Holland, 1975). To structure realistic interactions, ideally, parents or others who know the child's background and environment should be involved in the planning stages (Guess et al., 1978). These persons can provide information about topics that are of interest to the child.

It is not always possible to include parents or caretakers in planning. Most speech-language pathologists work in public school settings where persons who care for the child are seldom seen more than twice each year. Fortunately, we have the opportunity to confer with parents of children attending our clinic. The parents of the children described below participated in frequent short conferences about our treatment/management program.

## CASE STUDIES

All data that could identify the student clinicians and the children described below have been eliminated to protect their privacy. The ideas generated by the students were important to me in my growth as a supervisor. I am grateful for the information I gained during my experiences with them as we explored the impact of media on carryover.

### Case Study 1

$Child_1$ ($C_1$), a 5-year-old male who had received treatment for several semesters exhibited the typical behaviors associated with brain injury and autism during our first language training sessions. He crawled on the cubicle floor, manipulated the drapes, banged on the tape recorder, grunted and hummed, did not respond to the clinician's attempts at communication, seldom made eye contact, and licked the floor.

The clinician evaluated this last behavior as a demonstration of the child's desire to make oral contact with his environment. A tasting activity was developed with candies to gain the child's attention. Initially, each piece of candy was chosen for use if $C_1$ could name its flavor. Others were added as the activity was developed further. Intelligibility of the candy's name was not a critical element at first. To structure the child's attention, the candies were placed in cups and an "eyes closed" behavior was necessary before a piece was placed on his lips for tasting. A set-to-attend was established quickly through this procedure which was performed while standing. A short phrase which included the name of the flavor was verbalized by the clinician and soon was imitated by $C_1$. His speech, although largely unintelligible, seemed to contain sentence elements. At times he appeared to say, "This is lemon candy."

$C_1$'s constant movement and distractability began to decline as his interest in the above activity increased. Other positive changes in behavior were noted when the clinician began to use a soft, well-modulated, soothing voice during the session. This boy displayed a general tactile defensiveness which was seen in his refusal to be touched and his immediate retraction when he came into contact with objects. Noise also acted as a stimulus to produce negative behaviors. This defensiveness diminished as more candy flavors were introduced and described. Finally, the child was able to sit at a table long enough to look at a picture.

The clinician decided that this was the appropriate time to introduce her media approach. Multimedia were chosen to facilitate carryover of the intelligible phrases the child was developing. The student asked $C_1$ if he had ever gone to a movie (fortunately he had) and told him that they were going to make a movie in the clinic. She explained her method of "movie making" to him. First, they would write a script, and then they would record it, line by line, on language master cards to play later as they showed pictures. A series of colored sequence cards was introduced as the subject materials for the movie. Movie making began.

$C_1$ made up a sentence describing each card, and the clinician "wrote" it down. Each word was represented by slots. For example, in one "movie," entitled the "Cutting Grass Movie," the phrase "Daddy is pushing the mower" was represented by _____
____ _____ ____ _____ . The slots were touched by the child as he said the words. He then recorded these verbalizations on language master cards and listened to determine whether the sentence was clear enough for the movie sound track. At first, each picture had to be viewed separately as the child could not sequence a series of two events. The goal was to use at least two sequenced cards for a movie.

After two or more cards were recorded, the child had the responsibility of playing them on the language master as the clinician displayed the appropriate sequence card with an opaque projector. The clinic cubicle was darkened during this final step. Making movies encouraged much conversation which soon became understandable. Incidental modeling of correct articulation was interspersed whenever possible. The words used were of value to the child (Holland, 1975; Bloom and Lahey, 1978).

Increased communication in the home was reported by the mother, who wanted to know more about the movies which the child was talking about all of the time. The parents were encouraged by the increasing amount of speech the child initiated in the car traveling to and from the clinic. During the movie making process, the child gradually agreed to re-record difficult to understand phrases which he previously would have accepted as intelligible. Respect for materials was evident. He no longer banged on the tape recorder or threw the sequence cards on the floor. Correction of syntax was incorporated into treatment as content became more clear. The parents observed the child in the clinic, but home assignments did not seem appropriate during this semester.

The changes in the child's impulsive behavior, in his attention span, in his attitude toward the clinician, and in his articulation and language were extremely positive and exciting. He seemed concerned when the clinician expressed her feelings about his actions during his uncooperative periods. The clinician decided this concern demonstrated a readiness for more social interaction. Other clinicians were invited to visit during the language sessions, and the child explained the movie making process to them. Later, a young girl of his age was brought in to learn how to run the machines in order to make movies. $C_1$ demonstrated the media, and they decided to make a movie together. He corrected her when she did not use the machines in sequence or made other errors in the process. The social interaction and sharing were positive indications of progress.

Another incident also reflected $C_1$'s growth in socialization. One day, when the child had been working without interruption for a long period, the clinician said she needed a drink of water and asked if he wanted one. The boy said he was not thirsty, but he would go to the fountain with her so that she would not have to go alone. This interaction and numerous other verbalizations demonstrated this child's entrance into the world of natural communication. The roles of sender and receiver were being used interchangeably in the session. He carried these communication skills into his home and continued to make progress.

## Case Study 2

In contrast to $Child_1$, $Child_2$ ($C_2$), a 6-year-old female in the first grade, was a cooperative client. Her performance in school was beyond grade level. Her /l/ and /r/ misarticulations and occasional misuse of articles and verb tenses were not serious enough to influence intelligibility. For some reason, however, she avoided communicating. Her response to questioning was usually "I don't know," and she seldom initiated conversation in the clinic.

The clinician's initial goal was to encourage free verbal interchange. Transparencies (Newby) containing /l/ words were chosen as media. They were shown on an overhead projector by the clinician, who made up a sentence with each word. Then the sentences were woven into a story. This activity was short, but long enough to catch $C_2$'s attention and interest.

Transparencies were brought to the next session, and the child was asked to select some to show and describe following the clinician's pattern. $C_2$ attempted to use several transparencies in sequence in order to make up a story. This task turned out to be difficult, as relationships between the /l/ words were not sufficiently obvious to her. Her initial verbalizations were uncorrelated sentences, but gradually she learned to make thematic presentations. With help from the clinician, the child was successful in incorporating many key /l/ words into her stories. This media process was followed each day until a corpus of correctly articulated /l/ and /r/ words was collected. Although this activity took place early in the training sequence, carryover of these words was noted by the clinician.

At this point, the mother, who seldom observed her child in the clinic, was invited to watch her daughter go through a series of transparencies and weave the words into a story. The child talked freely and seemed very pleased with the praise she received from her mother for her success.

The next step was to involve the family in the media approach in order to facilitate carryover in the home. Clear pieces of 8" × 11" used X-ray film (another option would be clear acetate sheets available in educational supply centers) were given to the child to take home to draw her own pictures of sequences. The mother was instructed to encourage her to draw by talking with her about experiences they were to represent. In this way, the whole family became involved in the media activity and learned through the take-home assignment what was happening in treatment.

The mother reported an increase in correct sound production at home. She was pleased when her daughter began to play "speech school" with her young brother who also drew pictures on the X-ray film for our clinic sessions. Key words acquired in the clinic were used at home. Additionally, the child's willingness to continue working at home demonstrated to us that she had positive feelings about the media approach.

**Case Study 3**

Transparencies were also used to encourage carryover of /l/ for Child$_3$ (C$_3$), a 6-year-old, first grade male. This child had received speech instruction during the previous summer. When the child arrived for his first speech session, he presented the attitude: "I dare you to make me work." He seldom smiled or initiated a positive comment during the first few sessions. According to his mother, he did not wish to return to the clinic.

The progress report of the previous summer indicated that C$_3$ stuttered and that attention was centered on the correction of his /l/ and /r/ misarticulations. An auditory discrimination approach had not been successful in remediating /r/. Because C$_3$ was unable to discriminate between /r/ and distortions of this phoneme, the language master was introduced as an appropriate medium to identify correct and incorrect [r, ɝ, ɚ] productions. His response to the machine was catastrophic. We later learned that he had previously rejected this media procedure.

To offset this negative reaction, the clinician decided to use the media approach that she was using successfully with C$_2$. Because C$_3$ could produce /l/ in a few words, the clinician introduced transparencies in an effort to generalize these few correct instances of /l/ to short phrases and sentences. The child monitored and recorded his correct and incorrect /l/ productions on a chart as he attempted to articulate the /l/ words in longer utterances. He began to accept his failures as normal occurrences during this self-evaluative process.

C$_3$'s attempts to sequence stories using the /l/ words were like those of C$_2$. His stories were not logical, not sequenced properly, and often contained repetitious structures. As the percentage of correct sound productions increased, however, a similar increment was noted in spontaneous speech.

Stuttering behaviors began to disappear as confidence in talking during the carryover procedures became evident. The child laughed and communicated more naturally as sender and receiver in his communications with the clinician and with me. His stories became humorous and often absurd; they were typical of a happy 6-year-old. C$_3$ had finally joined in the game of language (Muma, 1978).

Most importantly, C$_3$ came to the clinic willingly and cooperated during the entire session. The transparency presentations were interesting descriptions of soccer games and other important events in the life of his family. He, like C$_2$, manipulated the overhead projector and was in charge of the carryover session. All of the pragmatic behaviors noted in the literature were incorporated into treatment. In addition, parental involvement increased. We learned that the child's request for a tape recorder to practice his speech at home would be granted at Christmas. His success and his positive reaction to and interest in the media were indications to us that the media process had produced many attitude changes which are difficult to document. His desire to use a tape recorder for home practice after violently rejecting the language master in the clinic was a positive change. We believe media had made the difference.

## ADVANTAGES OF USING MEDIA IN ARTICULATION AND LANGUAGE TRAINING

The children described above benefited from the media carryover activities. Without encouragement at home, however, it might not have been possible for them to have made such rapid gains in carryover of communication patterns and to feel successful about their communication efforts. Kazdin (1980) in his exceptionally readable text on behavior modification stated that future behaviors were most likely to occur if the person were in a situation similar to the one in which a behavior is learned. His theory was supported by our results. As $C_2$ and $C_3$ began to discuss daily activities at home in preparation for their training sessions, their successful communications increased in both places. They also began to monitor their errors as evidenced by the appearance of self-corrections of previously misarticulated sounds and the use of more advanced language form and content.

The opaque and overhead projectors presented a challenge to the children who easily learned the simple adjustments that are required for focusing the machines. The projectors served to motivate the children to work cooperatively with the clinician in the media activity. Also, inclusion of the other clinicians and children helped to expand the cubicle and to offset the problems of generalization that arise when only one interventionist works with a child (Siegel and Spradlin, 1978; Guess et al., 1978).

The media approach enabled the children to involve themselves in the learning process, to explore feelings, to get and give information, and to learn turn taking and other language strategies. Repetition of target behaviors was possible in varied contexts by using different media to illustrate the same theme. These repetitions presented old forms and content in new ways and new forms and content in old ways. The media provided stimuli for meaningful communication, an essential feature which should be sought in natural language training (MacDonald, 1976). They also created a bridge to the natural setting (Hart and Warren, 1978).

The following advantages of media are also worth mentioning. Learning can be enhanced when visual and acoustic input are presented simultaneously. Also with media, input can be varied in complexity, which according to Winitz (1981) is more natural than "linear" language processing which he describes as orderly, prescribed, straight-line language learning based upon developmental sequencing. We noted that the children integrated new and more advanced language into their conversations at home during the preparation of the transparencies even though these language forms were not directly taught according to a prescribed sequence. Nonlinear processing occurred because information from several levels of language complexity were integrated from an input which was rich and varied, yet meaningful, and within the child's ability to understand.

Cultural experiences and values, essential elements to consider in home intervention (Hubbell, 1981), can be shared if children and their caregivers prepare media to illustrate important holidays and cultural events. Children who are deprived of family sharing might also benefit from taking part in producing puppet shows which focus on family life and cultural activities. With this kind of emphasis, the clinician should no longer feel inhibited because of lack of knowledge about the child's life. Children who prepare media to express their needs, interests, and desires also have a reason to talk. The words they use match their cognitive level; thus, the stimuli will be more appropriate than those chosen by the clinician. Experimentation with learning styles is also possible as one tries different media. Children can perform actions to portray characters introduced through media, and they can change their responses or descriptions of a drawing, slide presentation, or movie sequence several times without tiring of the subject. Even TV, which is considered to be a passive teacher, is adaptable to an action format. Time moves quickly during action-packed media sessions. The child and clinician leave looking forward to the next session.

## GUIDELINES FOR MEDIA PLANNING

Chalfant and Foster (1976) present several guidelines that are helpful to the speech-language pathologist planning to develop media for carryover. They are adapted below:

1. State your objectives in terms of what the child must do for the media presentation to be considered successful.
2. Specify the attentional, motor, and/or vocal responses that the media are intended to elicit.

3.  Identify the psychological processing demands, such as memory, discrimination, formulation of concepts, and problem solving, that the media make on the child.
4.  Decide which topics should be broken down into smaller units and how these units can be further subdivided into smaller steps.

Speech-language pathologists who have not used media will find a book by Kemp (1968) to be an excellent source. Kemp offers instruction in media, crossmedia, and multimedia techniques. Also, local settings have media specialists who can be of assistance. For more information on the use of media the reader can contact the National Center on Education Media and Materials for the Handicapped, Special Education Instructional Materials Center in his/her area, Regional Media Centers for the Deaf, and Area Learning Resource Centers (Kemp, 1968).

## SUMMARY

This chapter presents an overview on the use of media as a method to expand the clinic cubicle to teach carryover of newly acquired speech and language skills. Media can bring the outside world into the clinic. Three children with varying degrees of speech and language problems made excellent progress when their clinicians utilized media consistently early in the carryover process.

## REFERENCES

Backus, O. L., and Beasley, J. 1951. Speech Therapy with Children. Houghton Mifflin, Boston.

Bangs, T. E. 1968. Language and Learning Disorders of the Pre-Academic Child. Appleton-Century-Crofts, New York.

Bernthal, J. E., and Bankson, N. 1981. Articulation Disorders. Prentice-Hall, Englewood Cliffs, NJ.

Bloom, L., and Lahey, M. 1978. Language Development and Language Disorders. John Wiley and Sons, New York.

Bosley, E. C. 1981. Techniques for Articulatory Disorders, Chapter 17. Charles C Thomas Publisher, Springfield, IL.

Chalfant, J. C., and Foster, G. E. 1976. Learners Needs. In: F. B. Withrow and C. J. Nygren (eds.), Language, Materials and Curriculum Management for the Handicapped Learner. Charles E Merrill Pub. Co., Columbus, OH.

Engel, D., Brandriet, S. E., Erickson, K. M., et al. 1966. Carryover. J. Speech Hear. Disord. 31:227–233. (1966).

Gerber, A. 1973. Goal: Carryover. Temple University Press, Philadelphia, PA.

Gray, B. B., and Ryan, B. P. 1973. A Language Program for the Nonlanguage Child. Research Press, Champaign, IL.

Guess, D., Sailor, W., and Baer, D. M. 1978. Children with limited language. In: Richard L. Schiefelbusch (ed.), Language Intervention Strategies, Vol. II. University Park Press, Baltimore.

Hart, B., and Warren, A. 1978. A mileau approach to teaching language. In: Richard L. Schiefelbusch (ed.), Language Intervention Strategies, Vol. II. University Park Press, Baltimore.

Holland, A. L. 1975. Language therapy for children: Some thoughts on context and content. J. Speech Hear. Disord. 40:514–523.

Holland, A. L., and Matthews, J. 1968. Application of teaching machine concepts to speech pathology and audiology. In: H. Sloane, and B. MacAulay (eds.), Operant Procedures in Remedial Speech and Language Training. Houghton Mifflin, Boston.

Hubbell, R. D. 1981. Children's Language Disorders, Prentice-Hall, Englewood Cliffs, NJ.

Kazdin, A. E. 1980. Behavior Modification in Applied Settings, Revised Ed. The Dorsey Press, Homewood, IL.

Keenan, J. S. 1975. A Procedure Manual in Speech Pathology with Brain-Damaged Adults. The Interstate Printers and Publishers, Danville, IL.

Kemp, J. E. 1968. Planning and Producing Audiovisual Materials, 2nd Ed. Chandler Publishing Co., Scranton, PA.

MacDonald, J. D. 1976. Environmental language intervention. In: F. B. Withrow and C. J. Nygren (eds.), Language Materials and Curriculum Management for the Handicapped Learner. Charles E. Merrill Pub. Co., Columbus, OH.

Muma, J. R. 1978. Language Handbook: Concepts, Assessment, Intervention. Prentice-Hall, Englewood Cliffs, NJ.

Prutting, C. A. 1979. Process: The action of moving forward progressively from one point to another on the way to completion. J. Speech Hear. Disord. 44:3–30.

Schiefelbusch, R. L. (ed.). 1978. Language Intervention Strategies, Vol. II. University Park Press, Baltimore.

Siegel, G. M., and Spradlin, J. E. 1978. Programming for language and communication therapy. In: Richard L. Schiefelbusch (ed.), Language Intervention Strategies, Vol. II. University Park Press, Baltimore.

Webster's New International Dictionary. 1959. 2nd Ed. Riverside Press, Cambridge, MA.

Weiss, C. E., Lillywhite, H. S., and Gordon, M. E. 1980. Clinical Management of Articulation Disorders. C. V. Mosby Co., St. Louis, MO.

Wepman, J. M., and Morency, A. 1963. Filmstrips in aphasia therapy. J. Speech Hear. Disord. 28:191–194.

Winitz, H. 1975. From Syllable to Conversation. University Park Press, Baltimore.

Winitz, H. 1981. Nonlinear learning and language teaching. In: H. Winitz (ed), The Comprehension Approach to Foreign Language Instruction. Newbury House, Rowley, MA.

Withrow, F. B., and Nygren, C. J. (eds). 1976. Language Materials and Curriculum Management for the Handicapped Learner. Charles E. Merrill Publishing Co., Columbus, OH.

Young, E. H., and Hawk, S. S. 1938. Motokinesthetic Speech Training. Stanford University Press, Stanford, CA.

## CHAPTER 12

# Effective Use of Parents and Others in Articulation Treatment

*Barbara Hartmann*

*Carryover is a difficult and troublesome area in articulation teaching. Hartmann reviews research on carryover and provides lesson plans and some important suggestions to improve carryover.*

1. *Hartmann indicates that parents and paraprofessionals should be used to improve effectiveness in teaching carryover. What reasons does she provide, and do you agree with these?*
2. *What are the essential characteristics of Hartmann's lesson plans for teaching carryover? What procedures, in particular, would seem to improve carryover? At what point in articulation training should this program be implemented? Do you think paraprofessionals can carry out these tasks?*
3. *What guidelines does Hartmann indicate should be provided to parents and paraprofessionals for them to be effective trainers?*

In 1969, WHEN 169 CLINICIANS WERE ASKED by Sommers to list their most serious clinical problem, 77% of them stated, "carryover." Recently, in an in-state workshop I asked 30 school speech-language clinicians the same question. The unanimous answer was again "carryover."

Because of time restrictions, few clinicians have time to work on carryover to assure that newly learned skills transfer to settings other than the clinical setting. A solution I recommend is the use of supportive personnel or paraprofessional aides as the primary teachers of children in the large disorder group of articulation problems.

In this chapter, I discuss why paraprofessionals should be used, who can serve as a paraprofessional, and how to train and use paraprofessionals most effectively and efficiently. I describe and report the results of a 2-year parent/paraprofessional administered articulation program developed at the University of Utah.

## Why Use the Parent/Paraprofessional Alternative?

1. *The administrator's reasons* Parents and other paraprofessionals can provide effective service at reduced cost. With their help, the number of children that can be serviced can be increased. In a 10-year study of 7000 children Barker (1981) found that the use of trained paraprofessionals in the public schools reduced by about 50% the cost of remediation per child, and a corresponding reduction in the clinician's case load.
2. *The clinician's reasons* The use of paraprofessionals enables clinicians to service additional children, and spend more time with children they are treating. At the University of Utah Speech-Language-Hearing Clinic, preschool children acquired a phoneme in spontaneous conversational usage at home and in the clinic in a mean of 5½ weeks. On the average, 3 hours of clinician time and 12 hours of parent/paraprofessional time were involved. Barker (1981) also found that it took an average of 3.3 hours of clinician time for school-age children to master a phoneme to the level of conversational speech when parents provided help at home. Most importantly, the persistent problem of poor carryover can be dealt with effectively when paraprofessionals conduct lessons in the clinic, in the child's home, and in other environments.
3. *The parent's reasons* Parents are pleased when the number of visits to the speech-language clinic is reduced because transportation costs and professional fees also are reduced. Furthermore, parents who serve as paraprofessionals show reduced frustration with their child's problem, according to Baker (1976).

Baker (1976) notes that parents' roles have changed over the years. Parents were originally considered objects of study, providers of information, and patients to be treated as part of the articulation problem. Later, parents became spectators, and recently, advocates for improved services for their children, volunteers in treatment settings, and paraprofessional teachers of their own children.

Parents are asked frequently to be carryover agents, but otherwise are not usually involved. My recommendation is that parents be considered *co*-teachers and responsible for their childs' improvement under the direction of the speech-language pathologist. Parents who actively participate in their children's treatment feel worthwhile and important as contributors to the solution of their child's problems.

4. *The child's reasons*   Children are pleased when more people become involved and more time is spent to improve their communication problem. Children seem delighted to have additional private and positive contact with a parent or favorite sibling.

5. *The author's reasons*   My experience with parents and other paraprofessionals who have worked with children's articulation problems helped convince my colleagues and me that paraprofessionals can be the primary teachers in articulation treatment. We know that parents and other paraprofessionals are effective as the primary teachers of children with behavior problems (Graziano, 1977; Johnson and Katz, 1973; Odell, 1974). Of seventeen studies from the speech pathology literature with parent/paraprofessional administered articulation remediation programs, only two failed to show significantly positive results from treatment provided by paraprofessionals (McCroskey and Baird, 1971; Shea, 1955). These studies are summarized in Table 1.

As we developed the University of Utah program, we carefully considered the procedural differences between the successful and the two unsuccessful programs. A program developed by Fahey (1976) was used as a model for the development of our program. The Fahey program consisted of nine structured lessons which parents administered to their children twice each day. Twenty-two of the 25 children in the study successfully completed the program and maintained 90% or better correct conversational usage of their target phoneme 6 weeks after the program's completion.

**A Specific Parent/Paraprofessional Administered Articulation Program**

The University of Utah's Home-Based Articulation Program is summarized in Table 2. The first University of Utah study was done with

Table 1. Empirical studies from speech-language literature concerned with parent/paraprofessional administered articulation programs

| Author | Location | Grouping | Population | Paraprofessionals | Initial training | Contact after initial training | Results |
|---|---|---|---|---|---|---|---|
| Sommers et al. (1959) | Clinic and home | 1. 36 children seen by clinician and trained parents<br>2. 36 children seen just by clinician | School age functional articulation, 60% substitutional errors; 5;8, and 5;5 mean ages of 2 groups | Parents | 30 min lecture 30 min observation daily plus clinician contacts | 4 days a week for 3½ weeks | Significantly more improvement in group involving parents |
| Tufts and Holliday (1959) | Preschool | 1. 10 parent trained<br>2. 10 clinician trained<br>3. 10 control no treatment | Preschool with articulation problems: 4–6 years | Parents | 30 min training in articulation problems and remediation techniques, plus 30 min group discussion | 1 hr weekly for 7 months | No difference between group 1 and 2 but significantly improved over third |

| Sommers (1962) | Clinic | 1. 10 mentally retarded, group treatment with help<br>2. 10 mentally retarded, group treatment no parents help<br>3. 10 mentally retarded, individual treatment with parent help<br>4. 10 mentally retarded, individual treatment, no parent help<br>5. Same groupings with 40 normals | 70–90 IQ = mentally retarded<br>90–115 IQ = normals 7- and 8-year old | Parents | 45 min | 45 min a day for 4 weeks | Significantly greater progress with groups when mothers were involved |
|---|---|---|---|---|---|---|---|
| Sommers (1969) | Clinic | 1. 20 children with trained mothers in top 35% of attitude scale<br>2. 20 with trained mothers in bottom 35%<br>3. 20 with untrained mothers top 35%<br>4. 20 with untrained mother bottom 35% | Children with articulation problems 7–10 years | Mothers | 15 min lectures<br>15 min discussion<br>15 min observing | 1 hr daily 4 days a week for 50 min concurrent with treatment of children for 4 weeks | Top 35% mothers' children significantly improved over bottom 35% mothers. All children of trained mothers, significantly improved over untrained mothers' children |

(*Continued*)

Table 1. (*Continued*)

| Author | Location | Grouping | Population | Paraprofessionals | Initial training | Contact after initial training | Results |
|---|---|---|---|---|---|---|---|
| Carrier (1970) | Home | 1. 10 children's mothers used Carriers structured program<br>2. 10 children's mothers only to correct child's errors as heard | 4–7 years | Mothers | All mothers shown how child should make target sound<br>Trained mothers were given written explanation of 6 lessons | No follow-up training | Significantly more improvement in children of trained mothers. 1½ hours of clinician time per phoneme |
| Evans and Potter (1974) | School | All taught with Mowrer S-Pack (Mowrer et al., 1968):<br>1. 8 taught by speech clinicians<br>2. 8 taught by 6th graders who had been previously treated for speech disorders<br>3. 8 taught by 6th graders who had not been previously treated for speech disorders | Functional frontal lisps 6–9 years | 6th graders | 4 1-hr sessions | 10 min of observation first day of training | No significant difference between groups |

| Study | Setting | Number served | Population | Aides | Initial training | Ongoing training | Results |
|---|---|---|---|---|---|---|---|
| Barker (1981) | School | Approximately 7000 children seen by aides over 10-year period | Grades K to 12 (80% in grades K–6) | Paid aides | 2 days of training | On-job training and supervision | Mean of 23 20-min sessions or 6.1 hr to master a phoneme. 98% or better in conversation at the end of the program and 6 weeks post-program |
|  | Home | 30 children | Grades preschool to 6 | Parents | 1 30-min session | 30-min sessions weekly, for 3 weeks only, for each phoneme | 3.1 hr of clinician time to master phoneme |
| Daum and Fisher (1975) | Public school preschool program | 39 children | Cleft palate children, birth to 6 years | Parents | Series of group sessions | Regular home visits for 1 year | 36 of 38 were within normal limits at end of the year |
| Galloway and Blue (1975) | School | 134 students who otherwise would not have been served | Grades 1–5 | 30 paid aides | 70 hr | 45 hr in-service each year and 2 weeks training in the summer | 134 students corrected total of 206 phonemes with 83.5% correct performance upon post-testing |

*(Continued)*

Table 1. (*Continued*)

| Author | Location | Grouping | Population | Paraprofes-sionals | Initial training | Contact after initial training | Results |
|---|---|---|---|---|---|---|---|
| Scalero and Eskenazi (1976) | Schools and 3 children centers | 125 children completed articulation program | K–6 | 15 paid aides, 6 hr a day; 15 volunteers, 2 hr, 2 days a week | 70 hr (both speech and language preparation) | Inservice training during year | 75% of 125 maintained carryover after 15 weeks; 71% or better at 6 months |
| Fahey (1976) | Clinic waiting list | 25 pairs of a child and parent | /r,s,l,θ/ errors 7–14 years | Parents | 2 hr with training tapes for target phoneme | Weekly 10–15 min clinician checks | 23 pairs of child and parent mastered phonemes and 6 weeks post-program the 90% or better rate maintained |
| Costello and Schoen (1978) | School | Children taught by: 1. 5 paraprofessionals plus Mower S-Pack (1968) on video 2. 5 paraprofessionals plus Mowrer on audio 3. 5 speech clinicians | Elementary school age, /θ, s/ errors | Paid aides | Average of 6.9 hr per paraprofessional Group session first session only | | No significant difference between groups |

| | | | | | | | |
|---|---|---|---|---|---|---|---|
| University Clinic of Utah I (Fahey-Ganz et al., 1981) | 18 child and trainer pairs | 3–8;11 years | Parents, 1 day care worker and 1 older sibling | 40 min training session | Weekly 25-min follow-up sessions | The average was 3 hr, 10 min or 6½ weeks of clinician time to master phoneme to spontaneous conversation | |
| University Clinic of Utah II (Fahey-Ganz et al., 1981) | 16 child and trainer pairs | 3;5–6;8 years | Parents | 1-hr group training session | Weekly, 25-min follow-up sessions | The average was 2⅔ hr clinician time or 5⅓ weeks. Ratio of parent time to clinician time 6:1 | |
| Shea (1955) | Schools | 1. Children whose parents volunteered to help 2. Children whose parents did not help | Functional articulation | Parents | No training | Supplemental home assignments for 16 weeks | No significant difference between groups |

*(Continued)*

183

Table 1. (*Continued*)

| Author | Location | Grouping | Population | Paraprofessionals | Initial training | Contact after initial training | Results |
|---|---|---|---|---|---|---|---|
| McCroskey and Baird (1971) | Schools | Random selection by clinician:<br>1. 20 children whose parents were trained<br>2. 20 children whose parents were untrained | Functional articulation problems 2nd graders | Parents | One hour-long meeting explaining problem and program | 2 follow-up meetings at school or at home; demonstration of program and instruction to help and then follow-up meeting | No significant effect of parental involvement |

Table 2. Summary of lessons—University of Utah Home-Based Articulation Program

| Lesson | Description | Trainer | | Child | Trainer | |
|--------|-------------|---------|---|-------|---------|---|
| 1[a] | 1 word | Imitation | "Say 'comb'" | (Show picture) | "comb" | + Praise and activity |
| 2 | 1 word | Spontaneous | "What's this?" | (Show picture) | "comb" | − Try again |
| 3 | 2 words | Imitation | "Say 'a comb'" | (Show picture) | "a comb" | + Praise and activity |
| 4 | 2 words | Spontaneous | "What's this?" | (Show picture) | "a comb" | − Try again |
| 5 | Repeat carrier phrase | Imitation | "Say 'I have a comb.'" | (Child takes picture card) | "I have a comb." | + Praise and activity |
| 6 | Repeats carrier phrase | Spontaneous | "What do you have?" | (Child takes picture card) | "I have a comb." | − Try again |
| 7 | Child-used sentences | Imitation | "Say 'Do you have a comb?'" | (Show card) | "Do you have a comb?" | + Praise and activity |
| 8 | Child-used sentences | Spontaneous | "What's going on here?" | (Put picture card in a purse, etc.) | "The comb's in your purse." | − Try again |
| 9 | Stories | Repeats trainer's story or tells own story | (The reference is to two to four picture cards which are made to move with small toys such as little doll, car, and doll house furniture.) This girl (doll) is cold (point to "cold" picture). Her mom said, "Where's your coat? Look in the car." So the girl looked. Then she found the coat under the bed." (coat picture under doll house bed). | | The child tells another story or retells the story the adult told. The adult may point to and move around the toys and dolls with the picture cards to help the child recall the story. | Mother counts good responses by raising fingers. She also asks "What happened then?" to keep story going. |

*(Continued)*

185

Table 2. (*Continued*)

| Lesson | Description | Trainer | Child | Trainer |
|---|---|---|---|---|
| 10 Place re-minders | Picture cards taped up in appropriate settings | The adults may need to remind the child to use words as he or she talks. | Words are to be used sponta-neously by the child as part of the activities of the settings. | The adults praise the child when a word is used cor-rectly, and make a small tear in the card. At the end of the week the number of tears in the cards are counted. |
| | | Consider new words for target phoneme or new phoneme | | |
| 11 Activity re-minders | The adult lists all target phoneme words which would be appro-priate to use in an activity often shared with the child. Visual re-minders (perhaps appropriate pic-ture cards taped together) are used. | 1. The trainer uses these words while participating in the activity.<br>2. The adult then reminds and cues the child prior to and during the *real* enactment of the activity to use his words as he talks. | The child sponta-neously uses the words as he goes through the activity. | The trainer praises correct responses and lets the child know the total number as it is re-corded on a data sheet. |

| 12 | Person reminder | The adult, child, and other people wear a special ring, sticker, or sign to remind the child its time to use his or her "new sound." | The adult may need to cue child to use his sound as he talks. | The child spontaneously uses the target sound in new situations and places. | The trainer praises as correct responses are counted. The child is informed of the total number as it is recorded on a data sheet. |

[a] When necessary, nonsense syllables are used in this lesson.

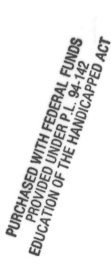

10 lessons. In the second there were two additional lessons. The lessons range from a child's imitation of single words or nonsense syllables in Lesson 1 to spontaneous conversation with target words in home and community settings in Lessons 10, 11, and 12. If a child can only produce a phoneme in isolation or with vowels the parent asks the child to imitate nonsense syllables or the isolated phoneme before starting words with Lesson 1.

The first eight lessons present 20 child-used words which include the target phoneme in progressively longer units of speech. Each unit is first imitated by the child (Lessons 1, 3, 5, and 7), then spontaneously produced by the child (Lessons 2, 4, 6, and 8). In the spontaneous response lessons, starting with Lesson 4 or 6, the children are asked to self-monitor and to self-correct their responses. In Lessons 8 and 9, small toys and objects are often used to help the children construct their utterances. Lesson 9 involves repetition or spontaneous telling of a story with emphasis on three to four of their target words. In Lesson 10 the practice cards are taped up in appropriate places in the child's home so they can serve as visual cues to remind him or her to use target words spontaneously in normal conversation. To prepare for Lesson 11, the parent and child list all the words containing the target phoneme that would be appropriate to talk about in an activity they regularly share, such as lunch or bedtime. They then place a visual reminder in the settings in which these activities take place. The parent counts and reinforces the child as he or she uses the words correctly. For Lesson 12, the parent, the child, or another important person wears some kind of visual cue, such as a sign or ring, to remind the child to use the target sound in a wide variety of settings.

All parents attend 1-hour-long group training sessions where they receive a written description of the program. They also receive a booklet that contains 60 motivating activities for them to use in their sessions. The parent and child come to the clinic weekly to participate together in 15–30 minute counseling and training sessions. Careful consideration is given to both the parent's and the child's motivational systems. Parents are advised to plan practice sessions to precede one of their child's highly desired, naturally occurring behaviors, such as watching television or eating a treat. Parents are encouraged to use some of the 60 activities given to them in the initial training session. If parents become discouraged, the clinician reviews for them their child's progress and may suggest the use of other family members as trainers. The parents use an arbitrarily established criterion for moving their child from lesson to lesson between visits to the clinic, such as if the child goes through a lesson three times at home responding correctly for 90% or more of their 20 representative words, he or she proceeds to the next lesson.

Table 1 includes the findings of the Utah program with 34 children who were normal in all respects except for their articulation errors. The first group of 18 children (mean age of 5 years 9 months) was administered 10 lessons and the second group of 17 children (mean age of 5 years) was administered all 12 lessons. The children entered the program at different times and participated for different lengths of time during the periods of study. The average time for a child to acquire spontaneous use of a target phoneme was 5.3 weeks, which was 2 hours and 40 minutes clinician time. The mean parental time was about 6 hours for each hour of clinician time.

We have also found our program to be successful when used in a public school setting even though the parents and their children participated on a bi-weekly basis for only 10 minutes with the school clinician. Our conclusions are tentative, however, because only a small number of parent-child pairs were involved. A large scale study of public school children is planned.

We have found that day care workers and older siblings, like parents, can work effectively with children who have articulation problems. Our experience has been confirmed by several research investigations which have shown that older children and adults, whether or not they are volunteers or paid paraprofessionals, provide an important service in training the children to acquire error phonemes. See Table 1 for a review of the following studies: Barker (1981); Carrier (1970); Costello and Schoen (1978); Daum and Fisher (1975); Evans and Potter (1974); Fahey (1976); Fahey-Ganz et al. (1981); Galloway and Blue (1975); McCroskey and Baird (1971); Scalero and Eskenazi (1976); Shea (1955); Sommers (1962, 1969); Sommers et al. (1959); and Tufts and Holliday (1959).

## Effective Methods of Training and Using Parent/Paraprofessional Help

Our experience and that of others with paraprofessional administered programs indicate that success often depends on the following:

1.   *The program is most effective if paraprofessionals volunteer or are willing to participate.* McCroskey and Baird (1971) have shown that when parents are selected by the clinician, serious motivational problems can arise. Often these individuals do not wish to participate in the program. One option the speech-language clinician has is to create a positive image of the paraprofessional role by developing a favorable public image. An explanation of the program should be prepared and presented to

parents and to volunteers. The message could be phrased as follows (use term in parentheses as appropriate):

We are fortunate to have a new program at our setting that has been shown to be very helpful to children with speech problems because parents (aides) are involved in the treatment. With their assistance children have additional opportunities to practice and improve their skills. There are also cost savings because the cost of the speech pathologist's time and transportation are reduced. Also, more children will receive service. The speech-language clinician sees the parent (aide) and child for brief, weekly feedback and counseling sessions. Parents are effective and active participants in their children's improvement and can see and enjoy the progress that is made.

An effective way to get this message to potential parent/paraprofessionals is to describe the program in a newspaper or television feature and a child's success with it. When our program was publicized in Salt Lake City there was a significant increase in telephone requests for involvement in the program.     .

The clinician may also contact parents by sending information home with the child or holding a meeting for parents. Finally, a telephone call or letter is useful. Specific choice of times when orientation meetings are to be held should be indicated. Some parents may decline, others may be unable to participate because of intellectual, motivational, or interpersonal deficits. Sometimes a grandmother or an older sibling is a suitable trainer. Although paraprofessionals who volunteer are the most effective, Sommers (1962) found that parents with "poor attitudes" provided a positive influence when they were actively involved in their child's articulation program. When parents were not involved, the improvement of the children was significantly less.

2. *Repeated contact with parent/paraprofessional is necessary during the administration of the program.* Shea (1955) observed that homework assignments made no significant impact on children's articulation improvement. Apparently, when parents are not seen by the speech-language pathologist and when the assignments are not spelled out, parents make no significant impact on their children's progress.

3. *Programmed steps carefully outlined and provided in writing were included in all of the 15 successful studies in which paraprofessionals were used.* Apparently, providing information about articulation problems (McCroskey and Baird, 1971) or demonstrating to parents how sounds are made (Carrier, 1970) is not sufficient to effect an improvement in children's articulation skills.

4.  *Parents/paraprofessionals can be trained in groups.* Baker (1976), summarizing the outcome of a number of projects in various fields, found parents could be trained equally as well in groups as when trained alone. We have found it effective to train as many as 20 parent/paraprofessionals at one time. Baker also reported that for parents of low socioeconomic status the use of demonstration and role-playing in training sessions is far more effective than lectures. No differences were found between parents of other socioeconomic groups. For this reason we used demonstrations and role-playing for all socioeconomic groups.

5.  *Children make progress between visits to the clinician when their paraprofessional trainer knows clearly what steps to follow and has specific criteria for movement from step to step.* Parents in the University of Utah program knew the steps of the program, and the success rate required before going to the next step. In this way, a parent often will let their child progress through one or more lessons between contacts with their clinician. Some children in the Carrier (1970) and Fahey (1976) investigations completed all lessons for a particular phoneme between weekly visits to their clinician. With the University of Utah program, some children completed as many as nine lessons in a week of home practice.

6.  *The child and paraprofessional become involved in training through development of their child's program.* At the University of Utah, both are involved in the preparation of stimulus cards. For example, the clinician, the parent, and the child use the book *30,000 Selected Words* (Blockcolsky et al. 1979) to select words that represent the target phoneme. Words meaningful to the child are selected. For example, we added the word "goal" to one child's list of /g/ words when his parent told us he was an avid soccer player. When a parent and child prepare their own stimulus materials, they care about them.

7.  *By not requiring parents to keep records during practice sessions their motivation is increased.* A parent and child will enjoy practice sessions if record keeping does not interfere constantly with their activities. We found that record keeping is minimal when the picture cards are numbered and then arranged in two separate piles as the words are said correctly or are missed. At the end of the training session the parent can quickly use the numbers to record the words that are missed. This simple accounting system will not interfere with other activities, and will enable the parent to note criteria of success for purposes of advancement to the next step in training.

8. *Critical to a program's success is careful consideration of the child's motivational system and ways for the parent/paraprofessional to appeal to it.* As part of the University of Utah's program, we give the parent general ideas as to how to make the practice sessions appealing to their child. Some parents prefer to conduct a home practice session before the involvement of their child in a highly desirable activity or treat. In this way, practice becomes associated with the pleasurable activity that follows it. Many parents designate their child's favorite television program as a pleasurable activity. A surprise or a choice of treats is a powerful motivator. If the treat is a known quantity, halfway through practice, a child may consider it an insufficient reward to motivate him or her to complete the work involved. Treats and rewards, of course, vary from child to child and, at times for a specific child, from session to session. An older child may be pleased to mark a chart, apply a sticker, whereas a younger child might like to go to the park, play with a favorite toy, or find a popsicle in the freezer.

   Some parents prefer to make each practice session inherently enjoyable by using simple games, such as Concentration or "hide the sticker." In our program we present each parent with a booklet containing 60 enjoyable yet simple games to use while practicing. The booklet is appropriately entitled "How Not To Get Bored Playing with Cards." At the weekly clinical sessions, the clinician demonstrates a few games so that the parents will be encouraged to use them at home.

9. *Letting the parents/paraprofessionals know that they are being effective teachers should be part of the weekly counseling sessions.* Corrective, constructive feedback to parents or aides is necessary to maintain their skills as well as their motivation. The clinician should point out to parents that their child's progress is due directly to their positive and consistent efforts. Helping parent's build positive feelings about themselves is a consideration that cannot be ignored (Webster and Weston, 1976).

10. *Careful programming of carryover for generalization to each child's home and to other environmental settings assures that carryover will be successful.* As soon as a child correctly produces a small set of words representative of the targeted phoneme in spontaneous stories, parents are encouraged to follow up with a variety of practice experiences in the home. Parents are to put up picture cards in appropriate locations in the home. For example, for the /k/ sound picture cards representing "cookie, cake, cook, and cup" would be taped up in the kitchen as visual reminders to use these words and other words that begin with /k/.

Another more slightly advanced activity involves the use of target phoneme words in activities shared by the parent and child, for example, eating dinner, preparing for bedtime, or driving in a car. The parent lists all the target phoneme words appropriate in a situation and then both the parent and child practice using them in conversation. At first the parent cues the child to use these sounds in words as he or she talks. Soon the situation itself becomes a cue for the use of particular sounds and words. We also recommend the use of visual reminders such as little signs or rings placed on the child or trainer as cues to use the sounds or words in a wide variety of places. These activities have proven to be effective ways to assure carryover of new articulation skills to environments outside of practice sessions.

Anne Porcella (1979, p. 2), in a report made for the Exceptional Child Center at Utah State University, summarizes our position well when she describes the contributing factors for a successful parent program as follows:

> The most concerned parents are usually those who run home programs. However, getting all parents to run home programs is not easy. What kind of home programming is apt to be successful? One that is easy to run, which fits into the routine of the day, that has been modeled clearly and practiced by the parent, and finally, one that is reinforced by the school staff. . . Those programs which are usually doomed to failure are ones which are hard to run, time consuming, . . . agreed to reluctantly by the parent, and those which once implemented in the home are never monitored and reinforced by staff members.

Our experience, in agreement with the research findings of others, has indicated that trained parents or other paraprofessionals can work under the direction of a speech-language clinician to effect improvement in the articulatory skills of children. Paraprofessionals are particularly important in effecting carryover objectives. With their help children improve more rapidly and learn to extend their training to real world settings. Careful planning and resourcefulness is necessary, however, to ensure that paraprofessionals are used effectively.

## REFERENCES

Baker, B. L. 1976. Parent involvement in programming for developmentally disabled children. In: L. L. Lloyd (ed.), Communication Assessment and Intervention Strategies. University Park Press, Baltimore.

Barker, K. 1975. ECHO. In: D. Alvord (ed.), Beyond Tradition. Iowa State Department of Public Instruction, Des Moines, IA.

Barker, K. 1981. Communication aide program. Unpublished report, Iowa State Department of Public Instruction, Des Moines, IA.

Blockcolsky, V. D., Frazer, J. M., and Frazer, D. H. 1979. 30,000 Selected Words. Communication Skill Builders, Tucsan, AZ.

Carrier, J. K. 1970. A program of articulation therapy administered by mothers. J. Speech Hear. Disord. 35:48–58.

Costello, J., and Schoen, J. 1978. The effectiveness of paraprofessionals and a speech clinician as agents of articulation intervention using programmed instruction. Lang. Speech Hear. Serv. Schools 9:118–128.

Daum, W., and Fisher, L. I. 1975. A comprehensive model for preschool communication services in the schools. Lang. Speech Hear. Serv. Schools 6:44–54.

Evans, C. M., and Potter, R. E. 1974. The effectiveness of the S-Pack when administered by sixth-grade children to primary-grade children. Lang. Speech Hear. Serv. Schools 5:85–90.

Fahey, V. K. 1976. Parent conducted program of articulation modification. Human Commun, Spring.

Fahey-Ganz, C., Hartmann, B., Hanson, M. L., et al. 1981. A brief summary of the Fahey and the University of Utah's Home-Based Articulation Program and research. Unpublished manuscript. University of Utah.

Galloway, H. F., and Blue, C. M. 1975. Paraprofessional personnel in articulation therapy. Lang. Speech Hear. Serv. Schools 6:125–130.

Graziano, A. M. 1977. Parents as behavior therapists. In: M. Hersen, R. M. Eisler, and P. M. Miller (eds.), Progress in Behavior Modification. Academic Press, New York.

Johnson, C. A., and Katz, R. C. 1973. Using parents as change agents for their children. A review. J. Child Psychol. Psych. Allied Disciplines 14:181–200.

McCroskey, R. L., and Baird, V. G. 1971. Parent education in a public school program of speech therapy. J. Speech Hear. Disord. 36:499–505.

Mowrer, D. E., Baker, R. L., and Schutz, R. E. 1968. Modification of the Frontal Lisp: Programmed Articulation Control Kit. Educational Research Associates, Palos Verdes Estates, CA.

Odell, S. 1974. Training parents in behavior modification: A review. Psychol. Bull. 81:418–433.

Porcella, A. 1979. Increasing parent involvement. Technical Report No. 43, Exceptional Child Center, Outreach and Development Division, Logan, UT.

Scalero, A. M., and Eskenazi, C. 1976. The use of supportive personnel in a public school speech and language program. Lang. Speech Hear. Serv. Schools 7:150–158.

Shea, W. L. 1955. The effect of supplemental parental procedures on public school articulatory cases. Unpublished doctoral dissertation, University of Florida.

Sommers, R. K. 1962. Factors in the effectiveness of mothers trained to aid in speech correction. J. Speech Hear. Disord. 27:178–186.

Sommers, R. K. 1969. The therapy program. In: R. Van Hattum (ed.), Clinical Speech in the Schools. Charles C Thomas, Springfield, IL.

Sommers, R. K., Shilling, S. P., Paul, C. D. et al. 1959. Training parents of children with functional misarticulation. J. Speech Hear. Disord. 2:258–265.

Tufts, L. C., and Holliday, A. R. 1959. Effectiveness of trained parents as speech therapists. J. Speech Hear. Disord. 24:395–401.

Webster, E. J., and Weston, A. J. 1976. Professional Approaches with Parents of Handicapped Children. Charles C Thomas, Springfield, IL.

CHAPTER **13**

# Public Law 94-142: Computerized Educational Programs

*James M. Caccamo*

> *Writing an individualized educational program (IEP) is not easy to do. Caccamo suggests that computer programs be utilized to facilitate this purpose, and describes his experience with this approach.*

> 1. *State the purpose and provisions of Public Law 94-142 (PL 94-142). In this regard, what is meant by an "adverse affect test" and deregulation?*
> 2. *Why are IEPs difficult to implement in clinical practice? Caccamo suggests that IEPs can be effectively administered by utilizing pre-established clinical objectives. Do you agree with this approach?*
> 3. *What are the advantages and disadvantages of computer programs for writing IEPs and for obtaining demographic data?*

IN 1975, THEN PRESIDENT GERALD FORD SIGNED Public Law 94–142 (PL 94-142). No single piece of legislation has had a greater impact on the profession of speech-language pathology in the public schools. Called The Education for All Handicapped Children Act, PL 94-142 requires that every handicapped child be provided a free, appropriate public education in the least restrictive environment. The law also contains provisions requiring written permission from the parents before the evaluation of a child who is, or who is suspected of being, handicapped; a multidisciplinary team evaluation of the child; the development of an individualized educational program (IEP); and written permission from the parent before changing the child's educational placement. The issue of the IEP has caused more controversy than any other provision. The controversy centers around the inordinate time (6.5 hours) it takes for teachers to write the IEP (Price and Goodman, 1980).

## PL 94-142: AN EVOLVING PROCESS

Implementation of PL 94-142 has been an evolving process over the years, partially due to our increasing understanding of the rules and regulations and partially due to litigation and case law that has been emerging since 1975. The change of administration in Washington has also brought about new interpretations of the law and a move to de-regulate PL 94-142. On February 5, 1981, the Comptroller General of the United States reported to Congress that "94-142 program was not designed for children receiving speech therapy only." They recommended that "Congress clarify whether, and under what conditions, children who are receiving only speech therapy or other services currently cited in the law as 'related services' are eligible for coverage under the 94-142 coverage" (U.S. Comptroller General, 1981). The report advises that the nearly 1.4 million speech and language handicapped children now being served in the public school setting not be funded under 94-142. The report indicates that most of the speech-impaired children would not meet an "adverse affect" test. That is to say, in order to be eligible under 94-142 as a primary handicapping condition, the handicap must adversely affect the child's education. What would happen to our speech- and language-handicapped youngsters should speech and language services be reduced to only a "related service"?

Deregulation is another threat to the Education for All Handicapped Children Act. In a briefing paper prepared by the Office of Special Education (1981), the recommendation was made to remove the regulations governing PL 94-142. By this action, the regulation of PL 94-142 would become a state issue. Would your state also deregulate or would it continue to support special education if no federal regulations were in place?

A third issue in the evolution of PL 94-142 has been how to make the IEP process work sufficiently well to allow a high level of parent participation, enable the setting of reasonable objectives, and not consume the professional teacher's time in writing the document (Office of Special Education, 1980).

## IEP

In attaining compliance in accord with PL 94-142, states and local school districts have faced many problems. These problems have been and are being solved. One specific area of difficulty with which all agencies are struggling is the time and cost required to develop the individualized educational program. Price and Goodman (1980) have presented the issue well. In their article, they report that the average amount of teacher time in the development of an IEP was 6.5 hours. The major portion of that time is in the actual mechanical process of writing the IEP.

It is quite apparent that the Office of Special Education (1980) is also concerned about IEPs, as evidenced by their Bulletin #64, of May, 1980. The purpose of the Bulletin was to clarify the requirements for public agencies to be in compliance with the IEP provision of PL 94-142.

The IEP is a significant part of an appropriate educational program and those in the field of speech-language pathology generally support the concept of the IEP. At the same time, clinicians are unwilling to consume innumerable hours in writing IEPs. They would rather spend their time teaching.

The School District of Independence, Missouri serves about 1700 youngsters with various handicapping conditions, of whom 645 are speech and language impaired. The problem of efficient and cost effective teacher utilization in special education is critical. Our teachers must teach. The ability to solve this dilemma, we feel, exists in the form of computer technology and objective instructional programming.

## ASSUMPTIONS

In order to utilize computer programming to write IEPs, a primary assumption must be made. The assumption is that there is a finite number of instructional objectives used to teach handicapped youngsters. If this assumption is true, then we can gather those objectives, store them on a computer, and call them up when needed.

## PROGRAM DEVELOPMENT

In the Independence Public Schools, we made the assumption that a finite number of instructional objectives can be identified. Our next step was to compile these objectives. This responsibility was completed with the help of many, including the Monroe County Special Education Cooperative of Indiana.

Each objective was written with either "can" or "will be able to" as prefix statements. With this two-part classification, each objective was stated either as a present level of performance or as an instructional objective. Table 1 contains the table of contents from the Manual of Instructional Objectives. In Table 2, a sample page of instructional objectives is provided. Each objective in the manual is given a code number which the computer uses to find the specific objective the clinician wishes to use. The speech and language section of the manual is coded "SPA." Each section under speech and language is coded in alphabetical order by adding an additional letter to "SPA." Thus, the first section under speech and language is coded "SPAA," the next, "SPAB," and the next "SPAC." Under each section, specific objectives are coded by number. Our code numbering system is arbitrary and the code numbers are used by the computer to retrieve the specific objective. The first code in Table 2 is "SPAH003," which refers to section H, objective three under the speech and language objectives. The Manual of Instructional Objectives is 167 pages and contains over 3,800 objectives in all areas of special education. There are over 500 objectives for speech and hearing.

## EFFECTIVE PRACTICE IN SPECIAL EDUCATION

The Department of Education, Office of Special Education, has established Regional Resource Center in each of the federal regions. Its purpose is to provide technical assistance to State Departments of Education and to Local School Districts. About a year ago the Office of Special Education instructed each Regional Resource Center to identify effective practices in the use of the IEP within their regions.

The Midwest Regional Resource Center, which serves federal region 7, reviewed our computerized IEP system. The information they collected was provided to a panel of professionals who reviewed its effectiveness and compliance with the law. The panel approved the system as an effective practice in IEP.

Table 1.   Table of contents from the manual of instructional objectives for speech, hearing, and language

## PROGRAMMING

It is important to remember that a computer does not develop an IEP. Each IEP is developed by a speech-language clinician and the parent after a multidisciplinary team evaluation.

When the evaluation is completed, and after the interpretation of test information is provided to the parent, the staff works cooperatively with the parents to develop an IEP to meet their child's educational needs. Instead of writing out each objective, the teacher simply writes a code number for each objective agreed upon by the parent and the professional team. If an instructional objective is not in the manual, it

Table 2.    Sample page from the manual of instructional objectives

Articulation
  Production of target phoneme in syllables
    SPAH003  Produce the following in CV$^a$ syllables _____.
    SPAH006  Evaluate the following CV syllables _____.
    SPAH009  Produce the following in VC syllables _____.
    SPAH012  Evaluate the following in VC syllables _____.
    SPAH015  Produce the following in CVC syllables _____.
    SPAH018  Evaluate the following in CVC syllables _____.
    SPAH021  Produce the following in CCVC syllables _____.
    SPAH024  Evaluate the following in CCVC syllables _____.
    SPAH027  Produce the following in CCVC syllables _____.
    SPAH030  Evaluate the following in CVCC syllables _____.

Articulation
  Production of target phoneme in words
    SPAJ003  Produce the following in initial position in words _____.
    SPAJ006  Evaluate self-production of the following in initial position in words _____.
    SPAJ009  Produce the following in final position in words _____.
    SPAJ012  Evaluate self-production of the following in final position in words _____.
    SPAJ015  Produce the following in medial position in words _____.
    SPAJ018  Evaluate self-production of the following in medial position in words _____.

Articulation
  Production of target phoneme in phrases
    SPAL003  Produce the following in two-word phrase _____.
    SPAL006  Evaluate self-production of the following in two-word phrase _____.
    SPAL009  Produce the following in three-word phrase _____.

$^a$ C, consonant, V, vowel.

is, of course, included in the IEP. However, most of the objectives needed for an IEP are in the manual. We have less than 1% write-in objectives.

After the IEP is completed, the teacher forwards the list of code numbers along with demographic and diagnostic information on the youngster to the Central Office. The data are entered on the computer and four copies of the IEP are reproduced. A summary of services is provided, and evaluation and review criteria are included along with identification information. Several objectives for training are listed under each long range goal. The Appendix to this chapter contains a sample IEP.

**ADDITIONAL COMPUTER SERVICES**

Although the IEP process was the primary reason for the development of a computerized program, other programs are also served. The Director of Special Education utilized the stored data on each child to gather information for the Missouri State Department of Education. At the touch of a button, we can determine child counts, demographic data, types of speech and language disorders, success rate, continuity of training, and much more information.

A list of youngsters in need of their third year evaluation and class lists are also stored in the computer to facilitate the selection of names and addresses of children and parents by school, handicapping condition, and type of program. For example, a workshop for parents of children in self-contained language disorders classes was conducted recently, and the computerized mailing list enabled us to invite only the parents of these children.

With our system we can determine quickly the number of IEP objectives established and met. In addition, this information can be determined for each child, clinician, and building so that we can review the instructional objectives for each child and clinician in our various settings.

Another set of advantages that a computerized IEP system can provide are:

1.  Parents can easily read each objective because they are printed clearly and neatly.
2.  The IEP's have district wide consistency and all the instructional objectives can be measured and taught.
3.  The system forces evaluation. In order to assess a child's level of performance, an in-depth competency based evaluation must be administered.

## SUMMARY

The Education of All Handicapped Children's Act, PL 94-142, states that every handicapped child is to be provided an appropriate education. As required by this law, each child must have an individualized educational program. Usually, it takes an inordinate amount of time to write an IEP, a feature disliked by most clinicians. The Independence Missouri Public School System has developed an efficient and easily applied computer system to write the IEP and to monitor the progress and goals of treatment.

## REFERENCES

Hayes, J., and Higgins, S. 1978. Issues regarding the I.E.P.: Teachers on the front line. Except. Child. 44.
Killen, J., and Myklebust, H. 1980. Evaluation in special education: A computer-based approach. J. Learn. Disabil. 13.

Lehrer, B., and Deiher, J. 1978. Computer based information management for professionals serving handicapped learners. Except. Child. 44.

Miller, S., Miller, K., and Madison, C. 1980. A speech and language clinician's involvement in a PL 94-142 hearing: A case study. Lang. Speech Hear. Serv. Schools. April.

Office of Special Education. 1980. Individual Education Programs (I.E.P.'s). Office of Special Education Policy Paper, U.S. Education Department, Washington, DC.

Price, M., and Goodman, L. 1980. Individualized education programs: A case study. Except. Child. 46.

U.S. Comptroller General. 1981. Report to the Congress: Unanswered Questions on Educating Handicapped Children in Local Public Schools, HRD-81-43. February.

**APPENDIX**

## Computer printout of Individualized Educational Programs for a sample IEP

### INDEPENDENCE PUBLIC SCHOOLS

IDENTIFICATION INFORMATION

    NAME                                   BIRTHDATE

    PARENT                               PHONE #

    ADDRESS                             HOME SCHOOL

                                      BEGIN. DATE     9/01/81

                                      ENDING DATE     5/01/82

    SCHOOL OF ENROLLMENT ON BEGIN. DATE

    SPECIAL EDUCATION PROGRAM AND LEVEL

    SPECIAL EDUCATION TEACHER

  DATE OF CONFERENCE COMMITTEE MEETING     5/27/81

  IEP TO BE IMPLEMENTED BY

  IEP CONFERENCE COMMITTEE


EDUCATIONAL SERVICES TO BE PROVIDED

    1. SPECIALIZED PROGRAMS AND SERVICES    PROGRAM    TYPE    MINS/WEEK

                                           SPEECH     RES

    2. REGULAR CLASSES AND PROGRAMS

       ALL ACADEMIC AREAS EXCEPT THOSE LISTED IN #1 ABOVE.

EVALUATION AND REVIEW

    1. APPROPRIATE CRITERION TESTS WILL BE ADMINISTERED FOR SHORT

    TERM OBJECTIVES THROUGHOUT THE SCHOOL YEAR. RECORDS WILL BE

    KEPT OF THE CRITERION TESTS AND THE DATE OF INITIATION AND

    COMPLETION OF EACH OBJECTIVE.

    2. DIAGNOSTIC TESTS IN APPROPRIATE SUBJECT AREAS WILL BE

    ADMINISTERED AS NEEDED TO DETERMINE PRESENT PERFORMANCE

    LEVEL AS WELL AS SERVE AS A BASIS FOR EVALUATION.

## INDIVIDUALIZED EDUCATION PROGRAM
## INDEPENDENCE PUBLIC SCHOOLS

% OF SUCCESS

SUBJECT   SPEECH, HEARING AND LANGUAGE
          ARTICULATION
          SOUND RECOGNITION


PRESENT PERFORMANCE LEVEL - STUDENT CAN

   SPAA009   RECOGNIZE THE FOLLOWING IN ISOLATION


LONG RANGE GOAL - STUDENT WILL IMPROVE SKILLS
IN THE AREA OF   SPEECH, HEARING AND LANGUAGE


OBJECTIVES - STUDENT WILL BE ABLE TO

   SPAA012   RECOGNIZE THE FOLLOWING IN CV SYLLABLE PATTERN.

   SPAA015   RECOGNIZE THE FOLLOWING IN VC SYLLABLE PATTERN

   SPAA018   RECOGNIZE THE FOLLOWING IN CVC SYLLABLE PATTERN

   SPAA021   RECOGNIZE THE FOLLOWING IN CVCC SYLLABLE PATTERN

   SPAA024   RECOGNIZE THE FOLLOWING IN CVCC SYLLABLE
             PATTERN        •

   SPAA027   RECOGNIZE THE FOLLOWING IN INITIAL POSITION IN
             WORDS       •

   SPAA030   RECOGNIZE THE FOLLOWING IN FINAL POSITION IN
             WORDS      •

   SPAA033   RECOGNIZE THE FOLLOWING IN MEDIAL POSITION
             IN WORDS      •

   SPAA036   IDENTIFY POSITION OF THE FOLLOWING IN INITIAL
             POSITION IN WORDS       •

   SPAA039   IDENTIFY POSITION OF THE FOLLOWING IN FINAL POSITION
             IN WORDS       •

   SPAA041   IDENTIFY POSITION OF THE FOLLOWING IN MEDIAL
             POSITION IN WORDS       •


SUBJECT   SPEECH, HEARING AND LANGUAGE
          ARTICULATION
          SOUND DISCRIMINATION

INDIVIDUALIZED EDUCATION PROGRAM
INDEPENDENCE PUBLIC SCHOOLS

% OF SUCCESS

SUBJECT   SPEECH, HEARING AND LANGUAGE
          ARTICULATION
          SOUND DISCRIMINATION

          CONTD


LONG RANGE GOAL – STUDENT WILL IMPROVE SKILLS
IN THE AREA OF   SPEECH, HEARING AND LANGUAGE


OBJECTIVES – STUDENT WILL BE ABLE TO

    SPAD003   DISCRIMINATE THE FOLLOWING FROM ERROR PHONEME IN
              ISOLATION          •

    SPAD006   DISCRIMINATE THE FOLLOWING FROM ERROR PHONEME IN
              CV SYLLABLES          •

    SPAD009   DISCRIMINATE THE FOLLOWING FROM ERROR PHONEME IN
              VC SYLLABLES          •

    SPAD012   DISCRIMINATE THE FOLLOWING FROM ERROR PHONEME IN
              CVC SYLLABLES          •

    SPAD015   DISCRIMINATE THE FOLLOWING FROM ERROR PHONEME
              IN CCV SYLLABLES          •

    SPAD018   DISCRIMINATE THE FOLLOWING FROM ERROR PHONEME IN
              CVCC SYLLABLES          •

    SPAD021   DISCRIMINATE THE FOLLOWING FROM ERROR PHONEME IN
              INITIAL POSITION IN WORDS          •

    SPAD024   DISCRIMINATE THE FOLLOWING FROM ERROR PHONEME IN
              FINAL POSITION IN WORDS          •

    SPAD027   DISCRIMINATE THE FOLLOWING FROM ERROR PHONEME IN
              MEDIAL POSITION IN WORDS          •

    SPAD030   DISCRIMINATE THE FOLLOWING FROM ERROR PHONEME IN
              SENTENCES          •


SUBJECT   SPEECH, HEARING AND LANGUAGE
          ARTICULATION
          PRODUCTION OF PHONEME IN ISOLATION

# INDIVIDUALIZED EDUCATION PROGRAM
# INDEPENDENCE PUBLIC SCHOOLS

% OF SUCCESS

SUBJECT   SPEECH, HEARING AND LANGUAGE
          ARTICULATION
          PRODUCTION OF PHONEME IN ISOLATION

               CONTD


   LONG RANGE GOAL - STUDENT WILL IMPROVE SKILLS
   IN THE AREA OF  SPEECH, HEARING AND LANGUAGE


   OBJECTIVES - STUDENT WILL BE ABLE TO

       SPAF003   RECOGNIZE PROPER PLACEMENT FOR PRODUCTION OF SOUND.

       SPAF006   PRODUCE THE FOLLOWING CORRECTLY WHEN PAIRED WITH
                 AT LEAST ONE CONSONANT        •

       SPAF009   PRODUCE THE FOLLOWING WHEN AUDITORY, VISUAL AND
                 KINESTHETIC MODELS ARE PRESENT        •

       SPAF012   PRODUCE THE FOLLOWING WHEN AUDITORY MODELS ARE
                 PRESENT       •

       SPAF015   PRODUCE THE FOLLOWING WHEN KINESTHETIC MODELS ARE
                 PRESENT       •

       SPAF018   PRODUCE THE FOLLOWING WHEN VISUAL MODELS ARE
                 PRESENT       •

       SPAF021   PRODUCE THE FOLLOWING IN ISOLATION IN THE ABSENCE
                 OF A MODEL        •

       SPAF024   EVALUATE SELF-PRODUCTION OF THE FOLLOWING IN
                 ISOLATION        •

       SPAF027   PRODUCE THE FOLLOWING AND ERROR PHONEME UPON
                 REQUEST        •


SUBJECT   SPEECH, HEARING AND LANGUAGE
          ARTICULATION
          PRODUCTION OF TARGET PHONEME IN SYLLABLES


   LONG RANGE GOAL - STUDENT WILL IMPROVE SKILLS
   IN THE AREA OF  SPEECH, HEARING AND LANGUAGE


   OBJECTIVES - STUDENT WILL BE ABLE TO

# INDIVIDUALIZED EDUCATION PROGRAM
# INDEPENDENCE PUBLIC SCHOOLS

% OF SUCCESS

SUBJECT  SPEECH, HEARING AND LANGUAGE
         ARTICULATION
         PRODUCTION OF TARGET PHONEME IN SYLLABLES

         CONTD

    SPAH003  PRODUCE THE FOLLOWING IN CV SYLLABLES          .

    SPAH009  PRODUCE THE FOLLOWING IN VC SYLLABLES          .

    SPAH015  PRODUCE THE FOLLOWING IN CVC SYLLABLES          .

    SPAH021  PRODUCE THE FOLLOWING IN CCVC SYLLABLES          .

    SPAH027  PRODUCE THE FOLLOWING IN CVCC SYLLABLES          .


SUBJECT  SPEECH, HEARING AND LANGUAGE
         ARTICULATION
         PRODUCTION OF TARGET PHONEME IN WORDS

    LONG RANGE GOAL - STUDENT WILL IMPROVE SKILLS
    IN THE AREA OF  SPEECH, HEARING AND LANGUAGE

    OBJECTIVES - STUDENT WILL BE ABLE TO

    SPAJ003  PRODUCE THE FOLLOWING IN INITIAL POSITION IN
             WORDS        .

    SPAJ006  EVALUATE SELF-PRODUCTION OF THE FOLLOWING IN INITIAL
             POSITION IN WORDS        .

    SPAJ009  PRODUCE THE FOLLOWING IN FINAL POSITION IN WORDS

    SPAJ012  EVALUATE SELF-PRODUCTION OF THE FOLLOWING IN FINAL
             POSITION IN WORDS        .

    SPAJ015  PRODUCE THE FOLLOWING IN MEDIAL POSITION IN
             WORDS        .

    SPAJ018  EVALUATE SELF-PRODUCTION OF THE FOLLOWING IN
             MEDIAL POSITION IN WORDS        .


SUBJECT  SPEECH, HEARING AND LANGUAGE
         ARTICULATION
         PRODUCTION OF TARGET PHONEME IN PHRASES

## INDIVIDUALIZED EDUCATION PROGRAM
## INDEPENDENCE PUBLIC SCHOOLS

% OF SUCCESS

SUBJECT   SPEECH, HEARING AND LANGUAGE
          ARTICULATION
          PRODUCTION OF TARGET PHONEME IN PHRASES

          CONTD

  LONG RANGE GOAL - STUDENT WILL IMPROVE SKILLS
  IN THE AREA OF   SPEECH, HEARING AND LANGUAGE

  OBJECTIVES - STUDENT WILL BE ABLE TO

     SPAL003   PRODUCE THE FOLLOWING IN TWO-WORD PHRASE        .

     SPAL009   PRODUCE THE FOLLOWING IN THREE-WORD PHRASE        .

     SPAL015   PRODUCE THE FOLLOWING IN FOUR-WORD PHRASE        .


SUBJECT   SPEECH, HEARING AND LANGUAGE
          ARTICULATION
          PRODUCTION OF TARGET PHONEME IN SENTENCES

  LONG RANGE GOAL - STUDENT WILL IMPROVE SKILLS
  IN THE AREA OF   SPEECH, HEARING AND LANGUAGE

  OBJECTIVES - STUDENT WILL BE ABLE TO

     SPAN003   PRODUCE ONE OF THE FOLLOWING IN A SIMPLE KERNEL
               SENTENCE   UNTRANSFORMED        .

     SPAN006   PRODUCE TWO OF THE FOLLOWING IN A SIMPLE KERNEL
               SENTENCE   UNTRANSFORMED        .

     SPAN009   PRODUCE MORE THAN TWO OF THE FOLLOWING IN A SIMPLE
               KERNEL SENTENCE   UNTRANSFORMED        .

     SPAN012   PRODUCE ONE OF THE FOLLOWING IN A SYNTACTICALLY
               COMPLEX SENTENCE CONTAINING AT LEAST ONE
               TRANSFORMATION        .

     SPAN015   PRODUCE TWO OF THE FOLLOWING IN A SYNTACTICALLY
               COMPLEX SENTENCE        .

     SPAN018   PRODUCE MORE THAN TWO OF THE FOLLOWING IN A
               SYNTACTICALLY COMPLEX SENTENCE

## INDIVIDUALIZED EDUCATION PROGRAM
## INDEPENDENCE PUBLIC SCHOOLS

% OF SUCCESS

SUBJECT    SPEECH, HEARING AND LANGUAGE
           ARTICULATION
           PRODUCTION OF TARGET PHONEME IN SENTENCES

           CONTD


SUBJECT    SPEECH, HEARING AND LANGUAGE
           ARTICULATION
           PRODUCTION OF TARGET PHONEME IN STRUCTURED
           SPEECH


   LONG RANGE GOAL - STUDENT WILL IMPROVE SKILLS
   IN THE AREA OF   SPEECH, HEARING AND LANGUAGE


   OBJECTIVES - STUDENT WILL BE ABLE TO

       SPAR003   PRODUCE THE FOLLOWING IN RESPONSE TO QUESTIONS

       SPAR009   PRODUCE THE FOLLOWING IN DESCRIBING A PERSON, PLACE,
                 THING, OR ACTION


SUBJECT    SPEECH, HEARING AND LANGUAGE
           ARTICULATION
           PRODUCTION OF TARGET PHONEME IN CONVERSATIONAL
           SPEECH IN THE SPEECH ROOM


   LONG RANGE GOAL - STUDENT WILL IMPROVE SKILLS
   IN THE AREA OF   SPEECH, HEARING AND LANGUAGE


   OBJECTIVES - STUDENT WILL BE ABLE TO

       SPAT006   USES THE FOLLOWING CORRECTLY IN RETELLING STORY

       SPAT009   USE THE FOLLOWING CORRECTLY IN SPEECH DESIGNED TO
                 INITIATE CONVERSATIONAL SPEECH


SUBJECT    SPEECH, HEARING AND LANGUAGE
           ARTICULATION
           PRODUCTION OF TARGET PHONEME IN CONVERSATIONAL
           SPEECH OUTSIDE THE SPEECH ROOM

## INDIVIDUALIZED EDUCATION PROGRAM
## INDEPENDENCE PUBLIC SCHOOLS

% OF SUCCESS

SUBJECT   SPEECH, HEARING AND LANGUAGE
          ARTICULATION
          PRODUCTION OF TARGET PHONEME IN CONVERSATIONAL
          SPEECH OUTSIDE THE SPEECH ROOM

          CONTD

LONG RANGE GOAL - STUDENT WILL IMPROVE SKILLS
IN THE AREA OF  SPEECH, HEARING AND LANGUAGE

OBJECTIVES - STUDENT WILL BE ABLE TO

    SPAV003   USE THE FOLLOWING CONSISTENTLY IN THE CLASSROOM WITH
              CLINICIAN PRESENT TO SERVE AS A VISUAL CURE

    SPAV006   USE THE FOLLOWING CONSISTENTLY IN THE CLASSROOM WHEN
              NOT AWARE OF THE PRESENCE OF THE CLINICIAN

    SPAV009   USE THE FOLLOWING CONSISTENTLY WHEN CONVERSING WITH
              FRIENDS AND FAMILY OUTSIDE THE CLASSROOM

    SPAV012   USE THE FOLLOWING CONSISTENTLY IN SITUATIONS OF
              STRESS, ANXIETY, EXCITEMENT, ETC.

# CHAPTER 14

# Types of Velopharyngeal Incompetence

*Hughlett L. Morris*

*A cleft palate disturbs normal velopharyngeal functioning and often causes speech production to be impaired. Morris provides guidelines for diagnosis and treatment by describing subgroups of patients according to velopharngeal competency, speech behavior, and prognosis for improvement.*

1.  *Distinguish between cleft palate, congenital palatopharyngeal competence, and submucous cleft of the palate.*
2.  *What are the speech disorders that we should look for when we examine velopharyngeal competence?*
3.  *With regard to velopharyngeal competence, Morris identifies four diagnostic groups. Discuss each group, taking into consideration velopharyngeal function and their respective speech deviations. In each case, what is the prognosis for recovery?*

THERE IS LITTLE DOUBT ABOUT the importance of the velopharyngeal mechanism in the physiology of speech production. In the normal individual the intact hard palate is a rigid partition between the oral and nasal cavities in the anterior two-thirds of the palate's dimension. The soft palate constitutes the posterior one-third of the palate's dimension and, together with the pharyngeal walls, must be capable of both partitioning and coupling these two cavities during speech (and also deglutition).

When coupling is desired for nasalized speech,[1] the soft palate rests against the dorsum of the tongue, the pharyngeal walls move distally, and the velopharyngeal port is opened. When oral speech is required, the soft palate is raised, the pharyngeal walls move mesially, and the velopharyngeal port is closed. Our understanding of velopharyngeal function indicates that the speaker must be able to open and close the velopharyngeal port in this manner and with some precision and consistency in order to obtain normal speech.

Several groups of speech-disordered patients show velopharyngeal dysfunction. Patients with pharyngeal structures that restrict velopharyngeal opening, such as hypertrophied adenoids, show less nasalization of speech than is normal, and we call such speech *denasal*. That may also be a problem when restriction in port size is the result of an excessively wide palatopharyngeal flap, originally constructed for velopharyngeal incompetence.

The major type of velopharyngeal dysfunction, however, is the result of inability to close the velopharyngeal port, so that nasalized speech is physiologically determined and cannot be prevented by the patient. This is a major finding, of course, in cleft lip and palate. Before palatal surgery, the patient is unable to separate the oral and nasal cavities because of the physical clefting. Velopharyngeal incompetence is found in about one-fourth of cleft palate patients even after the primary palatoplasty because of shortness and immobility of the soft palate. It may be found also in patients who have had secondary management, such as posterior pharyngeal flap, if the flap is too narrow.

Velopharyngeal incompetence may be found also in other orofacial disorders, congenital or acquired. *Congenital palatopharyngeal incompetence (CPI)* refers to a birth defect in which there is velopharyngeal insufficiency, resulting in nasalized speech (Morris et al., 1982). The patient's speech is very much like that following unsuc-

---

[1] The term *nasalized speech* is used here to refer to both voice quality that is excessively nasal and to consonant articulation that is characterized by nasal emission of oral air pressure.

cessful surgery for cleft palate, but the patient does not have a cleft palate nor has he or she ever had one. CPI is sometimes confused with submucous cleft palate, a form of cleft palate. The latter is more easily diagnosed because generally there are physical symptoms that can be clinically detected, such as absence of the posterior nasal spine or a notch in the hard palate, where the posterior nasal spine normally is found. Bifid uvula is often found also in patients with submucous cleft palate. Although CPI and submucous cleft palate are congenital defects, they sometimes are not detected until later in life. Typically, diagnosis is made because of nasalized speech from early childhood or nasalized speech after adenoidectomy. Adenoidectomy uncovers these defects as well as an incompetent mechanism in a cleft palate patient because before surgery the bulk of the adenoidal pad in the nasopharynx compensated for velopharyngeal deficit. After adenoidectomy, the velopharyngeal mechanism is unable to compensate for the abrupt change in physical status. In contrast, it appears that typically the mechanism can compensate for the changes in nasopharyngeal dimensions that occur with normal adenoidal atrophy, presumably because the changes take place so gradually. There is controversy about this sequence of events. There are isolated clinical reports about "developing" velopharyngeal incompetence as a result of normal adenoidal atrophy, but only one such case, a patient with cleft palate, has been reported (Mason and Warren 1980). Mason and Warren described an additional case in their report, but by most standards the patient (also cleft palate) had marginal velopharyngeal incompetence before the adenoidal involution. Further investigation of this interesting phenomenon is needed.

Velopharyngeal dysfunction is also sometimes found in patients with congenital craniofacial anomalies (CFA) such as Apert syndrome and Cronzon disease (Elfenbein, et al., 1981; Peterson, 1973), and in some patients with acquired neurological disease or disorder (Darley et al., 1975). The CFA and neurological disorders are substantially different in history and clinical findings from cleft palate and CPI, and will not be considered in this discussion.

## DIAGNOSIS OF VELOPHARYNGEAL COMPETENCE

Most clinical speech-language pathologists experienced in cleft palate and related disorders agree that there is no single technique preferred to all others for diagnosing velopharyngeal competence.[2] For most purposes, the diagnosis is a clinical judgment based on different kinds of

---

[2] See McWilliams et al. (1981) for an interesting study that is designed to compare several methods for assessing velopharyngeal competence.

information. Observations during typical speech production are necessary to determine the usual function of the mechanism in providing oral-nasal balance. Most of us do that by means of a word articulation test, and also by listening carefully to connected speech. As we evaluate speech production, we also must be alert for the probable contribution to the disordered speech by other factors, such as dentition, maturation, and compensation for any existing structural deficits. During this kind of testing we want to attend carefully to the speech production of the so-called pressure consonants (plosives, fricatives, affricatives) because they are most sensitive to velopharyngeal dysfunction. We also attend carefully to error type, because velopharyngeal incompetence results in errors that are nasalized (nasal emission of oral air pressure that characterizes these pressure consonants). Other types of etiological factors (for example, dental anomalies) result in oral, not nasal, distortion. Throughout all speech testing, we look for inconsistency. Evidence that patients on occasion can prevent nasal emission on a speech production task that they normally nasalize indicates that the oral response may indeed be in their speech production repertoire, an inference that is clinically significant for planning management.

We also must test further for possible inconsistency of speech performance by assessing how the patient responds to auditory-visual stimulation. Actually, this is trial speech training. Again, for these purposes, the focus is on whether with stimulation the patient can change a nasal speech performance to an oral one. If so, this observation is further evidence of flexibility of performance in the aerodynamics and resonance of speech production.

Most test batteries for velopharyngeal competence also include so-called physiological measures. The intent of these procedures is to provide information about velopharyngeal structures and their function either during speech or during nonspeech activities that require velopharyngeal function.[3] Procedures such as physical examination, radiography, and endoscopy enable the observer to examine the structures in a reasonably direct way; inferences about function can then be made. Aerodynamic measures provide information about velopharyngeal function; statements about structure can be made only as inferences. Both types of information are useful, but neither tells the whole story. Findings from both require careful interpretation by the speech pathologist when the patient is inconsistent in velopharyngeal function: for such patients these measures may indicate incompetence

---

[3] See Shelton and Trier (1976) for an excellent discussion of some issues to be considered in assessing velopharyngeal competence.

Table 1.   Clinical findings for Type I velopharyngeal function:
Velopharyngeal competence

| Type I    velopharyngeal competence |
| --- |
| 1. May show nasalization of speech, but also shows some oral speech or can be stimulated for oral speech. |
| 2. Connected speech may or may not be more nasalized than single word responses. |
| 3. No nares constriction. |
| 4. Aerodynamic and X-ray film results varies with the task. |
| Speech training is successful for generalization of the oral speech response. Patient should show improvement toward more oral speech after 10 hours of treatment. |

during typical behavior but competence when best efforts at oral speech are demonstrated.

**IDENTIFICATION OF DIAGNOSTIC GROUPS**

The experienced speech pathologist in general practice has little difficulty in identifying the two extreme groups of: 1) unmistakable velopharyngeal competence; and 2) gross velopharyngeal incompetence. These two groups are labeled Types I and III in this discussion and described in outline form in Tables 1 and 2.[4]

**Type I   Velopharyngeal Competence**

These patients sometimes show nasal emission during some pressure consonants but they usually also show some oralized pressure consonants or can be stimulated to do so. Voice quality typically is not hypernasal. There is no constriction of the nares. They usually are able to perform nonspeech blowing activities ("blow this tiny paper boat from the palm of my hand") without nasal emission. Connected speech may or may not be more nasalized than one-word responses.

   Physical examination gives generally negative findings: the palate is intact and appears normal in length and mobility. Aerodynamic and X-ray findings must be obtained and interpreted with care because the patient is probably inconsistent in performance.

   If the patient performs the tasks orally during the observations, then the findings will indicate adequate velopharyngeal function. On the other hand, if the patient performs the tasks with nasal emission, the findings will show velopharyngeal dysfunction. For this reason, careful attention must be given to task performance during the observation for reliable interpretation of findings.

---

[4] This discussion of diagnostic groups according to velopharyngeal function represents an expansion of an earlier paper on the subject (Morris, 1972).

Table 2.   Outline description of Type III velopharyngeal function:
Velopharyngeal incompetence

| Type III   velopharyngeal incompetence |
| --- |
| 1.   Consistent nasalization of speech, not stimulable. |
| 2.   One word responses and connected speech equally nasal. |
| 3.   May or may not show nares constriction. |
| 4.   All physiologic measures reflect velopharyngeal opening during activities that are normally oral. |

Prognosis: speech training is not successful in developing velopharyngeal closure. Trial speech framing may be provided but should be discontinued after 4 hours of training if no improvement is noted.

The clinical interpretation of these findings is that the patient with Type I competence is physiologically capable of velopharyngeal closure. The nasal emission errors observed during diagnosis, on an inconsistent basis, persist because of the influence of old behavior patterns and not because of physiological restrictions. Speech training is indicated, directed to the goal of generalization of oral speech responses. Training with these patients is successful, and there should be improvement toward oral speech after 10 hours of training, usually earlier.

## Type III   Velopharyngeal Incompetence

These patients (Table 2) are at the other end of the continuum: they show nasalized speech and in a highly consistent manner. There is nasal voice quality and nasal emission of oral air pressure during both speech and nonspeech tasks that normally are oral. Furthermore, attempts to stimulate their performance to be oral are not successful. They frequently, but not always, show constriction of the nares during pressure consonants. Physical examination may indicate short or immobile palate, but such examination is not sufficiently precise to be dependable.[5] X-ray films and endoscopic findings consistently show velopharyngeal opening during tasks for which there normally is closure, and aerodynamic procedures reveal the inability of the velopharyngeal mechanism to function properly in preventing nasal leakage.

The clinical interpretation of these findings is that these patients (Type III) show gross velopharyngeal incompetence that physiologically precludes normally oral speech. Furthermore, there are no treatment procedures other than surgery or in certain cases, dental pros-

[5] Interpret the findings from physical examination of the oral cavity with great caution. We now know that a frontal view of the velopharyngeal mechanism gives incomplete information about velopharyngeal function and cannot be trusted. Be particularly alert for a deep velopharynx and a short palate that shows mostly vertical, not posterior, movement.

thetics, that rectify the physiological deficit. Speech training is not useful for "teaching" velopharyngeal competence and is effective only for helping the patient minimize the effects of the physical deficit.[6] Trial speech instruction may be provided for several weeks but should not be extended for longer periods of time without a clear justification. Physical management of the deficit is needed, usually pharyngeal flap surgery. There are, of course, other reasons for treating these patients, such as language delay, for example.

### Type II    Marginal Velopharyngeal Incompetence

Unfortunately, many patients do not fit neatly into either of these extreme groups. Diagnostic findings are internally conflicting, and we find it difficult to categorize the patient neatly with regard to velopharyngeal competence. As a consequence, in clinical practice we use a third diagnostic category, marginal incompetence, for these patients. Not very much information is available about this group, however, and it seems reasonable to suppose that there is considerable variation within it.

The purpose here is to describe two major subgroups that are important in considering plans for treatment. In addition, these subgroups are defined mainly in terms of clinical findings from a conventional examination by a speech-language pathologist. The two groups are described in outline format in Table 3.

### Type IIA    The Almost-but-Not-Quite (ABNQ) Subgroup

The key words in describing velopharyngeal function in this ABNQ subgroup are *mild* and *consistent*. Although the extent of dysfunction is mild, the nasalization of speech resulting from the marginal incompetence is highly consistent among and within tasks. The patient is not stimulable for oral responses. Physiological measures indicate a small but consistent velopharyngeal opening, but these measures sometimes give results that are in apparent disagreement with observations about speech production. For example, if the opening is very small and if soft tissue delineation is not of highest quality, X-ray films may not reveal the very small velopharyngeal opening. In addition, on some aerodynamic measures, a deviated septum or other nasal obstruction may counteract the effect of the very small velopharyngeal opening, and the test results may indicate competence when indeed there is none for connected speech purposes. Finally, such small openings are dis-

---

[6] See Shelton (1963) for an excellent discussion of the theoretical implications of attempting to "teach" velopharyngeal competence to patients with physiological deficits. Also see Shelton et al. (1968) and Wells (1971) for suggestions about training intended to minimize the effects of a physical deficit.

Table 3.   Outline description of Type II velopharyngeal function: Marginal velopharyngeal incompetence

| Type IIA   marginal velopharyngeal incompetence, ABNQ[a] |
|---|

1. Slight but consistent nasalization of speech. Not stimulable.
2. Connected speech similar to single word responses in degree of nasalization.
3. Probably does not show nares constriction but might.
4. X-ray films show slight velopharyngeal opening if soft tissue delineation is good. NPF views show slight velopharyngeal opening by skillful examination.
5. Aerodynamic measures indicate slight nasal leakage of air pressure/flow during oral activities. Deviated septum or other nasal obstruction may partially counteract the slight velopharyngeal opening.

| Type IIB   marginal velopharyngeal incompetence, SBNA[b] |
|---|

1. Inconsistent nasalization of speech. Usually stimulable.
2. Connected speech generally more nasalized than are single responses.
3. Typically no nares constriction.
4. Findings from x-ray films, NPF examination, and aerodynamic measures vary with the performance of the task: oral performances indicated physiological closure, nasalized performances do not.

[a] Prognosis: speech training for extension of velopharyngeal activity is not successful. Trial therapy can be provided but should not be continued past 6 hours of treatment if no improvement is noted. Decision about physical management depends on judgment about severity.

[b] Training for generalization of oral responses is usually not successful. Discontinue speech training after 10 hours of treatment if no improvement noted. Decision about physical management depends on judgment about severity.

covered by nasopharyngeal fiberscope (NPF) or other endoscopic procedures only by a highly experienced examiner.

The major disability in these cases is one of structural deficiency. Generally, the problem is a short palate, but there may also be an unusually deep velopharynx. Typically, movement patterns of the palate, and probably other velopharyngeal structures, are within normal limits.

Speech training is not successful with the ABNQ group for the purpose of improving velopharyngeal function. That is because the patient apparently has already extended the mechanism to the physiologic limits and does so consistently. If trial training for that purpose is provided to confirm the diagnosis of ABNQ marginal incompetence, it should be discontinued after 6 hours of treatment if no improvement in velopharyngeal function is observed. As indicated before, there are other purposes for which training with this group is justified.

If normal oral speech is the goal, physical management of the velopharyngeal deficit will be needed. Pharyngeal flap surgery is a possibility; pharyngeal injection by Teflon paste or some similar nontoxic material is also successful, provided the velopharyngeal space is small and the soft palate is mobile.

Discussions of treatment for the ABNQ patient sometimes reveal differences of opinion about whether the severity of the nasalization of speech is sufficient to warrant surgery. In such a case, the role of the speech-language pathologist is to estimate the extent to which the nasalization is a deviation from normal and impairs communication. The surgeon has to justify whether the expected benefits are worth the risks, although certainly the risks of surgery are minimal under normal circumstances. All members of the team provide useful evaluations of degree of impairment; in this role they serve as a kind of sophisticated representative of the public. In the final analysis, however, it is the patient and the family who must make the decision, and members of the team must not forget that it is proper that they do so.

### Type IIB    The Sometimes-but-Not Always (SBNA) Subgroup

The key words in describing velopharyngeal function in this marginal incompetence subgroup are *inconsistency* and *response to treatment*: sometimes patients show signs of improvement and sometimes they do not. For example, they may give normal oral responses on single word tasks (such as during a traditional word articulation test) but their automatic connected speech is typically nasalized. Or the patient may give nasalized responses on an articulation test but can be stimulated to be oral. Or the patient may give oral responses on a syllabic train consisting of vowels and "pressure" consonants, but the entire response becomes nasalized when nasal consonants are interspersed among the pressure consonants in the task.

In the same way, physiological findings also are inconsistent. Observations taken by x-ray or aerodynamic measures during sustained production of single phonemes or blowing, single word tasks, or tasks that include only pressure consonants reflect velopharyngeal competence. In contrast, findings taken during connected speech, tasks that include nasals, or tasks performed at a fast rate, reflect incompetence.

The major disability for this group appears to be one of timing. The structures are adequate, in terms of size and relationship, but mobility is either restricted or, more probably, poorly coordinated. If we consider the ABNQ group to show a deficit primarily of structure, we must view the SBNA group as having primarily a neurologic deficit.

The lack of improvement from speech training is the major diagnostic finding for this group. These patients continue over time to demonstrate on certain tasks that they are capable of improvement and can achieve normal speech, because oral responses are clearly in their repertoire. But when treatment is provided for generalization of the oral response to responses that typically are nasalized, this generalization does not occur. A major distinguishing feature of the SBNA group, then, is the difference between diagnostic findings, which indicate velopharyngeal competence, and the results from treatment, which indicate incompetence. The speech-language pathologist should provide training for generalization purposes, for a sufficient period of time, to test the mechanism reliably. If there is no improvement in automatic connected speech after 10 hours of treatment, however, the SBNA diagnosis should be considered, and if there is none after 20 hours of treatment, the diagnosis is confirmed. In contrast, as indicated in Table 1, the patient with velopharyngeal competence shows positive response to treatment for this purpose after 10 hours of training.

Diagnosis of these patients is frequently controversial. Inexperienced speech pathologists fail to interpret correctly the lack of improvement from training. Parents are falsely optimistic about the outcome because they observe the variance in speech production that is typical of the group. Surgeons and dentists who work often with cleft palate patients over-interpret the observation that the SBNA patient can perform well on single word tasks or highly specific speech activities. As a consequence, it is vital that observations about response to speech training (or rather, lack of it) be included as part of the diagnostic findings for these patients.

Nor are decisions about physical management for the SBNA patient clear cut. These characteristic problems of timing persist even after pharyngeal flap surgery, for example, and so differences before and after surgery are not as dramatic for this group as they frequently are for the ABNQ group. A rationale for secondary surgery (usually pharyngeal flap) is that making the velopharyngeal space smaller in dimension will minimize the effects of the timing disorder. To the extent that rationale is sufficient to justify surgery, surgery is indicated. In instances in which that is not the case, surgery is not indicated and the patient may have to live with the problem. In such cases it is helpful to make the patients aware that they can use this physiological variability to their advantage. This is one instance in which "talking more slowly" really helps! Most SBNA patients, however, find it nearly impossible to maintain that kind of monitoring during all connected speech.

## DISCUSSION

The patient with cleft palate and related palatal disorders presents some interesting problems to the speech-language pathologist because of the interactions between physical structure and function. These patients show a variety of physical disorders that potentially prevent good speech production, but the primary one is velopharyngeal incompetence and that is our focus in this discussion.

Our understanding of the role of velopharyngeal incompetence and its effect on speech production has increased tremendously during the past 25 years. The speech-language pathologist is now able by careful use of conventional diagnostic procedures to diagnose with some confidence those who have physiologic competence and those who clearly do not. These decisions are generally sufficient for deciding, on the one hand, to provide training for generalization purposes and, on the other, to refer the patient to a specialty team at a teaching hospital for more precise diagnosis.

In the same way, described here is a model for identifying two subgroups of marginal incompetence by which clinical observations can be used for more careful diagnosis. These two subgroups have not been defined by research findings but by about 25 years of clinical practice. They are offered here for consideration by researchers in speech pathology in the hope that the questions about marginal velopharyngeal incompetence may be eventually easier to answer.

Correspondence about the models is welcomed, and research about their validity is encouraged.

## REFERENCES

Darley, F. L., Aronson, A. E., and Brown, J. R. 1975. Motor Speech Disorders. W. B. Saunders Co., Toronto.

Elfenbein, J. L., Waziri, M., and Morris, H. L. 1981. Verbal communication skills by six children with craniofacial anomalies. Cleft Palate J. 18:59–64.

Mason, R. M., and Warren, D. W. 1980. Adenoid involution and developing hypernasality in cleft palate. J. Speech Hear. Disord. 45:469–480.

McWilliams, B. J., Glaser, E. R., Philips, B. J., et al. 1981. A comparative study of four methods of evaluating velopharyngeal adequacy. Plastic Reconstr. Surg. 68:1–9.

Morris, H. L. 1972. Cleft palate. In: A. J. Weston (ed.), Communicative Disorders: An Appraisal. Charles C Thomas, Springfield, IL.

Morris, H. L., Krueger, L. J., and Bumsted, R. M., 1982. Indications of congenital palatal incompetence (CPI) before diagnosis. Ann. Otol. Rhinol. Laryngol. 91:115–118.

Peterson, S. J. 1973. Speech pathology in craniofacial malformations other than cleft lip and palate. In: R. T. Wertz, (ed.), Orofacial Anomalies: Clinical and Research Implications. ASHA Reports 8. The American Speech and Hearing Association, Washington, DC.

Shelton, R. L., Jr. 1963. Therapeutic exercise and speech pathology. Asha 5:855–859.

Shelton, R. L., and Trier, W. C. 1976. Issues involved in the evaluation of velopharyngeal closure. Cleft Palate J. 13:127–137.

Shelton, R. L., Jr., Hahn, E., and Morris, H. L. 1968. Diagnosis and therapy. In: D. C. Spriestersbach and D. Sherman (eds.), Cleft Palate and Communication. Academic Press, New York.

Wells, C. G. 1971. Cleft Palate and Its Associated Speech Disorders. McGraw-Hill, New York.

CHAPTER **15**

# Functional Velopharyngeal Incompetence: Diagnosis and Management

*John E. Riski*

> *Riski advances the position that a small number of children display nasal air emission and pharyngeal fricative substitutions because of a functional inability to achieve velopharyngeal closure. He terms this disorder* functional velopharyngeal incompetence, *and provides diagnostic and treatment procedures.*

> 1. *According to Riski, what clinical behaviors are present in functional velopharyngeal incompetence that distinguishes it from organic velopharyngeal incompetence?*
> 2. *Describe in detail the diagnostic procedures advised by Riski to assess functional velopharyngeal incompetence. Which test or tests do you regard as most important?*
> 3. *What particular strategies does Riski recommend for rehabilitating the deviant articulatory patterns of individuals with functional velopharyngeal incompetence? Are there any others that you would add?*

NORMAL ORAL-NASAL RESONANCE and adequate oral breath pressure for speech require competent velopharyngeal valving. Velopharyngeal valving may involve excursions of the soft palate, the lateral pharyngeal walls, and/or the posterior pharyngeal wall (Passavant's Ridge) (Skolnick et al., 1973). Without adequate velopharyngeal valving, speech is characterized by hypernasal resonance, nasal air emission, and misarticulations such as glottal stop and pharyngeal fricative sound substitutions. Whereas hypernasal resonance, or hypernasality, is the perception of too much nasal resonance on vowels and vocalic consonants, nasal air emission is the projection of the air stream through the nose on pressure consonants.

Organic velopharyngeal incompetence (VPI) results from several structural abnormalities that affect velopharyngeal valving. A cleft of the soft palate may cause the soft palate to be short or to have a limited range of motion (Mazaheri et al., 1964). A deep nasopharynx may result adventitiously from an adenoidectomy or congenitally from cervical spine anomalies (Osborne et al., 1971). Reduced velar movement may also result from a neuromotor insult as in dysarthria.

Nasal air emission is most frequently associated with organic VPI. Several studies, however, have described the presence of nasal air emission as an articulatory feature in some individuals without demonstrable organic VPI (Peterson, 1975; Peterson-Falzone, 1981; Riski and Paone, 1980). These authors speculated that faulty learning of velopharyngeal valving may be, in part, responsible for this aberrant misarticulation. Riski and Paone (1980) refer to this use of nasal air emission as "functional" VPI. This term is used to distinguish a functional misuse of the velopharyngeal valve from an organic structural velopharyngeal deficit.

The following pattern was observed in the individuals labeled functional VPI: 1) no generalized hypernasality, 2) nasal air emission is sound specific (i.e., confined to the sibilant and/or affricate sounds with no nasal air emission on other pressure consonants), 3) complete and consistent velopharyngeal closure demonstrated with radiographic films and/or pressure flow studies for all sounds except the sibilant and/or affricate sounds; and 4) the ability to learn to produce /s/ without any nasal air flow in connected speech (Peterson, 1975; Peterson-Falzone; 1981; Riski and Paone, 1980).

In the period from February, 1978, to June, 1981, eight individuals were diagnosed as demonstrating a functional VPI at the Center for Speech and Hearing Disorders of Duke University Medical Center. These patients included three males and five females who ranged in age from 3 years, 5 months to 23 years. The referring diagnoses ranged from "talks through nose" to "submucous cleft palate" to "short immobile palate." Two individuals had hearing losses of a magnitude to account for the articulation deficit. In two other individuals, an adenoidectomy performed before 2 years of age may have resulted in a transient VPI and the maladaptive misarticulations. The four remaining individuals seemed to acquire the defective pattern through faulty learning. One of these individuals underwent an adenoidectomy at 9 years of age, but it appeared not to affect the child's speech pattern, as the parents reported no speech change after surgery.

In each case there was no evidence of clefting or neuromuscular deficits. Clinical tests indicated adequate oral air pressure, normal velopharyngeal closure in connected speech, and no abnormal nasal air escape for any of the sounds but the sibilants. Two individuals substituted nasal air emission for /s/ in /s/ blends only. Three substituted nasal air emission for /s/ in single element environments as well as in blends, and two substituted nasal air emission only in /s/ nasal blends. Finally, the voiceless pharyngeal fricative, denoted [ħ], was substituted for /s/ in /s/ blends by one individual.

## DIAGNOSIS

A standard protocol for evaluation of velopharyngeal function can be used to distinguish between functional and organic VPI (Riski and Millard, 1979). This protocol includes simple noninvasive clinical tests as well as quantitative measures of velopharyngeal valving. Also, the consistency of articulatory deviations are examined. This assessment is used as a basis for direct management: physical, such as surgery, or behavioral, such as speech remediation.

Clinical tests are used to rate speech qualities perceived with the unaided ear, to screen for the presence or absence of a velopharyngeal opening, or to judge the consistency of the velopharyngeal opening. Physical examination of the oral structures aids the identification of any structural anomalies.

### Perceptual Evaluation

In the perceptual evaluation, the clinician is encouraged to focus attention on the amount of intraoral air pressure. For example, does the /b/ in "boy" have adequate pressure and sound like a /b/ or is it lacking in pressure and sound like /m/? The individual with a functional VPI will exhibit adequate breath pressure on /b/ as well as the remaining plosive phonemes.

Oral-nasal resonance may be rated on a three-point scale: 1) normal resonance; 2) borderline hypernasality; or 3) excessive hypernasality. The individual with a functional VPI will exhibit normal resonance.

The consistency of nasal air escape is also examined. The individual with a functional VPI will exhibit many sounds that are produced without nasal air emission or facial grimacing. Typically, these are the plosive and the nonsibilant fricative phonemes. Nasal air emission and/or pharyngeal fricatives are sound specific and occur typically on the sibilants, although the affricates may be affected also.

**Clinical Screening Tests**

Screening tests of velopharyngeal closure are simple noninvasive methods for determining whether the velopharyngeal valve is open or closed. These tests do not measure how open the valve might be. The presence of nasal air flow indicates that velopharyngeal closure is not complete. On the other hand, a lack of nasal air flow usually indicates complete velopharyngeal closure.

The nasal listening tube and See Scape (1978) are especially sensitive to air flow. A nasal listening tube may be constructed using an 18″ piece of rubber tubing with nasal tips attached to each end. A satisfactory tubing size is 12 mm outside diameter and 8 mm inside diameter. One nasal tip is placed at the patient's most freely breathing nostril while the other is held to the clinician's ear. Any nasal air flow will be detected by the clinician. One word of caution: the nasal listening tube, like the stethoscope, may require some experience to use most effectively.

The See Scape consists of an 18″ length of rubber tubing with a nasal tip attached to one end. The other end is attached to a glass tube that contains a styrofoam piston. The nasal tip is placed at the patient's most freely breathing nostril. Nasal air flow will cause the styrofoam piston to elevate in the glass tube.

Because our concern is velopharyngeal closure, the speech sample used for these screening tests should incorporate sounds that normally require velopharyngeal closure. The plosive, nonsibilant fricative, affricate, and sibilant phonemes fall into this category. Because another concern is the consistency of velopharyngeal closure, an individual's performance on a plosive and nonsibilant fricative speech sample (e.g., "puppy, people, father, and five") may be contrasted with a sibilant and affricate speech sample (e.g., "sixty-six, sister, and church").

The individual with a functional VPI will demonstrate nasal air flow while producing the sibilant, and possibly the affricate speech sample. There will be no nasal air flow for the plosive and nonsibilant fricative speech sample. In contrast, the individual with an organic VPI will typically demonstrate nasal air flow for both speech samples.

## Oral-Facial Examination

An oral-facial examination can indicate the presence of structural anomalies and help distinguish between a VPI of organic and functional origin. The hard and soft palate should be examined for an oral-nasal fistula that may provide communication between the oral and nasal cavities. Additionally, the soft palate should be examined for neuromuscular insufficiency. Ask the patient to say single syllables which normally require velopharyngeal closure and still allow observation of the velum, such as /ka/. After the tongue releases from its lingual-velar contact in this syllable, the occurrence of velar elevation is readily observed. On single vowel utterances the patient may not elevate the soft palate and the erroneous conclusion could be drawn that the patient is unable to elevate the velum.

One possible reason for an absence of velar movement is that the use of a tongue depressor, in some instances, may elicit a gag reflex which can restrict further movement. Before proceeding with the exam, ask the patient to breathe through the nose with the tongue depressor still in place. The soft palate will return to its rest position and testing can be continued.

Look for signs of a submucous cleft. Examine the uvula. Is it bifid? Mucous may join the bifid tags. Examine the posterior aspect of the hard palate. The change in color from the hard to soft palate should outline the hard palate in the shape of a chevron or shield. A notch in the posterior portion of the hard palate indicates a submucous cleft. Examine the coloration of the hard and soft palate. The color should be pink. A bluish tint in the midline suggests structural discontinuity and a submucous cleft.

## Pressure Flow Testing

The purpose of the instrumental examination is to quantify VPI. Quantitative measures are used to assess normal functioning and to compare an individual's performance before and after management. Pressure flow testing of velopharyngeal function is used to document differences in oral and nasal air pressures as well as to quantify the rate of nasal air flow (Warren, 1975, 1976). A pressure score without nasal air flow indicates complete velopharyngeal closure. An individual with functional VPI will generate normal differential oral-nasal air pressure values in the range of 3 to 7 cm $H_2O$ with no nasal air flow for plosive sounds. Additionally, there will be an absence of nasal air flow on

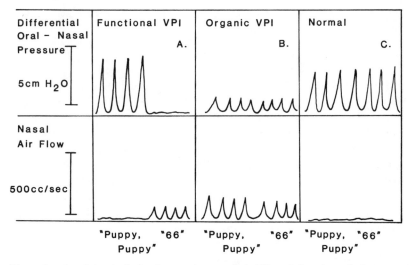

Figure 1. A print-out of simultaneously recorded differential oral-nasal air pressure (*top*) and nasal air flow (*bottom*). A, The individual with a functional VPI has normal pressure valves for plosives but substitutes nasal air emission for the sibilants. B, The individual with an organic VPI has reduced differential pressure scores throughout the speech sample and consistent nasal air flow accompanying all attempts at pressure sound production. C, The individual with normal velopharyngeal function has normal differential pressure valves and no nasal air escape throughout the speech sample.

nonsibilant fricative sounds. In contrast, excessive nasal air flow for sibilants and, possibly, affricates will be evident.

Figure 1 displays typical measures of differential oral-nasal air pressure and nasal air flow for individuals with functional VPI, organic VPI, and normal velopharyngeal closure. The individual with functional VPI has normal air pressure for the plosive-laden words without nasal air flow. The individual with organic VPI demonstrates reduced air pressure for both plosive and sibilant laden words and has nasal air flow for both speech samples. In contrast, the normal speaking individual has adequate oral pressure without nasal air flow for both the plosive and sibilant speech samples.

## MANAGEMENT

Functional VPI is an unusual articulation disorder. Unlike the management of organic VPI, for which surgery and/or a prosthetic appliance is usually recommended, functional VPI is treated by correcting the deviant articulation patterns. There is no evidence to suggest that surgery or palatal prosthetics will be beneficial without speech training.

Pharyngeal fricatives appear to be more resistant to treatment than nasal air emission for the following reason. Occluding the nostrils prevents nasal air escape and counteracts the physiological error of the velopharyngeal opening when nasal air emission is the target. The point of turbulence for a pharyngeal fricative is usually lingual-pharyngeal, however, and occurs, at times, as low as the epiglottis. Thus, a pharyngeal fricative has both an oral and a nasal outlet and its production cannot be prevented by occluding the nose. It follows, therefore, that occluding the nostrils is also a simple diagnostic technique to differentiate between nasal air emission and pharyngeal fricatives. These two types of misarticulations of course, can co-occur. For example, in a recent evaluation in our Center, a 9-year-old male with a repaired cleft substituted nasal air emission for /s/ and /z/, and substituted a pharyngeal fricative for /ʃ/, tʃ, and dʒ/.

## Facilitating Postures

An initial goal of treatment is to establish the correct articulatory posture for the oral sibilants. The lingual-alveolar phoneme /t/ is useful in initiating this process. The patient is instructed to say a /t/ and to continue into an /s/ (i.e., tsss). A drinking straw is used to increase the patient's perceptual awareness of oral turbulence. When the straw is placed in front of the mouth so that air passes through the straw, a perceptible turbulence is evident. During transition from the /t/ to an /s/, the patient is instructed to maintain the turbulent sound of /t/, which is perceptibly different from either nasal air emission or pharyngeal friction.

A second articulatory posture that will facilitate the production of /s/ is /ʃ/, provided of course that /ʃ/ is produced correctly. The individual imitates the examiner's production of /ʃ/, first, with the lips rounded and then with the lips retracted. The retraction of the lips will often cause tongue-palatal constriction for /ʃ/ to move anteriorly to form /s/.

A third technique for facilitating /s/ is to initiate oral air flow with the interdental /θ/. The individual is then asked to imitate the examiner who retracts the tongue to a postdental position. We have found this technique to be the most successful method for facilitating /s/ when a pharyngeal fricative sound substitution is present.

## Use of a Nose Clip

The use of a swimmer's nose clip to occlude the nares is another approach for obstructing nasal air and facilitating oral air flow early in the remediation program. Once the correct pattern of oral air flow for /s/ is established the use of the nose clip may be discontinued.

## Visual Feedback

The use of a See Scape provides visual feedback to a patient about nasal air flow. When the styrofoam piston remains at the bottom of the glass tube, it signals complete velopharyngeal closure and an accurately produced /s/. Coupled with ear training, it provides a basis for teaching the difference between correct and incorrect productions.

## Reverse Chaining

Once the /s/ has been established it may be chained appropriately into a series of phonemes. Chaining is especially useful in learning /s/ blends. For example, the word "spoke" may be divided into chains /s/ and /pok/. Each of these members of the chain is strengthened separately by a series of reinforced repetitions and then an attempt is made to construct the entire chain in reverse, or right to left, order. The patient is asked to repeat first /pok/ and then to preceed that production with an /s/ to produce /s::pok/.

## CASE STUDY

The following case study describes the use of the evaluation and management of functional VPI in a young female patient seen at the Duke University Center for Speech and Hearing Disorders. The patient, H.F., was 3 years, 3 months old when referred for evaluation of velopharyngeal function by her pediatrician because of a "nasal quality" in her speech. She had experienced numerous ear infections which prompted an adenoidectomy with bilateral myringotomy and tubes at 18 months of age. Subsequent audiometric testing at 3 years, 9 months indicated normal hearing bilaterally.

Evaluation revealed no hypernasality, no evidence of clefting, and no neuromuscular deficits. Clinical testing of velopharyngeal closure using the See Scape indicated complete closure for all phonemes except the /s/ in nasal blends. The /s/ phoneme was produced normally without nasal air escape when it appeared as a single element. Further testing indicated the omission of /s/ in other blends. Additionally, other developmental errors such as f/θ and w/r were noted. Initial testing indicated that correct /s/ nasal blends could be achieved easily using reverse chaining. A home treatment program was initiated and the patient was given a return appointment for 6 months.

On reevaluation, the home program was labeled a failure because the child had generalized the substitution of nasal air emission for /s/ to all /s/ blends. Pressure flow testing (Figure 2) indicated adequate oral pressure with no nasal air flow for correctly produced pressure phonemes. However, nasal air emission was consistently found in all

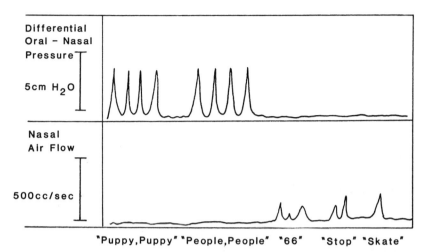

"Puppy,Puppy" "People,People"  "66"    "Stop" "Skate"

Figure 2.   Print-out for patient H.F. of differential oral/nasal pressure (*top*) and rate of nasal air flow (*bottom*). Note that for the plosive speech sample there is adequate differential pressure with no nasal air flow, which indicates complete velopharyngeal closure. Also note that for /s/ blends there is a spike of nasal air flow for each /s/. Differential pressure was not measured for the /s/ blend sample.

/s/ blends. A lateral radiograph, taken during sustained /i/ phonation in the syllable /pi/, demonstrated complete velopharyngeal closure (Figure 3).

At this point, the patient was enrolled in individual articulation remediation and attended a total of 16 one-half hour sessions before being discharged. Correct /s/ blend production was easily established using reverse chaining. Then /s/ production was taught in single words, short phrases, and long phrases. Imitation was used first, then speech was elicited spontaneously with picture stimuli. During the last treatment session, no instances of nasal air emission were noted in connected speech or in conversational speech.

**CONCLUSION**

The individual with a functional VPI is often regarded as a candidate for palatal surgery when first referred to the speech-language pathologist. Sometimes parents are told that their child has a cleft palate or a submucous cleft, when in fact, the velopharyngeal structure is normal and capable of normal function, but is used incorrectly. The correct treatment is articulation training and not surgery or a prosthetic appliance. The individual with a functional VPI is not to be confused with the individual with a borderline, or touch, velopharyngeal closure.

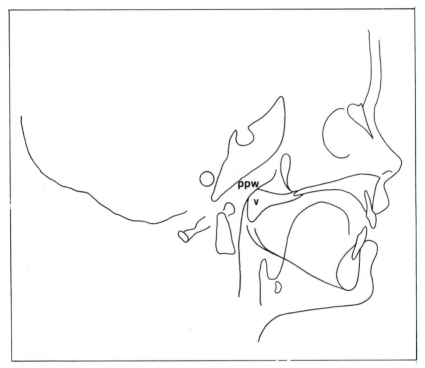

Figure 3.    A lateral cephalometric radiograph of patient H.F. She is sustaining the vowel /i/ which was preceded by the plosive /p/, in /pi:/. The velum (V) has elevated to make contact with the posterior pharyngeal wall (PPW).

These individuals are, typically, mildly hypernasal, and consistent nasal air escape may be evident for plosives as well as sibilants. The individual with a true organic VPI will not profit from articulation training without attention first being given to corrective surgery and/or the appropriate fitting of a prothesis (Van Demark, 1974).

The etiology of functional VPI remains open to investigation. For two of the eight individuals described above, a history of a hearing loss may have precipitated the articulation errors. In two others the VPI followed adenoidectomy. No etiology could be determined, however, in four of the cases. In those four cases we speculate that the misarticulation involves faulty learning in agreement with Peterson (1975).

The failure to identify any organic deficit responsible for the faulty use of the velopharyngeal valve does not preclude the presence of minimal organic incompetence during the formative years of articulation learning. Isshiki et al. (1968) have speculated that adequate velopharyngeal closure may be more important for acquisition of correct articulation than for its maintainence. Because sibilants require greater sustained air pressure flow requirements than plosives, it follows that the acquisition of correct sibilant production may place a great demand on physiological competence.

Several clinical observations seem to support the position that VPI can have a functional basis. On several occasions when teaching the /s/ sound to young children, we found that they produced nasal emission while trying to produce sibilants. This latter observation was also made by Smith (1973) who found that his young child produced "nasal lisps" in his effort to produce /sn/ clusters.

In summary, the articulation deficits of nasal air emission and pharyngeal fricative sound substitutions may be found in individuals with intact velopharyngeal mechanisms. This phenomenon has been termed functional VPI to distinguish it from organic VPI. A functional VPI is characterized by the absence of hypernasal resonance, by the presence of nasal air emission, and/or pharyngeal fricatives that are restricted to sibilant phonemes. Key diagnostic features that distinguish functional VPI from an organically based deficit are the ability of the patient to produce plosives and fricatives with complete velopharyngeal closure and to learn correct sibilant production with complete velopharyngeal closure. It is the responsibility of the speech-language pathologist to make an accurate differential diagnosis of organic versus functional VPI and to implement a management program to treat the associated articulatory defects.

## REFERENCES

Isshiki, N., Honjow, I., and Marimoto, M. 1968. Effects of velopharyngeal incompetence upon speech. Cleft Palate J. 5:297–310.

Mazaheri, M., Millard, R. T., and Ericson, D. M. 1964. Cineradiographic comparison of normal to noncleft subjects with velopharyngeal inadequacy. Cleft Palate J. 1:199–209.

Osborne, G. S., Pruzansky, S., and Koepp-Baker, H. 1971. Upper cervical spine anomalies and osseous nasopharyngeal depth. J. Speech Hear. Res. 14:14–22.

Peterson, S. J. 1975. Nasal emission as a component of misarticulation of sibilants and affricates. J. Speech Hear. Disord. 40:106–114.

Peterson-Falzone, S. J. 1981. Nasal distortions and compensatory articulations in velopharyngeal competent speakers. Paper presented at IV International Congress on Cleft Palate and Related Craniofacial Anomalies. May, Acapulco, Mexico.

Riski, J. E., and Millard, R. T. 1979. Processes of speech: Evaluation and treatment. In: H. K. Cooper et al. (eds.), Cleft Palate and Cleft Lip: A Team Approach to Clinical Management and Rehabilitation of the Patient. W. B. Saunders, Philadelphia, PA.

Riski, J. E., and Paone, C. A. 1980. Functional velopharyngeal incompetency: Diagnosis and management. Paper presented at American Speech-Language-Hearing Association. November, Detroit, MI.

See Scape. 1978. C. C. Publications, Gladstone OR.

Skolnick, M. L., McCall, G., and Barnes, M. 1973. The sphincteric mechanism of velopharyngeal closure. Cleft Palate J. 10:286–294.

Smith, N. V. 1973. Acquisition of Phonology. Cambridge University Press, Cambridge.

Van Demark, D. R. 1974. Some results of speech therapy for children with cleft palate. Cleft Palate J. 11:41–49.

Warren, D. W. 1975. The determination of velopharyngeal incompetence by aerodynamic and acoustic techniques. Clin. Plastic Surg. 2:299–304.

Warren, D. W. 1976. Aerodynamics of speech production. In: N. Lass (ed.), Contemporary Issues in Experimental Phonetics. Academic Press, New York.

# CHAPTER 16

# Management of Acquired Articulation Disorders in Adults

*Jeri A. Logemann*

> *Logemann directs her attention to clinical management decisions for the adult with an acquired articulatory disorder. Diagnostic goals and options for treatment are discussed for patients with degenerative and nondegenerative vocal tract impairments.*

1.  *What are the universal proposals Logemann advances as important considerations in the treatment of acquired articulation problems in adults?*
2.  *What procedures does Logemann recommend for the evaluation of vocal tract control? Are there additional evaluations that you would recommend?*
3.  *What philosophy does Logemann put forward with regard to treatment? In your answer include Logemann's reference to intelligibility and the status of the impairment.*
4.  *Describe the compensatory strategies that can be used with patients with degenerative and nondegenerative disorders.*

ACQUIRED ARTICULATION PROBLEMS in the adult result most frequently from two etiologies: neurological damage of sudden or progressive origin (Canter, 1967; Darley et al., 1975), and damage to vocal tract structures caused by trauma or surgery for head and neck cancer (Logemann et al., 1977; Logemann and Bytell, 1978). Although these two groups differ markedly in the speech symptomatology they display, there are many similarities in their evaluation and management. This chapter defines a single model, in the form of a decision tree, that the speech-language pathologist may find to be useful in handling adult patients with newly acquired articulation deficits. It is based upon universal assumptions about the management of adults with these disorders.

The first universal assumption in handling adult patients with a history of new speech disturbances pertains to an assumption clinicians need to make about adult patients without cortical damage. It is that the phonological structure underlying their articulatory production or performance deficit is normal, and that whatever etiology caused changes in anatomy or neuromotor control has not affected linguistic competence. Obviously, if cortical damage is suspected, this assumption cannot be made.

The second universal assumption lies in the approach used to evaluate and treat articulation deficits in these populations. These articulation disorders should be thought of as disruptions in vocal tract control rather than changes in function of a single articulator. Unfortunately, much of the literature on articulation disorders acquired in adulthood can be misleading. Often, investigators have examined one isolated aspect of vocal tract control, such as lingual and/or labial functioning of patients with particular neurological lesions, without defining the effect of the disorder on control of the entire vocal tract (Dworkin et al., 1980; Leanderson et al., 1972; Logemann and Fisher, 1981; Meyerson, 1973). These studies have a narrow focus and require the reader to have sufficient background information to place the results in the larger context of motor control of the entire vocal tract. This type of focused analysis can leave the reader with the erroneous impression that these authors conceptualize acquired articulation disorders in the adult in the narrow sense. Viewed within this narrow perspective, articulation disorders are a disruption of the behavior of particular articulators rather than a disorder in neuromotor control or structural competence of the vocal tract which can include any or all of the following: respiratory, laryngeal, pharyngeal, palatal, lingual, buccal, labial, and mandibular movement patterns in the production of a sequence of phonetic targets (Canter, 1963, 1965a, 1965b; Georgian and Logemann, 1982; Kent and Netsell, 1975; Linebaugh, 1979; Netsell et al., 1975). In fact, the constraints of complexity and availability of subjects often encourage investigators to compromise, that is, either to examine one aspect of vocal tract control in a large number of patients (Dworkin et al., 1980; Logemann and Fisher, 1981) or all aspects of vocal tract control in a small number of patients (Georgian and Logemann, 1982; Kent and Netsell, 1975).

In some respects, the communication disorders in these adults might appropriately be described as intelligibility problems, because the term *articulation* sometimes triggers the narrower view of select involvement of articulators, whereas *intelligibility* forces the clinician to examine the impact of all aspects of vocal tract function on the ultimate outcome of speech production: its understandability to the listener. For this reason, the clinician should examine thoroughly the structural competence and functional capacity of all aspects of the speech production system, from labial to respiratory, and their coordination, as indicated in the decision tree in Figure 1 (Darley et al., 1975; Netsell and Daniel, 1979; Netsell and Hixon, 1978).

## EVALUATION OF VOCAL TRACT CONTROL

The details of the anatomical and neuromotor test battery will not be discussed here except to highlight three important aspects of evaluation that are often excluded: detailed phonetic analysis, radiographic examination of speech and swallowing, and careful assessment of respiratory and laryngeal function, as they may contribute to speech intelligibility.

A detailed phonetic analysis of speech production should be made, and should include the listener's perceptions of labial and lingual articulatory placements, hypernasality and nasal emission, aspiration, voicing and devoicing, and intonation and juncture patterns. A careful analysis of speech production, perhaps best achieved with narrow phonetic transcription, will provide information on the coordination of laryngeal, palatal, lingual, labial, and respiratory function in connected speech, and assist the clinician in identifying which components of vocal tract control significantly impair the patient's speech production.

Also included in the battery should be a radiographic examination of vocal tract control for speech and swallow, as comparison of motor patterns for the two functions can provide valuable information on location of the neurologic lesion, stage of deterioration in neuromotor control in degenerative disease processes, and treatment planning (Logemann et al., 1977). The radiographic "test battery" should consist of videofluoroscopic studies of the vocal tract, including lateral

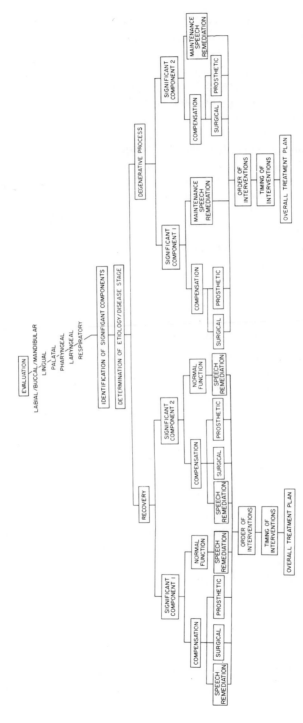

Figure 1.   Decision tree in the management of adults with acquired articulation disorders.

views of the entire vocal tract (from the lips anteriorly to the pharyngeal wall posteriorly, from the roof of the nasal cavity superiorly to the subglottal area inferiorly) with the patient seated. The recording should take place while the patient produces sentences that contain all places of articulation and all manners of production. Additionally, all places and manners of articulation should be placed in VCCV (vowel, consonant, consonant, vowel) context to examine coarticulatory abilities, such as in the phases *up to, up key, if so, is he, I'd know,* and so on.

After completion of the speech samples, the patient should remain seated in the lateral plane for videofluoroscopic assessment of deregulation. Particular attention is given to the oral preparatory, oral, and pharyngeal stages of deglutition. Two swallows should be examined after taking each of the following: 1) one-half teaspoon of a liquid barium; 2) one-quarter teaspoon barium paste of pudding-like consistency; and 3) a cookie or other material coated with barium requiring mastication. Recording of these radiographic studies on videotape permits detailed motion analysis at slow motion and frame by frame. Comparison of the range, speed, and pattern of motion of vocal tract structures during speech and deglutition can provide significant information on the etiology of the patient's disorder, particularly if it is of neurologic origin (Logemann et al., 1977). After the studies in the lateral plane are completed, the patient should be turned and the examination should continue in the anterior-posterior plane. In this view the patient should be asked: 1) to prolong the /s/ and /ʃ/ phonemes for several seconds; 2) to repeat several swallows of whichever materials were most difficult in the lateral study; and 3) to prolong the vowel /a/ for several seconds with the head tilted backward. On the prolonged consonant productions, the gross symmetry of lingual function can be examined. Asymmetry in filling and emptying of the valleculae and the pyriform sinuses can be evaluated during swallowing. During prolonged vocal production with the head backward, the gross symmetry of vocal fold movement can be assessed.

Examination of laryngeal function should include indirect laryngoscopy by an otolaryngologist so that vocal cord mobility and degree of vocal fold adduction can be defined. Laryngeal diadochokinetic rates and phonation times are also informative. During phonation time trials, the clinician should observe the movement patterns (rate, range, smoothness) of the upper chest, mid-lower chest, and upper abdomen during inhalation and exhalation. Effects of postural changes on chest and abdominal movements during phonation should be noted. Tests of postural modifications might include standing, sitting without back support, side lying, and leaning on the arms of a chair while sitting or standing. Improved control of respiratory movements during phonation may also be achieved when the patient resists the pressure of the clinician's hand against his abdominal or upper chest wall. Instrumental techniques for measuring pressure, air flow, and patterns of respiratory movement are also helpful, and may be used to provide feedback/monitoring information in treatment (Becker, 1973; Hardy, 1965; Iwata et al., 1972; Netsell and Hixon, 1978). For example, patients may be asked to watch instrumental write outs and maintain certain levels by changing muscle control.

From this detailed evaluation, the speech-language pathologist will have identified: 1) those structures or aspects of neuromotor control of the vocal tract that are affected; 2) the exact nature of the abnormality; and 3) those components of vocal tract dysfunction that have the greatest impact on the patient's intelligibility. These data may also be compared to existing information on vocal tract dysfunctions in specific neurological diseases to assist in diagnosis of particular medical conditions, such as multiple sclerosis and amyotrophic lateral sclerosis (Berry et al., 1974; Blonsky et al., 1975; Critchley, 1981; Darley et al., 1968, 1969; Farmakides and Boone, 1970; Linebaugh, 1979; Logemann et al., 1977).

### ESTABLISHMENT OF TREATMENT GOALS

As indicated in the decision tree in Figure 1, the etiology of the patient's disorder and the data on abnormalities in vocal tract structures or neuromotor controls most responsible for intelligibility disturbances should be used by the clinician to determine potential goals of management and the ordering of these goals. A treatment goal should be established for each of the vocal tract components which have been identified by the clinician as playing a significant role in the patient's low intelligibility, even if the decision is that no type of treatment is viable.

The etiological classification can be used to assign patients to one of two groups: those whose lesion or damage can be expected to improve with recovery, and those whose disease process will entail progressive impairment in vocal tract control. Among the degenerative diseases are untreatable cancer, a number of neurological diseases, and muscular deterioration. When planning management goals, the clinician would find it helpful to predict the pattern of change from the available information on sequence of recovery or degeneration in vocal tract structures associated with certain lesions or diseases. Unfortunately, such information has been reported on only a few subgroups of patients (Brown et al., 1970; Dworkin and Hartman, 1979; Kent et al., 1979; Logemann et al., 1973; Mackay, 1963; Mawdesley, 1973).

Table 1.    Example of a coarticulation exercise

| Target production | | Feature differences |
|---|---|---|
| but | CVC | |
| but can | CVCCVC | 1 feature different (place) |
| but dot | CVCCVC | 1 feature different (voice) |
| but said | CVCCVC | 1 feature different (manner) |
| but bite | CVCCVC | 2 features different (place, voice) |
| but not | CVCCVC | 2 features different (manner, voice) |
| but fat | CVCCVC | 2 features different (place, manner) |
| but vote | CVCCVC | 3 features different (adjacent place) |
| but run | CVCCVC | 3 features different (disparate place) |

This paucity of information is probably related to the fact that it is difficult to locate a sufficient number of patients with identical disease sites or lesion locations in each carefully defined stage of recovery or degeneration. And such research requires time consuming data collection and analysis procedures. However, the clinician can use information on the patient's own pattern of recovery or deterioration to date as an indicator of the potential for continued improvement or degeneration in particular aspects of vocal tract control.

### Definition of Management Goals and Strategies
### When Some Degree of Recovery Is Anticipated

For those patients whose articulatory deficits result from trauma or surgery, some improvement is likely as they show recovery. For some of these patients, a return to normal function in a particular aspect of vocal tract control is a viable goal of treatment. An intervention program is then designed to improve these selected aspects of motor control. For example, speech remediation to restore normal function in the tongue generally includes range of motion exercises, tongue placement exercises for target phonemes, phonetically controlled articulation drills to develop accuracy of tongue placement and coarticulation, and speed of movement drills. Providing patients with additional information on the positioning and rate of movement of articulatory structures or air flow through instrumental techniques, such as EMG and pneumography, is rapidly increasing in use (Daniel and Guitar, 1978; Hand et al., 1979; Hanson and Metter, 1980; Netsell and Cleeland, 1973). In the advanced stages of treatment, when isolated speech production gestures have been established, but coordination of lingual, labial, and palatal movements with voicing and respiration needs improvement, co-articulatory drills are recommended, such as those in Table 1.

An alternative goal for these patients is to develop compensatory strategies for permanent deficits in structure and/or function. As indicated in Figure 1, three types of compensatory strategies are available to the patient whose vocal tract control will not deteriorate: 1) speech remediation directed toward teaching alternate speech production strategies, such as bilabial productions of phonemes normally produced in the tongue tip and blade alveolar ridge places of articulation; 2) surgical compensations, such as injecting teflon into the posterior pharyngeal wall to create an anterior-projecting mass for the velum to contact (Furlow et al., 1982), injecting teflon into one vocal fold to improve laryngeal adduction (Dedo et al., 1973; Goff, 1969; Von Leden et al., 1967), constructing a pharyngeal flap to reduce nasal emission (Karpetansky, 1975), or surgically reconstructing or freeing the tongue (Logemann et al., 1977); and 3) prosthetic interventions such as palatal lift prostheses to improve velopharyngeal closure (Schweiger et al., 1970) or hard palate augmentation prostheses to lower the palatal vault and facilitate tongue to palate contacts (Cantor et al., 1969; Wheeler et al., 1980).

### Definition of Management Goals and
### Strategies in the Presence of Degenerative Processes

Patients with changes in vocal tract control resulting from degenerative processes present the speech-language pathologist with two choices in the selection of management goals for each aspect of vocal tract control which is significantly reducing intelligibility. Because the patient's functioning can be expected to worsen over time, it is important for the clinician to work with the patient's physician to determine anticipated progression and rate of deterioration in functional capacity of each aspect of vocal tract control. In most instances, these decisions are clinical judgments based on the experience of the professionals involved rather than calculations based on available research data.

When the clinician determines that degeneration of vocal tract control will be slow, compensatory strategies may be used to overcome particular problems such as reduced laryngeal adduction or reduced tongue elevation. These compensatory strategies may be successful for long periods of time. In some cases, as the patient's disorder progresses, one compensatory strategy may need to be traded for another. Surgical and/or prosthetic compensations may be appropriate for these patients, and may sometimes be used sequentially as deterioration progresses. For example, a Parkinson patient with reduced laryngeal adduction who initially received a teflon injection into one vocal fold (a surgical procedure) to improve glottal closure, may find that after several years, vocal fold movement begins to deteriorate further. At this point the patient may be fitted with a voice amplifier (a prosthetic compensation). As a patient's speech production approaches anarthria, a severe involvement of multiple components of vocal tract control, alternate communication systems become necessary. Training in use of these devices is usually the responsibility of the speech-language pathologist. Teaching muscular compensations is often unsuccessful in these patients with degenerative diseases because of the progressive nature of the dysfunction and, in some particular conditions such as Parkinson's disease, the patient's inability to carry over gains made in the structured therapy sessions to daily communication. For this reason, muscular compensations are not listed among treatment choices in Figure 1.

Maintenance of current function for some aspects of vocal tract control may be a viable goal of speech remediation for some patients with degenerative disease processes. For example, patients with a diagnosis of Parkinsonism may benefit from an exercise program that is designed to maintain range, rate, and precision of movement of certain vocal tract structures for speech. These programs generally focus on labial, lingual, laryngeal, and respiratory controls. In these cases the speech-language pathologist can provide the patient with a home program of exercises that is to be completed one to three times daily. Little attention has been given to the development and evaluation of intervention strategies designed to maintain vocal tract function for particular types of patients, although clinical experience indicates such programs may be warranted.

## SEQUENCE AND TIMING OF INTERVENTIONS

Before the overall treatment plan has been initiated for any adult patient with acquired articulation disorders, the speech-language pathologist must determine the order and timing of the various interventions, if more than one parameter of vocal tract functioning is affected. Frequently, a team of professionals which includes the patient's physician, otolaryngologist, maxillofacial prosthodontist, and speech-language pathologist must evaluate the potential intervention strategies in relation to the patient's overall medical treatment and medication schedule and then outline together the best sequence of therapies.

Effects of various medications on speech functioning have been examined by only a few investigators whose findings are inconclusive. Clinically, however, patients with degenerative processes often make maximum gains in vocal tract control at the time of introduction of a new medication, when medication dosage is being regulated, or other treatment is being implemented (Birkmayer and Hornykiewicz, 1961; Critchley, 1981; Nakano et al., 1973; Rigrodsky and Morrison, 1970).

## SUMMARY

This discussion presents a sequence of clinical decision making in diagnosis and intervention for acquired articulatory disorders in adults. It is based upon the recognition of these articulation disorders as disruptions in vocal tract control rather than dysfunction of a single articulatory structure. Some important components of the diagnostic test battery are described and choices of treatment to improve disordered intelligibility are defined according to the etiology of the patient's problem. Intervention options to improve communication are outlined for the patient who may be anticipated to recover, as well as the patient whose vocal tract control will continue to deteriorate. The model of decision making presented here is based on our current knowledge of acquired articulatory disorders in adults and the impact of currently available treatment approaches. Unfortunately, some information which would ease the decision making process for the clinician is not available. For example, details of recovery from vocal tract dysfunction related to specific neurological lesions are not documented for all types of lesions. Nor is the rate and nature of progressive deterioration in vocal tract control in particular neurological diseases completely defined. The impact of various instrumentation techniques such as EMG or pneumography in the assessment and treatment of articulatory disorders in adults is just beginning to be evaluated systematically.

These important details are not yet completely understood. The model presented here, however, assists the clinician seeing adult patients with acquired articulatory disorders to structure the decision-making process in diagnosis and treatment so that a maximum amount of accurate and pertinent information is available upon which to base management procedures to assure the patient optimal treatment.

## REFERENCES

Becker, N. 1973. A study of the effects of posture on durational and rate measures of breathing of athetoid cerebral palsied children and normal children. Unpublished doctoral dissertation. Northwestern University, Evanston, IL.

Berry, W., Darley, F., Aronson, A., and Goldstein, N. 1974. Dysarthria in Wilson's Disease. J. Speech Hear. Res. 17:169–183.

Birkmayer, W., and Hornykiewicz, O. 1961. Der L-3,4-Dioxyphenylalanin (-Dopa)-effekt bei der Parkinson-akinese, Wien. Klin. Wochnschr. 73:787–799.

Blonsky, E., Logemann, J., Boshes, B., and Fisher, H. 1975. Comparison of speech and swallowing function in patients with tremor disorders and in normal geriatric patients: A cineradiographic study. J. Gerontol. 30:299–303.

Brown, J., Darley, F., and Aronson, E. 1970. Ataxic dysarthria. Int. J. Neurol. 7:302–318.

Canter, G. 1963. Speech characteristics of patients with Parkinson's disease. I. Intensity, pitch and duration. J. Speech Hear. Disord. 28:221–229.

Canter, G. 1965a. Speech characteristics of patients with Parkinson's disease. II. Physiological support for speech. J. Speech Hear. Disord. 30:44–49.

Canter, G. 1965b. Speech characteristics of patients with Parkinson's disease. III. Articulation, diadochokinesis and overall speech adequacy. J. Speech Hear. Disord. 30:217–224.

Canter, G. 1967. Neuromotor pathologies of speech. Am. J. Phys. Med. 46:659–666.

Cantor, R., Curtis, T., Shipp, T., et al. 1969. Maxillary speech prostheses for mandibular surgical defects. J. Prosthet. Dent. 22:253–357.

Critchley, E. 1981. Speech disorders of Parkinsonism: A review. J. Neurol. Neurosurg. Psych. 44:751–758.

Daniel, B., and Guitar, B. 1978. EMG feedback and recovery of facial and speech gestures following neural anastomosis. J. Speech Hear. Disord. 43:9–20.

Darley, F., Aronson, A., and Brown, J. 1968. Motor speech signs in neurologic disease. Med. Clin. North Am. 52:840–844.

Darley, F., Aronson, A., and Brown, J. 1969. Differential diagnostic patterns of dysarthria. J. Speech Hear. Res. 12:462–496.

Darley, F., Aronson, A., and Brown, J. 1975. Motor Speech Disorders. W. B. Saunders, Philadelphia.

Dedo, H., Urrea, R., and Lawson, L. 1973. Intracordal injection of teflon in the treatment of 135 patients with dysphonia. Ann. Otoloaryngol. 82:661–667.

Dworkin, J., Aronson, A., and Mulder, D. 1980. Tongue force in normals and in dysarthric patients with amyotrophic lateral sclerosis. J. Speech Hear. Res. 23:828–837.

Dworkin, J., and Hartman, D. 1979. Progressive speech deterioration and dysphagia in amyotrophic lateral sclerosis. Arch. Phys. Med. Rehabil. 60:423–425.

Farmakides, M., and Boone, D. 1970. Speech problems of patients with multiple sclerosis. J. Speech Hear. Disord. 25:385–390.

Furlow, L., Williams, W., Eisenbach, C., and Bzoch, K. 1982. A long-term study on treating velopharyngeal insufficiency by Teflon injection. Cleft Palate J. 19:47–56.

Georgian, D., and Logemann, J. 1982. Compensatory articulation patterns of a patient after 20% glossectomy. J. Speech Hear. Disord. 47:77–82.

Goff, W. 1969. Teflon injection for vocal cord paralysis. Arch. Otolaryngol. 90:99–102.

Hand, C., Burns, M., and Ireland, E. 1979. Treatment of hypertonicity in muscles of lip retraction. Biofeedback Self Regulation 4:171–181.

Hanson, W., and Metter, E. 1980. DAF as instrumental treatment for dysarthria in progressive supra nuclear palsy: A case report. J. Speech Hear. Disord. 45:268–276.

Hardy, J. 1965. Air flow and air pressure studies. ASHA Rep. 1:141–152.

Iwata, S., von Leden, H., and Williams, D. 1972. Air flow measurement during phonation. J. Commun. Disord. 5:67–69.

Karpetansky, D. 1975. Transverse pharyngeal flaps: A dynamic repair for velopharyngeal insufficiency. Cleft Palate J. 12:44–50.

Kent, R., and Netsell, R. 1975. A case study of an ataxic dysarthric: Cineradiographic and spectrographic observation. J. Speech Hear. Disord. 40:115–134.

Kent, R., Netsell, R., and Abbs, J. 1979. Acoustic characteristics of dysarthria associated with cerebellar disease. J. Speech Hear. Res. 22:627–648.

Leanderson, R., Meyerson, B., and Persson, A. 1972. Lip muscle function in Parkinsonian dysarthria. Acta Otolaryngol. 74:271–278.

Linebaugh, C. 1979. The dysarthrias of Shy-Drager syndrome. J. Speech Hear. Disord. 44:55–60.

Logemann, J., and Bytell, D. 1978. Articulation patterns of five groups of head and neck surgical patients. Paper presented at the Annual Convention of the American Speech and Hearing Association. November, San Francisco.

Logemann, J., and Fisher, H. 1981. Vocal tract control in Parkinson's disease: Phonetic feature analysis of misarticulations. J. Speech Hear. Disord. 46:348–352.

Logemann, J., Boshes, B., and Fisher, H. 1973. The steps in the degeneration of speech and voice control in Parkinson's disease. In: J. Siegried (eds.), Parkinson's Disease. Hans Huber, Vienna.

Logemann, J., Boshes, B., Blonsky, E., and Fisher, H. 1977. Speech and swallowing evaluation in the differential diagnosis of neurologic disease. Neurol. Neurochirigia, Psych. 18:71–78.

Logemann, J, Fisher, H., and Bytell, D. 1977. Functional effects of reconstruction in partially glossectomized patients. Paper presented at the Annual Convention of the American Speech and Hearing Association, November, Chicago.

Mackay, R. 1963. Course and prognosis in amyotrophic lateral sclerosis. Arch. Neurol. 8:117–127.

Mawdesley, C. 1973. Speech in Parkinsonism. In: D. Calne (ed.), Advances in Neurology 3: Progress in the treatment of Parkinsonism. Raven Press, London.

Meyerson, B. 1973. EMG characteristics of labial articulatory muscles in Parkinsonism. In: J. Siegfried (ed.), Parkinson's Disease. Hans Huber, Vienna.

Nakano, K. Zubick, H., and Tyler, H. 1973. Speech defects in Parkinsonian patients. Neurology 23:865–870.

Netsell, R., and Cleeland, C. 1973. Modification of lip hypertonia in dysarthria using EMG feedback. J. Speech Hear. Disord. 38:131–140.

Netsell, R., and Daniel, B. 1979. Dysarthria in adults: Physiologic approach to rehabilitation. Arch. Phys. Med. Rehabil. 60:502–508.

Netsell, R., and Hixon, T. 1978. Noninvasive method for clinically estimating subglottal air pressure. J. Speech Hear. Disord. 43:326–330.

Netsell, R., Daniel, B., and Celesia, C. 1975. Acceleration and weakness in Parkinsonian dysarthrias. J. Speech Hear. Disord. 40:467–480.

Rigrodsky, S., and Morrison, E. 1970. Speech changes in Parkinsonism during L-Dopa therapy: Preliminary findings. J. Am. Geriatr. Soc. 18:142–151.

Schweiger, J., Netsell, R., and Sommerfield, R. 1970. Prosthetic management and speech improvement in individuals with dysarthria of the palate. J. Am. Dent. Assoc. 80:1348–1353.

Von Leden, H., Yanagihara, N., and Werner-Kukuk, E. 1967. Teflon in unilateral vocal cord paralysis—Preoperative and postoperative function studies. Arch. Otolaryngol. 85:666–671.

Wheeler, R., Logemann, J., and Rosen, M. 1980. Maxillary reshaping prostheses: Effectiveness in improving speech and swallowing of postsurgical oral cancer patients. J. Prosthet. Dent. 43:313–319.

# CHAPTER 17

# Selected Alternatives to Articulation Training for the Dysarthric Adult

*John C. Rosenbek*

*Rosenbek discusses a number of training procedures for the patient with dysarthria. As he indicates, the current strategies for treatment are largely experimental and, therefore, the clinician should be open minded and resourceful.*

1. *What does Rosenbek regard as the essential first step in the treatment of dysarthria? Although he regards it as an essential first step, why must it be applied continuously throughout treatment?*

2. *Explain why attention is given to posture in the treatment of dysarthria? Describe the prosthetic devices and their application recommended by Rosenbek that may be used to alter the posture of the dysarthric patient?*

3. *What does Rosenbek mean by "increasing effort" while speaking? Do you agree with this approach?*

4. *What procedures does Rosenbek recommend for use to alter the speaking rate and prosody of the dysarthric patient? What rational does he provide for their use? Would you use these procedures?*

DYSARTHRIA IS A neuromotor speech disorder. The structures of respiration, the larynx, the velopharynx, the tongue, the lips, and the jaw are usually involved unless the lesion is outside the central nervous system where more limited deficits are possible. Optimum care involves speech treatment, not just articulation treatment, even when the deficit is limited. Indeed, traditional articulation treatment alone is seldom salutary for the dysarthric talker even if the impairment involves only his tongue, lips, or jaw. Of course, elements of articulation treatment are included, but more is involved. Other components for the treatment of dysarthria include: counseling, postural adjustment, increasing effort, and altering speaking rate, rhythm, and stress. These elements are featured in this chapter.

## COUNSELING

For dysarthric speakers to improve, they must want to. Unfortunately, even a severe dysarthria does not guarantee that a patient will have this desire, and clinicians should eschew thinking that it will. Assessment, then, should include finding out how important improved speech is to each dysarthric speaker. The indifferent or undecided ones should be counseled about the methods and goals of treatment, and the importance of their active participation in their own recovery should be underlined. If they do not make a commitment to treatment after a few sessions, they should be spared treatment's rigors. If they do make a commitment, management can begin. This is not to say that counseling stops at this point. Most dysarthric speakers, regardless of their enthusiasm, require additional counseling and emotional support as treatment progresses.

## POSTURAL ADJUSTMENT

Specific management of dysarthria usually begins with attention to postural adjustment. Good posture, as used here, includes alignment of the head, neck, and trunk; position of the arms and legs; and position of the speech structures. Normal talkers are indifferent to any but the most extreme postures; dysarthric speakers are not. Some dysarthric speakers talk best while in normal postures; some talk best in atypical postures, as when the head is tilted to one side. The clinician's responsibility is to measure the influence of a variety of postures on each patient's speech. Of the talker's general posture we ask, does he or she sound better standing up, sitting up, lying down, leaning over? We

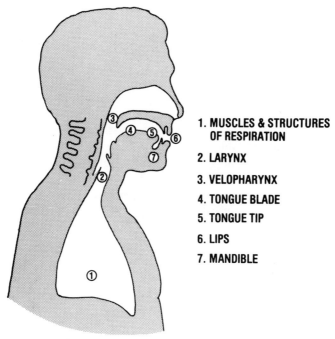

1. MUSCLES & STRUCTURES
   OF RESPIRATION

2. LARYNX

3. VELOPHARYNX

4. TONGUE BLADE

5. TONGUE TIP

6. LIPS

7. MANDIBLE

Figure 1.   Selected functional components of the speaking mechanism (adapted from
Netsell, 1973).

also evaluate, as appropriate, the posture of each functional component. After Netsell (1976, 1978), and Netsell and Daniel (1979), the
functional components are defined as those structures that generate or
valve the air stream, and are comprised of the diaphragm, abdominal
musculature, chest, larynx, velopharynx, tip and back of tongue, lips,
and jaw. Figure 1 displays the functional components.

A variety of prosthetic and positional manipulations may alter the
posture of each functional component, and improve speech as a result.
Posture for respiration may be improved in several ways (Hixon, 1975).
A "respiratory paddle" is displayed in Figure 2. This device is nothing
more than a board attached to a wheel chair, and appropriately posi-
tioned so that the patient can press up against it while he or she speaks.
The board acts to reinforce the abdominal muscles. A patient with
reasonable arm control can get the same effect by grasping himself
around the waist.

Posture for phonation may be improved by tilting the head or by
wrapping the neck. Posture for resonation may be improved by a palatal
life (Gonzalez and Aronson, 1970; Schweiger et al., 1970). A palatal
lift is an oral prosthetic device which consists of an anterior portion

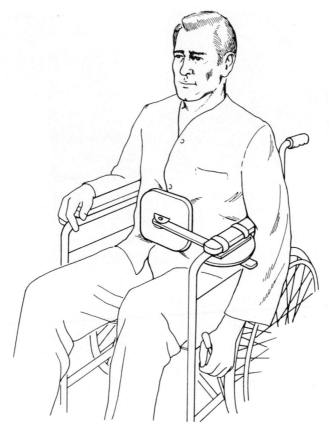

Figure 2.   Prosthetic device for improving the respiratory support of the dysarthric speaker.

with hooks that anchor it to the patient's teeth, and a posterior extension that elevates the soft palate to the posterior pharyngeal wall. The palatal lift produces a mechanical obstruction between the oral and nasal cavities. Another way to improve velopharyngeal function is to have the speaker recline so that gravity moves the soft palate toward the posterior pharyngeal wall (Luchsinger and Arnold, 1965).

Posture for articulation may be improved by using a bite block (Figure 3) to stabilize the jaw (Netsell, 1976). The typical bite block is made of pliable substances, such as silicone dental impression material. The clinician positions the bite block between the patient's upper and lower teeth, and instructs him or her to bite down gently. It is thick enough so that the patient's mouth is propped partly open (Figure 4). The patient is instructed to hold the block in place thereby immobilizing

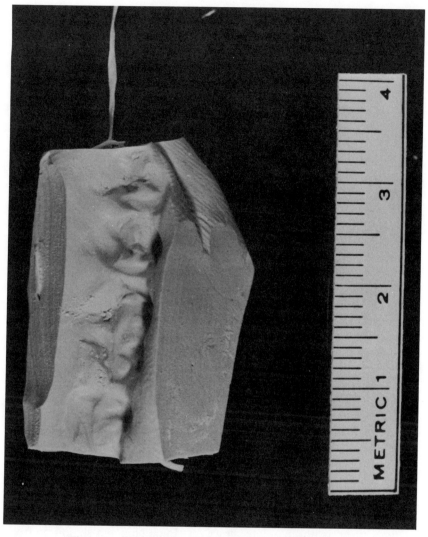

Figure 3.   Bite block made of a silicone base dental material.

his jaw, and then to talk. Appropriate postural changes can be more palliative than a month's practice on word and sentence lists.

Postural adjustments for both stable and degenerating patients can begin immediately. Timing is critical for the patient with a reasonable expectation of physiological improvement. Netsell (personal communication), for example, recommends as a general rule that a palatal lift should not be fitted while a patient is in a period of substantial neu-

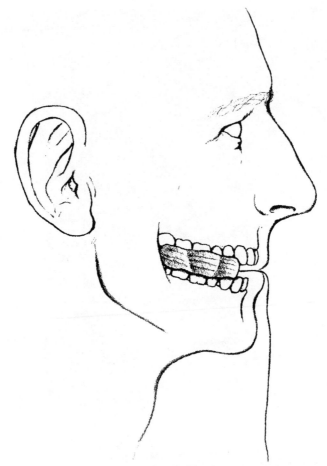

Figure 4.   Bite block in place.

rological recovery. This principle, like so many others in the treatment of dysarthria, is not inviolate, however. Each clinician should be free to make decisions about lifts or other prostheses, and even about simple behavioral, postural adjustment in response to each patient's unique circumstances.

## INCREASING EFFORT

Many dysarthric speakers sound better with an increase in bodily effort while they speak. We show them two ways to do this. First, we urge them to concentrate on going slowly, and to be as precise as they can

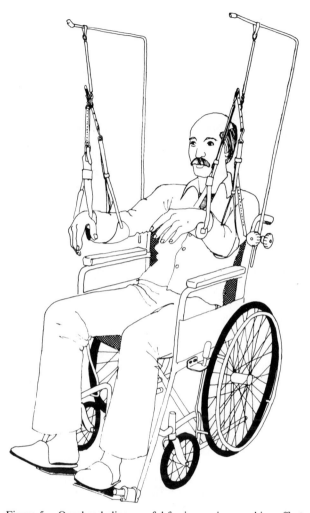

Figure 5.    Overhead slings useful for increasing speaking effort.

be each time they speak. Next, we teach them to talk while bearing down with their hands, arms, or entire body against a table top, lap board, or any other appropriate surface. Overhead slings (Figure 5) can be used by patients with severe problems. Even speakers with weakness in both arms can bear down by using gravity and their body's weight. We begin training by placing our hands, palm upwards, underneath the speaker's arms. We instruct patients to bear down when they feel our upward pressure. By comparing each patient's speech during increased effort to that when effort is not increased, the clinician can judge the maneuver's palliative effect. If the maneuver works, the speaker can be taught to do it with progressively less help from the clinician.

The reason this maneuver works, given our present state of knowledge, can only be guessed at. Our conjecture is that innervations from the arms and trunk of the body overflow to the speech musculature and cause them to work better. Unfortunately, the method does not work for all dysarthric speakers. And just as we do not know why neither can we predict for whom. Our clinical experience has been that speakers with muscular weakness are most likely to profit. Also we do not know the relative contribution of concentration and bearing down to improved speech. Probably, both contribute. Until we know, we will continue to use both simultaneously.

## ALTERING SPEAKING RATE, RHYTHM, AND STRESS

Dysarthric speakers have not forgotten how to make sounds, and they have no phonemic disorder unless a significant aphasia accompanies the dysarthria. Therefore, they do not need to relearn speech. Instead they need to participate in activities that will help them do what they mightily want to do: talk intelligibly. Although treatment of specific speech sounds is important, it is far less important than treatment of the prosodic factors of rate, rhythm, and stress. When rate, rhythm, and stress are improved, the dysarthric person's speech will also improve. There are several procedures for improving the dysarthric patient's prosody.

### Contrastive Stress Drill

To heighten control of stress, Fairbanks (1960) developed a technique called *contrastive stress drill*. Contrastive stress drill can be used with the dysarthric speaker to modify rate, rhythm, and stress to improve articulatory movements and intelligibility (Rosenbek, 1978; Rosenbek and LaPointe, 1978).

We first explain to patients that the drill involves a series of questions and answers that employ specially selected words and sentences. For example, a severely dysarthric talker may need to practice plosive, nasal, and vowel combinations, such as in "I do," "I can," "Me too," and "I got it." The clinician follows this explanation with a demonstration. He or she selects an utterance and tells the client to use it in answer to a series of questions. Example utterances are: "*Who* got it?" "*I* got it!" "*What* did you get?" "I got *it*." Sometimes the clinician will need to model both question and answer. At other times the patient will respond by answering appropriately.

When the goal is to change the dysarthric's overall speech pattern, a variety of verbal material can be used to encourage improvement in prosody. If the goal is improvement of particular sounds or movements, the use of verbal material must be focused. For example, if word-initial /k/ is the target for training, sentences can be addressed to the patient which encourage him or her to respond with heavy stress on certain target words. An illustration is "You bought a new what?" "I bought a new car."

When a patient's speech fails to improve, the clinician responds by offering encouragement and repetition, by modeling the patient's responses, by encouraging more dramatic rate, rhythm, or stress changes, or by changing the stimuli to make them easier. Typical changes include making the practice words and sentences shorter and by adding more sounds to the stimuli that the speaker can say easily. If even the simplest responses are still inadequate, practice with heavy stress on each word and with a slow overall rate can be tried. As speech improves, the clinician can make the drill more difficult in a number of ways.

First, the clinican can move the patient toward greater independence by requiring him or her to judge the adequacy of each response, and to repeat the inadequate ones. Second, the complexity of the drills can be increased. Short words and sentences can be replaced by longer ones, for example, and more difficult sounds and sound combinations, such as affricatives and consonant clusters can be introduced. Third, the speaker is encouraged to use normal rate, rhythm, and stress.

In time, we may learn how effective contrastive stress is with certain patients, and why it works only under certain conditions. Kent and Netsell (1971, p. 43) remark that "increases in stress are associated with increases in the muscular activity of the peripheral speech apparatus." Perhaps, there is similar effect on the peripheral speech system of the dysarthric speaker.

### GESTURAL REORGANIZATION

Another way to reduce articulatory distortion and improve intelligibility is to combine speech with simple, repetitive gesturing. The program is called *gestural reorganization* because it is based on Luria's (1970) concept of intersystemic reorganization. According to Luria, intersystemic reorganization occurs when an impaired activity is improved by pairing it with another, more intact activity. For that form of intersystemic reorganization, gestural reorganization, to work, the gesture should be simple and the pairing of it and speech should wait until the gesture can be predictably and confidently performed. Nothing is accomplished when dysarthric speakers are made to perform two activities simultaneously if they perform both of them poorly. We usually have patients tap with their finger or hand against a table top. Once the tapping is adequate, the speaker is taught to use it as an accompaniment to his or her spoken production of each syllable of the practice material. If necessary, the clinician provides extra help by talking and/or tapping along with the patient. When speech improves, the gestural accompaniment is diminished. If speech does not improve, the use of gestures may be necessary for a speaker's entire life. A lifetime of gesturing does not mean the program has failed as long as speech accompanied by gesture is better than speech without gesture.

## Combining Gestures and Contrastive Stress

The combination of gestural reorganization with contrastive stress drill is potentially more effective than using either approach alone. A question and answer dialogue can be used, as outlined above, and in addition, the patient can be trained to answer with gestural accompaniment. In some cases, gestural accompaniment further slows speaking rate and enhances the rhythm and stress of the answers, so that speech increases in intelligibility and precision. In addition, the use of gestures may remind the patient to utilize skills acquired in the clinic in environments outside the clinic.

The relative contribution of contrastive stress and gestural reorganization to improved speech functioning has not been thoroughly investigated. Our clinical procedure is to begin with contrastive stress and add gestures only if contrastive stress causes no improvement, we delay introducing them until we have to. On the other hand, if gestures spell the difference between adequate and inadequate speech, clinicians would be remiss if they did not introduce them. Of course, the patient deserves the opportunity to refuse them or any other treatment.

## The Pacing Board

The pacing board (Helm, 1979) (Figure 6) can also be used to slow speech and to heighten rhythm and stress. Helm's original pacing board is divided by partitions into separate squares. Each square is painted a different color to heighten its distinctiveness. A prosaic use of the board involves having patients touch successive portions of the board as they say each syllable or word in a target utterance. Creative use of the pacing board will depend on the severity of the dysarthria and, of course, on the clinician's goals. Patients can touch each of the portions in varying rhythm and stress patterns on every syllable, on stressed syllables only, on target syllables only, or the touching can be restricted to difficult syllables or words. Touch patterns can be hard

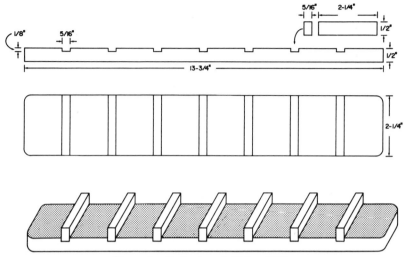

Figure 6.    Pacing board (Helm, 1979).

or soft, slow or fast. As the speaker improves, the use of the board can be gradually withdrawn. The board's superiority over other methods, if indeed it is superior, may be that patients cannot use it correctly without slowing down. Its drawbacks are that it requires considerable limb control and, unless the clinician is alert, can result in stereotyped patterns of rate, rhythm, and stress.

### Delayed Auditory Feedback

Delayed auditory feedback (DAF) is increasingly popular as a treatment for dysarthria (Hanson and Metter, 1980; Rosenbek et al., 1976) becuase it seems to slow speech and improve intelligibility and articulation. DAF appears to be superior to simple gestural reorganization or to the use of the pacing board because accompanying limb movements are not required. The potential shortcomings of DAF are that the speaker remains less active than is true of other methods, and in some cases speech does not improve and may even become worse. Furthermore, unless a portable DAF is used, transfer from treatment to functional communication may be difficult. As part of a total behavioral program, however, the DAF has its place in treatment especially for those dysarthric speakers who are unable to slow their speech by other methods.

Treatment begins with an explanation of the equipment and of the short- and long-range activities and goals of the program. Next comes a trial period for the clinician to discover the best loudness and delay interval, and for the speaker to adjust to the unusual sensation of voice delay. Delay intervals of 50 (Rosenbek et al., 1976) to 100 msec (Hanson and Metter, 1980) are likely to be optimum. Before treatment is begun, the clinician must select a delay interval that is appropriate for each individual speaker, and help to make the speaker familiar with DAF. With the help of the clinician the patient learns to recognize improved speech performance. Then the clinician systematically fades DAF by using alternating periods of feedback and no feedback. DAF programs are regarded as successful when they improve intelligibility, even if the patient must wear a portable model forever (Hanson and Metter, 1980). A lifetime of prosthetic management is a better fate than a lifetime of being misunderstood.

## PUTTING IT TOGETHER

The clinician begins by creating a willingness on the patient's part to undergo the rigors of treatment. Next, the clinician gets him or her into the appropriate posture(s) and teaches methods for increasing effort. With posture and effort adjusted, any one of several methods for achieving a palliative rate, rhythm, and stress profile can be implemented. We usually use contrastive stress drill first because it is the least invasive. We add gestures or the pacing board if contrastive stress drill fails. DAF is usually the last resort, but sometimes it is used initially to determine the influence of rate on intelligibility or to enable the patient to experience early success.

Regardless of the method, as the patient improves, assistance from the clinician is gradually reduced. We do not advise withdrawal of prostheses, however, or elimination of gestures, the pacing board, or DAF if the speaker cannot learn to function without them. If permanent compensations, such as a gestural accompaniment for speech, are necessary for patients to let other people know what is on their minds, we encourage their use. Patients must decide how much they cherish their "normal," untreated condition.

## CONCLUSION

Dysarthria is not just an articulation disorder, and dysarthria treatment is not just articulation treatment. That impaired articulation is common in dysarthria means only that articulation treatment is part of the total treatment package. The purpose of this chapter was to shift emphasis away from the tongue and its treatment and toward the total speech mechanism and methods for managing all its parts more or less simultaneously. The shift away from articulation training may make dysarthria treatment more efficient, and efficiency is especially critical for some dysarthric speakers. Efficiency is critical because many conditions causing dysarthria, such as Parkinson's disease and multiple sclerosis, require only short, infrequent hospitalization so that dysarthric speakers seldom are available for long-term treatment. Also, unless profound, dysarthria is only mildly handicapping; most dysarthric speakers with some effort make themselves understood. For this reason, dysarthric speakers are likely to tolerate only a short period of treatment. The methods described here will provide these patients with an understanding of what they can do to sound better. If pursued, these methods can give them better speech.

### REFERENCES

Fairbanks, G. 1960. Voice and Articulation Drillbook. Harper & Row, New York.

Gonzalez, J., and Aronson, A. 1970. Palatal lift prosthesis for treatment of anatomic and neurologic palatopharyngeal insufficiency. Cleft Palate J. 7:91–104.

Hanson, W., and Metter, E. 1980. DAF as instrumental treatment for dysarthria in progressive supranuclear palsy: A case report. J. Speech Hear. Disord. 45:268–276.

Helm, N. 1979. Management of palilalia with a pacing board. J. Speech Hear. Disord. 44:350–353.

Hixon, T. 1975. Respiratory-laryngeal evaluation. Paper presented at the Veterans Administration Workshop on Motor Speech Disorders, Madison, WI.

Kent, R., and Netsell, R. 1971. Effects of stress contrasts on certain articulatory parameters. Phonetica 24:23–44.

Luchsinger, R., and Arnold, G. 1965. Voice-Speech-Language. Wadsworth Publishing Company, Belmont, CA.

Luria, A. 1970. Traumatic Aphasia: Its Syndromes, Psychology and Treatment. Mouton, The Hague.

Netsell, R. 1973. Speech physiology. In: F. D. Minifie, T. J. Hixon, and F. Williams (eds.), Normal Aspects of Speech, Hearing, and Language. Prentice-Hall, Engelwood Cliffs, NJ.

Netsell, R. 1976. Physiological bases of dysarthria. Research Grant, NS 09627. National Institutes of Health, Rockville, Maryland.

Netsell, R. 1978. Physiologic recordings in the evaluation and rehabilitation of dysarthria. Communicative Disorders: An Audio Journal for Continuing Education. Grune & Stratton, New York.

Netsell, R., and Daniel, B. 1979. Dysarthria in adults: Physiologic approach to rehabilitation. Arch. Phys. Med. Rehabil. 60:502–508.

Rosenbek, J. 1978. Treating apraxia of speech. In: D. Johns, (ed.), Clinical Management of Neurogenic Communicative Disorders. Little, Brown and Co., Boston.

Rosenbek, J., and LaPointe, L. 1978. The dysarthrias: Description, diagnosis and treatment. In: D. Johns (ed.), Clinical Management of Neurogenic Communicative Disorders. Little, Brown and Co., Boston.

Rosenbek, J., Wertz, R., and Collins, M. 1976. Delayed auditory feedback in dysarthria therapy. Paper presented at the American Speech & Hearing Association Convention, Houston.

Schweiger, J., Netsell, R., and Sommerfeld, R. 1970. Prosthetic management and speech improvement in individuals with dysarthria of the palate. J. Am. Dent. Assoc. 80:1348–1353.

CHAPTER **18**

# Specific Characteristics and Treatments of the Dysarthrias

*James Paul Dworkin*

*The different dysarthrias and their treatment are outlined by Dworkin. A noteworthy feature of this chapter is Dworkin's extensive illustration of clinical principles.*

1. *Define and describe the five major types of dysarthrias.*
2. *According to Dworkin, what are the four basic clinical principles that should be considered in the treatment of dysarthria? Contrast these basic principles with the nine procedural principles Dworkin suggests for the patient with dysarthria.*
3. *What patients with significant tongue weakness may not benefit from tongue strengthening exercises? In this regard, identify what Dworkin considers to be five important procedures to follow when using tongue strengthening exercises. What are the specific strengthening exercises that he recommends?*
4. *With what type of dysarthria are "resistance to passive movement" exercises recommended? Are there techniques you might add to Dworkin's list of procedures?*
5. *What procedures does Dworkin recommend to increase range of movement of the forward part of the tongue in the dysarthric patient? Do you think the suggestions he recommends can also be applied to the posterior portion of the tongue?*
6. *How is timing and rhythm taught to a dysarthric patient according to Dworkin? Do you believe the skills learned in these exercises are helpful in relearning the timing relations required in natural conversational speech?*

DYSARTHRIA IS NOT a neurological disease. Rather, it is a speech diagnostic term which should only be used in reference to disorders of phonation, articulation, resonation, and prosody which occur, either singly or in combination, as a result of weakness, paresis, incoordination, and/or abnormalities in the tone of the muscles of the speech mechanism. These neuromuscular inadequacies underlying dysarthria are due to impairment of the central nervous system, peripheral nervous system or both, and they may vary in nature and degree from patient to patient.

There are five major types of dysarthria, each of which bears the name of its salient neuromuscular feature. These are: 1) *flaccid*, resulting from muscular flaccidity; 2) *spastic*, resulting from muscular spasticity; 3) *ataxic*, resulting from muscular incoordination or ataxia; 4) *hypokinetic*, resulting from muscular rigidity and reduced (hypo) mobility; and 5) *hyperkinetic*, resulting from uncontrollably excessive (hyper) muscular activities. When signs of two or more types are evident in the speech of an individual, the term *mixed* dysarthria is used.

A brief review of the differential neuromuscular and speech characteristics of the dysarthrias is presented below, and is followed by specific clinical intervention suggestions.

**DYSARTHRIAS**

### Flaccid Dysarthria

Flaccid dysarthria chiefly results when cranial nerves and/or spinal nerves (lower motor neurons, denoted *LMN*) are damaged and the muscles of the speech mechanism they supply become hypotonic, weak, atrophic (shrunken), and paralytic. These neuromuscular inadequacies, often labeled *bulbar palsy*, may occur unilaterally or bilaterally and may be observed in one or more muscles, depending on the extent of LMN damage. Consequently, the degree and nature of the speech difficulties exhibited by a patient with this type of dysarthria are generally proportional to which LMNs and how many are damaged. Articulatory imprecision most often occurs when the XIIth and/or VIIth cranial nerves are damaged because they normally supply the tongue and lip musculature, respectively; hypernasality and nasal air emission occur when the IXth and Xth cranial nerves are damaged because they normally supply the velopharyngeal musculature; and hoarse, breathy phonation occurs when the Xth cranial nerve is damaged because its recurrent and external branches normally supply the intrinsic laryngeal musculature.

## Spastic Dysarthria

Spastic dysarthria results when the corticobulbar tracts (upper motor neurons, denoted *UMN*) are damaged and the muscles of the speech mechanism become hypertonic, spastic, weak, and paretic. When damage is bilateral, these resultant neuromuscular inadequacies, often labeled *pseudobulbar palsy* because of their superficial resemblance to bulbar palsy, are generally widespread throughout the speech mechanism and cause moderate to severe articulatory imprecision, hypernasality and strained, strangled phonation. Unilateral UMN damage, on the other hand, may result in mild spasticity and weakness of the tongue and lower two-thirds of the face on the side opposite that of lesioning which may cause mild articulatory imprecision.

## Ataxic Dysarthria

Ataxic dysarthria results when the vermis of the cerebellum is bilaterally damaged and the majority of the speech musculature becomes hypotonic and incoordinated in its timing, range, speed, and force of movements. These neuromuscular inadequacies result in variable articulatory imprecision, prolongations of sounds and intervals between words, inappropriate patterns of stress and harsh, monopitch phonation. Patients with this type of dysarthria often sound inebriated. With more extensive lesioning of the cerebellum, signs of gait ataxia (wide based and reeling) and generalized dyssynergia (muscular incoordination) may also be observed.

## Hypokinetic Dysarthria

Hypokinetic dysarthria results from depigmentation of the substantia nigra in the upper brainstem and/or deficiency of dopamine, a neurotransmitter substance located in the upper brainstem and basal ganglia. These neuropathologic changes classically result in Parkinson's disease or parkinsonism and cause generalized rigidity (hypertonus) and marked limitations in the range and speed of movement of body musculature. Involvement of speech muscles chiefly results in articulatory imprecision and harsh, monopitch and monoloud phonation. Nonspeech signs of Parkinson's disease may include flexed truncal posture, mask-like facies, shuffling gait, and a "pill-rolling" tremor of the hands at rest.

## Hyperkinetic Dysarthria

Hyperkinetic dysarthria may result from focal as well as multifocal lesions of the extrapyramidal system, the characteristics of which will vary depending upon the nature and site(s) of lesioning. Interestingly, whereas lesions in certain areas may cause excessive and involuntary movement disturbances of various body musculature that are characteristically quick, unsustained, and jerky, as observed in individuals with chorea and myoclonus, other areas of lesioning produce predominantly slow, sustained, and writhing hyperkinesias as seen in individuals with dystonia and dyskinesia.

In chorea, muscles of the head, face, limbs, and trunk are usually affected. The quick, unpatterned, and jerky movement disturbances within the speech mechanism produce variable slowness and imprecision of articulation, accompanied by prolonged phonemes, and harsh, monopitch, and monoloud phonation. In myoclonus, involved musculature is characterized by sudden, rhythmic (2–4 Hz), and pulsating contractions that are present at rest. Palatal, pharyngeal, and laryngeal myoclonus is the classic complex of speech musculature involvement, the rhythmic effects of which are most notable during vowel prolongation. Mild to moderate hypernasality and tremor-like vocal quality are the salient speech features. In dystonia, the abnormalities of movement are slow and twisting in appearance, and may involve muscles throughout the body or they may be focal to speech musculature. Articulation is imprecise with prolongations of individual sounds and intervals between words, and voice is harsh and breathy in quality with excessive variations in loudness. In dyskinesia, abnormal movements may involve many body muscles or just speech muscles, and vary from quick and jerky to slow and writhing in nature. Speech characteristics may vary between those typical of chorea and dystonia.

It is interesting to note that a diagnosis of a hyperkinetic disorder may be reached when any form of abnormally excessive musculoskeletal movements is observed. When speech musculature are hyperkinetic and speech is impaired, the diagnosis of hyperkinetic dysarthria may be justified whether or not the condition is caused by extrapyramidal system impairment.

### Mixed Forms

Mixed forms of dysarthria result from multiple motor system impairments as occur in specific types of neurologic disease, such as amyotrophic lateral sclerosis (ALS) and multiple sclerosis (MS), and diffuse nervous system injuries and pathologies. Of course, the combined speech characteristics of mixed dysarthrias vary in accordance with the components of the mixture and their severity and underlying cause; one component may, and often does, predominate.

In ALS, progressive degeneration of corticobulbar tract fibers and cranial nerve nuclei results in a mixed spastic-flaccid dysarthria. Speech may range from mildly impaired in the early stage of the disease to severely unintelligible in the terminal stage. In MS, demyelination and scarring throughout the nerve tracts of the cerebrum, brainstem, cerebellum, and/or spinal cord result in a variably mixed spastic-ataxic dysarthria. In some individuals, the dysarthria may be moderate to severe, yet in others it may be episodic (paroxysmal) and mild; normal speech is not uncommon. In diffuse neuropathologies and injuries, the possible combinations of motor system impairments are highly variable as are the resultant mixed dysarthrias.

Table 1 summarizes the salient neuromuscular signs and specific speech (musculature) characteristics of the dysarthrias.

**CLINICAL INTERVENTION**

Because articulatory imprecision may significantly affect speech intelligibility in virtually all patients with dysarthria, and often can be improved through clinical treatments, it has been chosen as the major topic for this section. Naturally, other salient speech features in patients with dysarthria may also be responsive to clinical treatments, but space limitations restrict this review.

The primary objective when treating articulatory imprecision usually is to train compensatory articulation skills because normal speech patterns may no longer be possible to achieve. Such training includes not only phonetic exercises, but neuromuscular facilitation techniques designed to improve the tone, strength, and mobility of the tongue and lip musculature, in particular, so as to enhance their physiological potential for articulation. These latter techniques only are addressed here.

This section is divided into two subsections. These are: 1) general considerations, under which initial strategies, philosophies, and basic techniques of dysarthria treatments are briefly discussed; and 2) differential neuromuscular treatments, under which treatment approaches for tongue musculature dysfunctions specifically are detailed. The information presented is not meant to be a treatise, but a general guide for speech-language pathologists. Those who are interested in more extensive reviews of these topics are referred to the references at the end of the chapter.

**General Considerations**

*Initial Strategies*    In treating the dysarthrias, the speech pathologist should consider four important clinical principles. First, the type of dysarthria the patient has and its neuromuscular and speech signs must be determined so that treatments can focus economically on the client's speech disorders and their pathophysiological substrates. Second, the etiology and medical diagnosis may dictate the nature and timing of treatments. The treatment plan for a dysarthria caused by a

Table 1. Speech musculature characteristics underlying the dysarthrias

| Dysarthria type | Respiratory | Tongue | Lips | Larynx | Velo-pharynx |
|---|---|---|---|---|---|
| **Flaccid** 1. Lesion site(s): a) Lower motor neurons (variable) 2. Signs a) Hypotonia b) Weakness c) Paralysis d) Atrophy e) Fasciculations f) Unilateral or bilateral g) Hyporeflexes | 1. Lesion site(s): a) Spinal cord (LMNs) b) Respiratory muscles 2. Speech characteristics: a) Short phrase lengths b) Reduced loudness c) Inhalatory gasps | 1. Lesion site(s): a) Hypoglossal nerve (XII) b) Neuromuscular junction c) Tongue muscles 2. Speech characteristics: a) Lingual articulatory imprecision b) Slow lingual alternate and sequential movement rates | 1. Lesion site(s): a) Facial nerve (VII) b) Neuromuscular junction 2. Speech characteristics: a) Labial articulatory imprecision b) Slow labial alternate and sequential movement rates | 1. Lesion site(s): a) Recurrent and/or external laryngeal nerves (X) b) Neuromuscular junction c) Laryngeal muscles 2. Speech characteristics: a) Hoarse, breathy quality b) Aphonia (with bilateral involvement) c) Reduced phrase length during phonation d) Inhalatory stridor | 1. Lesion site(s): a) Pharyngeal plexus (IX and X) nerves b) Neuromuscular junction c) Velo-pharyngeal muscles 2. Speech characteristics: a) Hypernasality and nasal air escape b) Articulatory imprecision on pressure consonants |
| **Spastic** 1. Lesion site(s): a) Corticobulbar tracts 2. Signs: a) Hypertonia b) Weakness c) Paresis d) Typically bilateral e) Hyperreflexes | Speech characteristics: a) Short and choppy phrases b) Excessive loudness variations and outbursts | Speech characteristics: a) Lingual articulatory imprecision b) Slow, labored lingual alternate and sequential movement rates | Speech characteristics: a) Labial articulatory imprecision b) Slow, labored alternate and sequential movement rates | Speech characteristics: a) Strained, strangled quality b) Reduced phrase length (increased glottal resistance to air flow) | Speech characteristics: a) Hypernasality and nasal air escape b) Articulatory imprecision on pressure consonants |
| **Ataxic** 1. Lesion site(s): a) Cerebellum 2. Signs: a) Incoordination of timing, range, force, speed, and direction of movements | Speech characteristics: prolonged and explosive intonation variations | Speech characteristics: a) Lingual articulatory imprecision b) Phoneme and interval prolongations c) Variably slow and irregular lingual alternate and sequential movement rates | Speech characteristics: same as tongue, only on labial sound productions | Speech characteristics: a) Loudness outbursts b) Tremor-like and hoarse, harsh quality | Speech characteristics: no significant features |
| **Hypokinetic** 1. Lesion site(s): a) Substantia nigra b) Striatum | Speech characteristics: a) Short rushes and phrase lengths | Speech characteristics: a) Lingual articulatory imprecision | Speech characteristics: same as tongue, only on labial sound productions | Speech characteristics: a) Monopitch b) Monoloudness | Speech characteristics: no significant features |

| | Speech characteristics | Speech characteristics | Speech characteristics | Speech characteristics | Speech characteristics |
|---|---|---|---|---|---|
| **Hypokinetic**<br>1. Lesion site(s):<br>  a) Substantia nigra<br>  b) Striatum<br>2. Signs:<br>  a) Hypertonia (rigidity)<br>  b) Reduced range of movement<br>  c) Rest tremor | a) Short rushes and phrase lengths<br>b) Reduced loudness<br>c) Abrupt interruptions of speech (silences) | a) Lingual articulatory imprecision<br>b) Variably slow and irregular lingual alternate and sequential movement rates<br>c) Short rushes of lingual sound productions | same as tongue, only on labial sound productions | a) Monopitch<br>b) Monoloudness<br>c) Hoarse, harsh quality | no significant features |
| **Hyperkinetic**<br>**Chorea:**<br>1. Lesion site(s):<br>  a) Striatum<br>2. Signs:<br>  a) Variable hypertonia<br>  b) Quick-jerky involuntary movements<br>  c) Reduced range<br>**Dystonia:**<br>1. Lesion site(s):<br>  a) Extrapyramidal system<br>2. Signs:<br>  a) Variable hypertonia<br>  b) Repetitively slow-twisting movements<br>  c) Reduced range<br>**Athetosis:**<br>1. Lesion site(s):<br>  a) Extrapyramidal system<br>2. Signs:<br>  a) Variable hypertonia<br>  b) Slow-writhing movements<br>  c) Reduced range | Chorea:<br>a) Excessive loudness variations<br>b) Forced inspiratory and expiratory sighs<br><br>Athetosis/Dystonia:<br>a) Jerky and groaning voice<br>b) Inhalatory and exhalatory noise | Same as ataxic dysarthria | same as tongue, only on labial sound productions | a) Harsh quality<br>b) Variable loudness and pitch control | no significant features |
| **Mixed**<br>ALS    Spastic-flaccid<br>MS    Spastic-ataxic<br>       Non-specific | respective mixtures from above | respective mixtures from above | respective mixtures from above | respective mixtures from above | respective mixtures from above |

269

malignant neoplasm, for example, may be different from the same dysarthria caused by trauma. Third, the prognosis for improvement depends upon the severity and etiology of the dysarthria and whether it can be treated medically. For example, a patient with a moderate degree of dysarthria caused by a (medically responsive) neuropathology with a static (stable) course generally has a better prognosis than another dysarthric patient with a degenerative (dynamic) neuropathology which is not or has not been responsive to medical treatment. Fourth, when the treatment of dysarthria is aimed at improving speech intelligibility by training the patient to compensate for motor speech difficulties, the short- and long-term objectives are usually more realistic and attainable than the treatment plan which focuses on restoring normal motor skills and speech proficiency; albeit, those patients with the physiological potential to achieve speech proficiency should be encouraged and trained to advance to that level if possible.

*Philosophies of Treatment*     Treating symptoms in a standard or general fashion, irrespective of etiology, is called the *symptomological treatment approach*. Treating symptoms differentially, as a function of their underlying cause, is referred to as the *type-specific* or *etiological treatment approach*. Although it may seem theoretically reasonable to treat the dysarthrias using the former approach, because these (etiologically) diverse disorders are characterized by similar symptoms (articulatory, resonatory, and/or phonatory impairments), it is clinically justifiable to identify not only the symptoms of a dysarthria, but also their cause and pathophysiological characteristics so that type-specific treatments may be provided whenever indicated. An eclectic approach, one sensitive to the applications of symptomological as well as etiological treatments, is perhaps the most prudent of all.

*Basic Treatment Techniques*     Clinical, instrumental, medico-surgical, and prosthetic approaches have been used in various combinations, to treat the dysarthrias. Generally, these treatment approaches focus on improving the strength, mobility, and/or coordination of affected speech musculature. Clinical treatments may include behavioral tasks such as neuromuscular facilitation exercises of the tongue, lip, jaw, and respiratory muscles (Froeschels, 1952; Mysak, 1963; Rembisz and Gribin, 1975) and articulation, voice, and speech breathing drills (Hartman et al., 1979; Ince and Rosenberg, 1963; Robbins, 1940; Rosenbek and LaPointe, 1978; Wertz, 1978; Westlake, 1951). Instrumental treatments may include use of various types of appliances, such as auditory, visual, and EMG biofeedback devices (Amato et al., 1973; Leanderson et al., 1971; Netsell and Cleeland, 1973; Rubow et al., 1981), DAF units (Hanson and Metter, 1980), force transducers (Dworkin and Hartman, 1979), bite blocks (Dworkin, 1978,

1980b), non-oral communication systems (Beukelman and Yorkston, 1977; Dworkin et al., 1982; Hagen et al., 1973; McDonald and Schultz, 1973; Shane and Bashir, 1980) and pacing boards (Helm, 1979). Medico-surgical treatments may include drug prescriptions (Angel et al., 1971; Berry et al., 1974; Greer, 1970; Nakano et al., 1973; Osserman and Genkins, 1966; Rigrodsky and Morrison, 1970), muscular implantations (Arnold, 1962; Cosman and Folk, 1975; Dworkin and Johns, 1980; Johns and Salyer, 1978; Kiehm et al., 1965; Rubin, 1965, 1975), and neurosurgical procedures (Allan et al., 1966; Daniel and Guitar, 1978; Darley et al., 1975; Samra et al., 1969). Prosthetic treatments may include use of palatal lift devices (Dworkin and Johns, 1980; Gonzalez and Aronson, 1970; Hardy, 1967; Johns and Salyer, 1978; Kerman et al., 1973), neck, mandible, and trunk braces, and dummy hard palate appliances. It is most strategic for the speech pathologist to be familiar with the indications and contraindications of all of the above treatment techniques before designing an intervention program for a given patient. Inherent in the design of most dysarthric treatment programs is the ongoing cooperation and interaction between many different practitioners including speech-language pathologists, physicians, dentists, and physical therapists.

**Differential Neuromuscular Treatments**

Here we focus on basic neuromuscular facilitation techniques for tongue dysfunctions of patients with dysarthria. The treatment suggestions are mostly clinical in orientation, in view of the fact that many facilities are not equipped with elaborate instrumentation for treating patients with dysarthria, and therefore speech-language pathologists must often resort to treatment techniques that are clinically feasible and practical for their setting. It should be borne in mind, however, that if those medico-surgical and/or prosthetic treatments that may be indicated for a given patient are not identified and administered along with clinical treatment, the prognosis for improvement may decline significantly. Of course, determining which treatment suggestions are worth attempting with a given patient and whether these techniques should precede, coincide with, or follow other treatments that also are indicated is the responsibility of the entire rehabilitation team.

In designing the articulation intervention plan for a patient with dysarthria, the speech pathologist will find nine procedural principles helpful: 1) treatments of the underlying neuromuscular deficits of the tongue should coincide with, and in severe cases precede, compensatory articulation training; 2) demands that exceed the physiological potential of this musculature are generally counterproductive because they may frustrate the patient and undermine his aspirations for improvement; 3) training the patient to articulate with a slower than normal speed almost always improves speech intelligibility; 4) whenever possible, incorporate visual, auditory, tactile, and/or kinesthetic feedback in the treatment plan to enhance the patient's perception of these musculature during compensatory movements; 5) if respiratory, phonatory, and/or resonatory impairments coexist with articulatory imprecision they may compound the problem of speech unintelligibility and, possibly, limit the success of compensation training; 6) the results of an articulation test battery are used to classify the type of each misarticulation of "lingual" target sounds into one of three traditional categories: a) distortions, b) substitutions, and c) omissions; 7) begin phonetic training on those target sounds listed in category "a" and proceed with sounds in category "b" after criteria are met with all sounds in category "a" and so on; 8) as the prognosis for speech improvement increases, remains constant, or decreases as treatment is attempted, either as a response to the treatment, nature of the neurologic condition or both, the treatment objectives and criteria for improvement should be sensibly modified; and 9) if these treatments are unsuccessful, the efficacy of nonverbal communication systems should be explored, especially with the unintelligible patient.

As can be seen from Table 1, the speech characteristics of the tongue musculature for the different dysarthrias are similar; however, their underlying causes and neuromuscular abnormalities (signs) are generally different. The treatment suggestions below aim not at the lingual articulation characteristics themselves, but at their neuromuscular roots.

*Weakness*   Some speech pathologists use strain gauge transducers to measure the strength of the tongue musculature in patients with dysarthria because its use seems to ensure the most accurate measurements by eliminating examiner subjectivity. Others whose budgets prohibit purchase of such costly instrumentation may use a rating scale of −4 to 0 to +4 to measure tongue strength in a subjective manner, as shown in Figure 1. On this scale, −4 represents marked weakness, 0 represents normal strength, and +4 represents exceptional strength. The procedures for measuring tongue strength using this scale are discussed later in this section. The consensus is that the lingual articulatory disorders of virtually all patients with dysarthria may be attributable, in part, to an underlying weakness of the tongue musculature (Dworkin, 1980a; Dworkin and Aronson, 1982; Dworkin et al., 1980), and, therefore, tongue strength should be measured routinely in all patients who present lingual articulatory imprecision.

If tongue weakness is detected in a patient with dysarthria, the first clinical impulse may be to treat this weakness by administering a

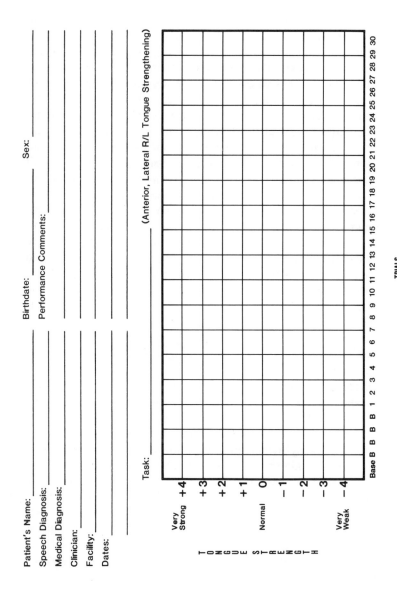

**TRIALS**

Figure 1.   Form for rating changes in the strength of the tongue musculature. A relatively straight line across the graph, at the zero (0) level, would signify normal tongue strength and, of course, is the ideal treatment goal for all patients. Indicate the task—anterior, right or left lateral—in the space provided and record patient performance for each trial.

regimen of muscle strengthening exercises, with hopes of increasing the physiological potential of the tongue for articulation training. I find that routine incorporation of tongue strengthening exercises in the speech training program is not clinically practical for all patients with tongue weakness. In fact, such exercises have proven to be counterproductive for certain patients with tongue weakness due to central nervous system pathology. The best route for improving lingual articulation skills in these types of patients has been one which combines phonetic practice with treatments to decrease hypertonicity and improve overall movement control of the tongue musculature. These treatment techniques are addressed later. Here, we focus on strengthening exercises for patients with hypotonic tongue weakness and associated flaccid dysarthria due to damage of the XIIth cranial nerve (peripheral nervous system), because these patients often respond favorably to such treatments. It should be mentioned, however, that some patients with flaccid dysarthria may not be good candidates for tongue strengthening exercises, despite the fact that they have significant tongue weakness. They include: 1) the patient with ALS who has a rapidly progressive form of this disease, the effects of which will override the results of such exercises; 2) the patient with myasthenia gravis who may become fatigued more quickly by exercises that require maximum and prolonged musculature contractions; and 3) the patient whose weakness and paralysis appear irreversible due to bilateral and complete XIIth nerve damage. Additionally, these types of patients may not benefit from compensatory articulation training either, but such training ought to be at least attempted.

The following five factors and procedures are important to consider in the utilization of the treatment plan below, which concentrates on strengthening the tongue musculature. These are: 1) if a patient has lingual articulation difficulties, routinely measure and record anterior and lateral tongue strength using instrumental or subjective rating procedures as mentioned above; 2) if weakness is detected and is due to XIIth nerve damage, as evidenced by coexisting paralysis, atrophy, and (possibly) fasciculations of one or both sides of the tongue, then strengthening exercises should be incorporated in the treatment plan provided the underlying neuropathology does not contraindicate their inclusion; 3) if strengthening exercises are indicated they should not be administered without the advice and approval of the physical therapy and medical team members, nor should they necessarily precede or take precedence over treatment of lingual articulation; rather, they should be incorporated at the beginning and end of every treatment session until such time that they are found to be insignificant or possibly counterproductive to the progress of the patient; 4) the amount of time the patient may need or be able to spend on these exercises is usually dictated by the nature and severity of the underlying neurological condition as well as progress made during such exercises, and should be adjusted accordingly; and 5) although the ideal goal in a strengthening regimen is to restore tongue strength to a normal level, most patients will not be able to advance to this level, and will benefit more if a less strict criterion is used in determining when they may progress to the next step in the treatment regimen.

At the beginning of the session, prop the patient in an upright position and hold the flat edge of a wooden tongue blade against the upper and lower incisor teeth and urge that the patient push as hard as possible against the blade with the tip of the tongue, and maintain maximum effort for as long as possible. Do not allow more than 7 seconds to elapse. As the patient pushes, the clinician should provide varying degrees of counter force or resistance with the blade. Score the patient's performance on the $-4$ to $0$ to $+4$ rating scale suggested above, wherein $-4$ is markedly weak and $+4$ is very strong. Because this task is dynamic, in that the patient may be pushing as hard as possible for several seconds, rate only the maximum force exhibited in the trial, regardless of when it is perceived. Repeat this strengthening task four times, allowing an interval of at least 30 seconds between trials. Somewhere near the end of the treatment session, repeat all five trials and score each one accordingly. If the patient demonstrates improvement in strength of at least two scale values from the onset of such treatment (baseline disability) through 30 consecutive trials (three treatment sessions equivalent), proceed to the next step. It is advisable that this first step (or 10 trials) be repeated once every five sessions for maintenance purposes.

Next, the clinician should place the index and middle fingers of one hand on one side of the cheek and urge that the patient push as hard and long as possible with the tongue tip against the inside of that cheek as counter force is applied with the fingers. Rate the patient's performance as suggested in the first step. Repeat the same procedure against the opposite cheek and rate that performance. Thereafter, alternate cheeks and repeat the task on each side four times for a total of 10 trials, allowing an interval of at least 30 seconds between each trial. Near the end of the session repeat this procedure, alternating from side to side and rate each trial in the usual way. Follow the same criteria for progress as suggested in the first step and design a strengthening maintenance program in accordance with the patient's level of improvement. If and when the strengthening regimen is successfully completed with the hypotonic and weak tongue musculature, measure the resistance of the tongue to passive movement, as suggested in the next section. If the rating obtained is −2 or worse, administer the tone therapy program as described below for the hypertonic tongue musculature, but adjust the treatment objectives to increase rather than decrease muscle tone. Use of a response form, like that shown in Figure 2, may facilitate this treatment regimen by enabling the clinician to record as well as analyze patient performance.

*Resistance to Passive Movement*   This neuromuscular deficit of the tongue may take the form of diminished resistance as in the hypotonic muscle state of the patient with XIIth nerve damage, or excessive resistance, as in the hypertonic states of patients with spastic, hypokinetic, and/or hyperkinetic disorders. Associated with and related to these tone abnormalities may be other deficits such as reduced range, slowness, and imprecision of tongue movements which virtually all dysarthric patients with articulation difficulties exhibit. Some speech pathologists may be of the opinion that exercises designed specifically to improve the tone of the tongue musculature should be included from the outset in the overall treatment plan because any improvement in tone promoted by these exercises may facilitate concurrent compensatory articulation treatments. Others may be of the opinion that treatments aimed directly at improving muscle tone may not need to be an integral component of the treatment plan because tone may be improved indirectly through compensatory articulation treatments. This writer supports the former position that direct muscle tone treatments may facilitate phonetic learning and should be incorporated in the intervention program whenever they are indicated for a given patient. They should be designed with the advice and consent of other team members, most notably the physical therapist and physician, and should be administered routinely in every treatment session.

Hypotonia of the tongue musculature may be improved through strengthening exercises, as described above. Strengthening exercises are not appropriate for improving hypertonia, however, even though weakness may be a salient feature of hypertonic musculature. Rather, treatments of hypertonia should be designed to relax involved musculature and improve their ease, range, and control of movement. The five sequential treatment steps described below may facilitate these clinical objectives, irrespective of the neurological condition causing the hypertonia, and ought to be considered in the daily treatment plan.

At the beginning of the session prop the patient upright, if possible, because this sitting position induces a more relaxed tongue posture than lying down (step 1). Second, instruct the patient to relax as much as possible. Place a gauze pad between the thumb and index finger, request the patient to open his or her mouth, and then gently grasp and pull the tongue tip forward with a steady and moderate degree of

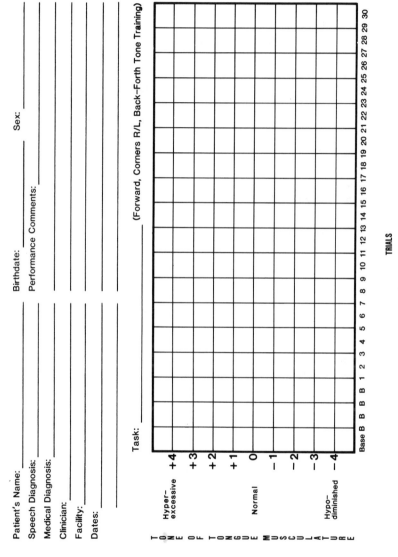

Figure 2.   Form for rating changes in the tone of the tongue musculature. A relatively straight line across the graph, at the zero (0) level, would signify normal tone, and, of course, is the ideal treatment goal for all patients. Indicate the task—forward, right or left corner, back-forth—in the space provided and record patient performance for each trial.

force (step 2). Although there likely will be initial, inherent muscle resistance to this passive movement technique, the clinician should maintain the pulling force until the tongue yields forward and/or 10 seconds have elapsed. Using a −4 to 0 to +4 rating scale, wherein +4 represents markedly excessive resistance, 0 represents normal tone, and −4 represents markedly diminished resistance, rate the degree to which the tongue resisted forward movement over the 10-second trial. Repeat this technique four times, allowing a 30-second interval between trials. Repeat this step later in the session, so that a total of 10 trials are administered, five in the beginning (baseline) and five at the end, and rate the level of resistance perceived on each trial. When the level of resistance decreases from the plus mark baseline level two or more scale values, or reaches the normal level, on 90% of 30 trials (three consecutive sessions) proceed to the third step. Next, grasp the tongue and pull it forward as in the second step. Then slowly and forcibly (moderate degree) move it toward one corner of the mouth and hold it there for 10 seconds (step 3). If the tongue resists movement do not try to force it over for more than 10 seconds per trial. Rate the level of resistance and repeat this technique four times with an interval of 30 seconds between trials. Later in the session, repeat this entire procedure, so that a total of 10 trials, five in the beginning (baseline) and five at the end are administered and rated. Follow the same criteria for progression to the next step as suggested in the second step. Administer the same techniques as in the above step, but this time move the tongue to the other corner of the mouth (step 4). Do not proceed to the next step until criteria are met in the direction of each corner of the mouth.

Next, grasp the tongue and pull it forward as indicated in the second step. Once it is maintained in the forward position for 10 seconds, slowly move it to the right corner of the mouth, hold it there for 3 seconds, and then slowly move it to the left corner. Next, slowly glide the tongue back and forth from the left to the right corner of the mouth, without hesitation along the way, for 30 seconds (step 5). Rate the overall level of resistance perceived during the 30-second continuum. Repeat this procedure four times and rate each trial accordingly. When the tongue can be moved passively, that is with no greater than +1 resistance 90% of the time over six consecutive treatment sessions (30 trials), the entire five-step program may need to be repeated only once every five sessions thereafter. Should the clinician feel that a more stringent maintenance program is indicated for a given patient, however, then the interval between review sessions can be adjusted accordingly. If criteria on any step are not achieved, treatments should continue from that step on until they are achieved. A response form like the one in Figure 3 may be used to record and analyze patient performances.

If and when the five-step treatment plan above is successfully completed with the hypertonic tongue musculature, measure the patient's tongue strength using the subjective rating scale as before. If this rating is $-2$ or worse, administer the tongue strengthening exercise regimen as described earlier.

Icing, brushing, stroking, and other neuromuscular facilitation techniques should be left to the physical therapist to administer if they are deemed appropriate for improving hypertonia of the tongue.

*Reduced Range of Movement*    This neuromuscular inadequacy of the tongue is evident in most dysarthric patients who exhibit lingual articulatory imprecision. It results from and is proportional to the degrees of abnormally decreased or increased tone and associated weakness of the tongue musculature. The hypertonic tongue of the severe spastic patient, for example, may be as limited in its movement potential and as impairing to speech production as the hypotonic tongue of the severe flaccid patient; yet, the underlying pathophysiology of these cases is dissimilar.

The chief objective with this deficit, regardless of its cause, usually is to increase as much as possible the tongue's range of movement so as to facilitate compensatory articulation training. Because abnormal tone and strength usually underlie movement limitations of the tongue, however, these deficits also need to be treated as discussed above, either before (in severe cases) or concurrent with treatments for reduced range.

Before proceeding with treatments for improving range of movement, the clinician should consider some important guidelines: 1) it is always wise to demonstate the task first and then request the patient to perform it; 2) use of a mirror can be helpful in feeding visual information about tongue positioning and movements; 3) proceed at a pace that is commensurate with the patient's performances and physiological potential; 4) be fairly lenient when judging the patient's performances, because compensatory movements are often the best that can be achieved; 5) if severe lip and jaw involvement coexist with tongue difficulties, certain tasks may have to be modified or eliminated; 6) whenever indicated and feasible, the clinician should assist the patient's tongue, either manually or with a wooden tongue blade, in its movement effort; and 7) some patients who are severely involved may not improve, and therefore, may benefit from use of compensation devices, such as prosthetic dummy hard palates and/or nonverbal communication systems.

280 Dworkin

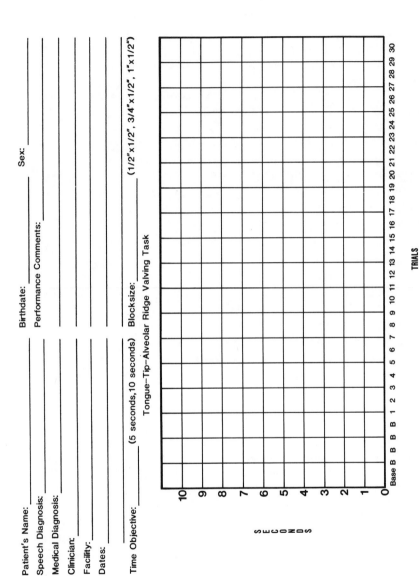

Figure 3. Form for rating changes in lingual alveolar valving skills. Relatively straight lines across the graph, at the 5-second and 10-second levels, would signify normal range and control of such movements, and, of course, is the ideal treatment goal for all patients. Indicate the block size used in the space provided and record the patient performance for each trial.

After muscle relaxation and/or strengthening treatments have been administered to the patient, the clinician should proceed in the session with the following clinical treatment plan. First, obtain three corks ($\frac{1}{2}'' \times \frac{1}{2}''$, $\frac{3}{4}'' \times \frac{1}{2}''$, and $1'' \times \frac{1}{2}''$), three 6" pieces of string, and a supply of latex finger cots (coverings). Tie a loop around the corks so that each cork has its own string attachment. Roll a latex finger cot over the $\frac{1}{2}'' \times \frac{1}{2}''$ cork so that it covers the cork and part of the string. Second, sit in front of a mirror with the patient and position the ends of the $\frac{1}{2}''$ cork between the left or right upper and lower bicuspid teeth, request the patient to bite down gently so that the jaws are stabilized while holding on to the connecting string to prevent accidental swallowing of the cork. This position not only sets the stage for tongue movement exercises, but also inhibits the mandible from assisting the tongue during these exercises. As a visual biofeedback device, the mirror may help increase control of tongue movements and decrease extraneous jaw movements. Third, request the patient to maintain a gentle biting force on the cork, lift the tongue tip to the alveolar ridge, hold it there for 5 seconds, and then lower it. Repeat these steps four times. It is important to note that patients with hyperkinetic movement disorders, such as dystonia and chorea, may dislodge the cork if the mandible or head involuntarily twists or jerks during this exercise. If this occurs, reposition the cork and try again using the mirror as an instructional aid for better jaw and head control. When the patient can demonstrate the ability to maintain tongue tip to alveolar ridge contact for 5 seconds over five consecutive attempts in the same session, proceed to the fourth step. Some patients may achieve these criteria in the first treatment session and consequently may be permitted to progress to the fourth step or beyond in the same session. As with other treatments, it is unwise to proceed to more complex movement tasks until criteria are met at simpler levels. Fourth, follow the same technique and trial guidelines as suggested in the first three steps, only this time request that tongue tip to alveolar ridge contact be maintained for 10, not 5 seconds. Proceed to the fifth step when the patient can perform this task five consecutive times. Fifth, follow the same technique and trial guidelines suggested in the first through fourth steps, only this time use the $\frac{3}{4}''$ cork. Proceed to the sixth step when the patient can perform the 10-second task five consecutive times. Sixth, use the 1" cork as you have the other corks. Once the patient achieves criteria on the 10-second task with this cork, design a maintenance program wherein practice with the 1" cork is repeated only once every five treatment sessions. Seventh, using the 1" cork again, request the patient to raise and lower the tongue tip 10 times without delay within or between trials. This task will train increased control and speed of tongue movement and should be practiced every treatment session after its introduction until the patient demonstrates proficiency of tongue tip to alveolar ridge movements. Thereafter, a maintenance program may be designed wherein the seventh step is practiced once every five treatment sessions. If corks do not seem appropriate, plastic bite blocks and a compatible handle may be used successfully and are described by Dworkin (1978, 1980b). Proceed to the eighth step after the patient has mastered the seventh step. Eighth, request the patient to stick out the tongue as far as possible, maintain protrusion for 5 seconds and then retract it. Repeat this task four times and proceed to the ninth step when the patient demonstrates success on five consecutive trials in the same session. Ninth, have the patient alternately and repeatedly protrude and retract the tongue without delay between movements for 10 seconds. When the patient can perform this task five consecutive times without signs of hesitation or inaccuracy proceed to the next step. Tenth, have the patient stick out the tongue and wiggle it with moderate speed from one side of the mouth to the other for 10 seconds. When the patient can perform this task five consecutive times with the tongue tip reaching the extreme corners of the lips and without signs of hesitation or inaccuracy, move on to the eleventh and last step. Eleventh, design a maintenance program wherein steps nine and ten are each repeated once every five treatment sessions along with the sixth and seventh steps. A response form like that given in Figure 4 may be used to record and analyze patient performances.

*Irregular Timing or Rhythm*    Neuromuscular deficits of the tongue in timing and rhythm underlie the articulatory difficulties of many patients with dysarthria, but should not be treated until coexistent abnormalities in the tone, strength, and/or range and control of tongue movements have been improved, as prescribed in the above treatment plans. If and when timing treatments are indicated, they should be administered in concert with compensatory articulation training.

A 4/4 time scale (designed according to the rhythm or beat of quarter notes, wherein each note or numeral represents a specific length of time) is simple for patients to follow. The numerals 1, 2, 3, and 4 are used to signify timing; 1 represents one beat, 2 represents two beats, and so on. The speed of the beat may be regulated according to the potential of each patient. Only the clinician need see these numerals; however, the patient may benefit from seeing the measures below and even from hand tapping along with tongue movements.

At the beginning of the session, instruct the patient that the first series of tasks will involve movements of the tongue tip from the rest position up to or toward (in the case of moderate to severe immobility)

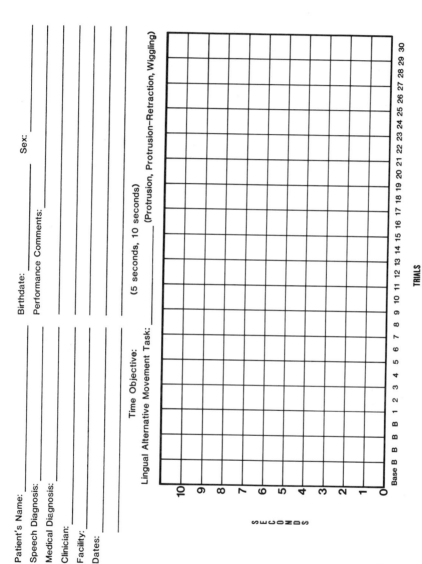

Figure 4.   Form for rating changes in lingual alternate motion skills. Relatively straight lines across the graph, at the 5-second and 10-second levels, would signify normal alternating tongue movement control, and, of course, is the ideal treatment goal for all patients. Indicate the task—protrusion, protrusion-retraction, wiggling—in the space provided and record patient performance for each trial.

the alveolar ridge and then down again, and that these movements will vary in terms of the length of time the tongue may have to remain in either position. Next, position the ¾″ cork or bite block between the patient's teeth as indicated above and request that the tongue-tip be moved up and down in response to your forthcoming verbal commands. The timing of these up (U) and down (D) verbal commands should follow the beat of the "musical score" below; remembering that "4" gets a silent count of four beats, and so on:

$$\left\|\begin{array}{c|c|c|c|c|c|c|c} \frac{4}{4}\ U & D & U & D & U\ D & U\ D & U\ D & U\ D \\ 4 & 4 & 4 & 4 & 2\ 2 & 2\ 2 & 2\ 2 & 2\ 2 \end{array}\right\| :$$

Have the patient repeat this entire score four times consecutively. Proceed to the next step when the patient learns to perform this entire score without errors in timing (errors in range of movement may be accepted) on 30 consecutive trials (six sessions).

Next, introduce the score below, making certain that your verbal commands are synchronized according to the prescribed beat or timing of each measure:

$$\left\|\begin{array}{c|c|c|c|c|c|c|c} \frac{4}{4}\ U\ D & U\ D & U\ D & U\ D & U\ D\ U\ D & U\ D\ U\ D & U\ D\ U\ D & U\ D\ U\ D \\ 2\ 2 & 2\ 2 & 2\ 2 & 2\ 2 & 1\ 1\ 1\ 1 & 1\ 1\ 1\ 1 & 1\ 1\ 1\ 1 & 1\ 1\ 1\ 1 \end{array}\right\| :$$

Have the patient repeat the entire score four times consecutively and proceed to the next score:

$$\left\|\begin{array}{c|c|c|c|c|c|c|c} \frac{4}{4}\ U\ D & U\ D & U\ D & U\ D & U\ D & U\ D & U\ D & U\ D \\ 2\ 2 & 3\ 1 & 2\ 2 & 3\ 1 & 2\ 2 & 1\ 3 & 2\ 2 & 1\ 3 \end{array}\right\| :$$

Have the patient repeat the entire score four times consecutively and proceed to the next score below:

$$\left\|\begin{array}{c|c|c|c|c|c|c|c} \frac{4}{4}\ U\ D\ U & D\ U\ D & U\ D\ U & D\ U\ D & U\ D\ U & D\ U\ D & U\ D\ U & D\ U\ D \\ 2\ 1\ 1 & 2\ 1\ 1 & 2\ 1\ 1 & 2\ 1\ 1 & 1\ 2\ 1 & 1\ 2\ 1 & 1\ 2\ 1 & 1\ 2\ 1 \end{array}\right\| :$$

Have the patient repeat the entire score four times consecutively and proceed to the sixth step and the criteria guidelines of the second step.

At this point, instead of tongue tip to alveolar ridge commands, instruct the patient to stick the tongue out and then pull it in. Follow the same scores and criteria for progress as suggested in the previous steps, but adjust the verbal commands from up/down to "out/in." Naturally, the cork should not be used here. Proceed to the next step when criteria on the last score are met. Now, instead of commands of tongue "out/in," instruct the patient to stick the tongue out and move it to one corner of the mouth and then to the opposite corner. Follow the same scores and criteria for progress as suggested in the second through fifth steps, but adjust the verbal commands from "up/down" or "out/in" to "over/over."

*Lingual Articulation Training: Some Considerations*   Not only are corks or bite blocks helpful in improving the physiological potential of the tongue, for articulation, as described above, they can also be used concurrently to facilitate training of lingual alveolar sounds (/t, d, n, l/) in patients whose prognosis is good for learning tongue tip to alveolar ridge productions. The technique described below may not be of use, however, with patients who must learn tip down and blade up productions of these sounds, because these compensations require the mandible to assist the tongue in its movements and the use of a bite block essentially inhibits such assistance.

At the beginning of the session, position the ½″ × ½″ cork or block between the patient's upper and lower bicuspid teeth on one side and request that the tongue tip be lifted to the alveolar ridge, pressed firmly against that area and then released abruptly to facilitate production of the /t/ sound. Repeated demonstrations of this approach and use of a mirror for visual biofeedback of tongue tip activity may be helpful. Sometimes a tissue held in front of the patient's lips, as productions are attempted, can provide additional information about the manner of /t/ production. Have the patient observe the fluttering of the tissue in response to the exploded airstream. Have the patient repeat /t/ attempts 25 times with the ½″ cork or block. Score each attempt as correct or incorrect and proceed with the second step when 90% of 25 consecutive trials are produced correctly. Next, repeat the same tasks as suggested in the above step, but this time use the ¾″ cork or block. Proceed with the third step when the 90% criterion is achieved as suggested above.

Now, combine the /t/ with the vowel /a/ and request that the patient repeat this consonant-vowel (CV) syllable 10 times without the aid of a block or cork; however, use the tissue once again for visual biofeedback of air explosion. When the patient can produce this CV syllable with acceptable intelligibility on 90% of 25 trials, change the vowel to /u/, then /i/, and so on. Follow the same strategy for each CV syllable, as suggested for /ta/. When all CV syllable combinations have been practiced and criteria have been met for each in isolation, the patient is ready to practice the syllables together. Have the patient take a deep breath and produce the entire list rapidly and without hesitation between syllables, and on one breath if possible. If the patient can produce the entire list as required on 90% of 25 trials, repeat the third and fourth steps above, but this time place the vowels in the initial position and the /t/ in the final position (VC). Ultimately, CVC and CVCV words are incorporated in the treatment plan as the patient demonstrates articulatory readiness for more complex sound combinations. When this training is completed, the patient is ready to receive training on the remaining lingual-alveolar sounds /d, 1, and n/.

The information in this chapter is not meant to suggest that treatment of tongue musculature abnormalities for improving the speech of patients with dysarthria should be done without systematic treatment of the neuromuscular disturbances that underlie the dysarthrias. Additionally, when an holistic neuromuscular facilitation approach is not successful, alternate nonverbal communication systems may prove helpful for many patients.

## REFERENCES

Allan, C. M., Turner, J. W., and Gadeacira, M. 1966. Investigations into speech disturbances following stereotaxic surgery for parkinsonism. Br. J. Disord. Commun. 1:55–59.

Amato, A., Hermsmeyer, C. A., and Kleinman, K. M. 1973. Use of electromyographic feedback to increase inhibitory control of spastic muscles. Phys. Ther. 53:1063–1066.

Angel, R. W., Alston, W., and Garland, H. 1971. L-Dopa and error correction time in Parkinson's disease. Neurology 21:1255–1260.

Arnold, G. E. 1962. Vocal rehabilitation of paralytic dysphonia 1X. Technique of intercordal injection. Arch. Otolaryngol. 76:358–365.

Berry, W. R., Aronson, A. E., Darley, F. L., and Goldstein, N. P. 1974. Effects of Penicillamine therapy and low-copper diet on dysarthria in Wilson's disease (hepatolenticular degeneration). Mayo Clin. Proc. 49:405–408.

Beukelman, D. R., and Yorkston, K. 1977. A communication system for the severely dysarthric speakers with an intact language system. J. Speech Hear. Disord. 42:265–270.

Cosman, B., and Folk, A. 1975. Pharyngeal flap augmentation. Plastic Reconstruct. Surg. 55:149–155.

Daniel, B., and Guitar, B. 1978. EMG feedback and recovery of facial and speech gestures following neural anastomosis. J. Speech Hear. Disord. 43:9–20.

Darley, F. L., Brown, J. R., and Swenson, W. M. 1975. Language changes after neurosurgery for parkinsonism. Brain Lang. 2:65–69.

Dworkin, J. P. 1978. A therapeutic technique for the improvement of lingua-alveolar valving abilities. J. Lang. Speech Hear. Serv. Schools 9:162–175.

Dworkin, J. P. 1980a. Tongue strength measurement in patients with ALS: Qualitative vs. quantitative procedures. Arch. Phys. Med. Rehabil. 61:422–424.

Dworkin, J. P. 1980b. Instructional use for bite blocks. In: J. P. Dworkin and R. A. Culatta (eds.), Dworkin-Culatta Oral Mechanism Examination. Edgewood Press, Nicholasville, KY.

Dworkin, J. P., and Aronson, A. E. 1982. Tongue strength and alternate motion rates in normal subjects and patients with different types of dysarthria. Unpublished manuscript.

Dworkin, J. P., and Hartman, D. E. 1979. Progressive speech deterioration and dysphagia in ALS. Arch. Phys. Med. Rehabil. 60:423–425.

Dworkin, J. P., and Johns, D. F. 1980. Management of velopharyngeal incompetence in dysarthria: A historical review. Clin. Otolaryngol. Allied Sci. 5:61–74.

Dworkin, J. P., Aronson, A. E., and Mulder, D. W. 1980. Tongue strength in normal subjects and dysarthric patients with amyotrophic lateral sclerosis. J. Speech Hear. Res. 23:828–837.

Dworkin, J. P., Bandur, D., and Hudson, A. J. 1982. Communication problems in ALS. In: D. Goldblatt (ed.), Management of ALS. ALS Society of America through the Muscular Dystrophy Association, Los Angeles, CA.

Froeschels, E. 1952. Dysarthric Speech. Expression Co., Magnolia, MA.

Gonzalez, J. B., and Aronson, A. E. 1970. Palatial lift prosthesis for treatment of anatomic and neurologic palatopharyngeal insufficiency. Cleft Palate J. 7:91–104.

Greer, M. 1970. L-Dopa therapy in Parkinson's disease. J. Florida Med. Assoc. 57:23–27.

Hagen, C., Porter, W., and Brinks, J. 1973. Nonverbal communication: An alternate mode of communication for the child with severe cerebral palsy. J. Speech Hear. Disord. 38:448–455.

Hanson, W. R., and Metter, E. J. 1980. DAF as instrumental treatment for dysarthria in progressive supranuclear palsy: A case report. J. Speech Hear. Disord. 45:268–276.

Hardy, J. C. 1967. Suggestions for physiologic research in dysarthria. Cortex 3:128–156.

Hartman, D. E., Day, M., and Pecora, R. 1979. Treatment of dysarthria: A case report. J. Commun. Disord. 12:167–173.

Helm, N. A. 1979. Management of palilalia with a pacing board. J. Speech Hear. Disord. 44:350–353.

Ince, L. P., and Rosenberg, D. N. 1963. Modification of articulation in dysarthria. Arch. Phys. Med. Rehabil. 54:233–236.

Johns, D. F., and Salyer, K. E. 1978. Surgical and prosthetic management of neurogenic speech disorders. In: D. F. Johns (ed.), Clinical Management of Neurogenic Communicative Disorders, pp. 311–331. Little, Brown and Co., Boston.

Kerman, P. C., Singer, L. S., and Davidoff, A. 1973. Palatal lift and speech therapy for velopharyngeal incompetence. Arch. Phys. Med. Rehabil. 54:271–276.

Kiehm, C. L., Des Prex, J. D., Tucker, A., and Malone, M. 1965. Activation of the incomplete soft palate by means of muscle transplants: A preliminary report on sixteen cases. Cleft Palate J. 2:133–140.

Leanderson, R., Meyerson, B. A., and Persson, A. 1971. Effect of L-Dopa on speech in parkinsonism. An EMG study of labial articulatory function. J. Neurol. Neurosurg. Psych. 34:679–681.

McDonald, E. T., and Schultz, A. R. 1973. Communication boards for cerebral palsied children. J. Speech Hear. Disord. 38:73–88.

Mysak, E. D. 1963. Dysarthria and oropharyngeal reflexology: A review. J. Speech Hear. Disord. 28:252–260.

Nakano, K. K., Zubick, W., and Tyler, H. R. 1973. Speech defects of parkinsonian patients: Effects of Levodopa therapy in speech intelligibility. Neurology 23:365–370.

Netsell, R., and Cleeland, C. S. 1973. Modification of lip hypertonia in dysarthria using EMG feedback. J. Speech Hear. Disord. 38:131–140.

Osserman, K. E., and Genkins, G. 1966. Critical reappraisal of the use of edrophonium (Tensilon) chloride tests in myasthenia gravis and significance of clinical classification. Ann. N.Y. Acad. Sci. 135:312–334.

Rembisz, L. S., and Gribin, S. A. 1975. Neuromuscular facilitation therapeutic techniques in treating the dysarthric patient. Scientific exhibit at Annual Convention of American Speech-Language-Hearing Association, Washington, DC.

Rigrodsky, S., and Morrison, E. B. 1970. Speech changes in parkinsonism during L-Dopa therapy: Preliminary findings. J. Am. Geriatr. Soc. 18:142–151.

Robbins, S. D. 1940. Dysarthria and its treatment. J. Speech Disord. 5:113–120.

Rosenbek, J. C., and LaPointe, L. L. 1978. The dysarthrias: Description, diagnosis and treatment. In: D. F. Johns (ed.), Clinical Management of Neurogenic Communicative Disorders, pp. 251–310. Little, Brown and Co., Boston.

Rubin, H. J. 1965. Pitfalls in treatment of dysphonias by intercordal injection of synthetics. Laryngoscope 75:1381–1397.

Rubin, H. J. 1975. Misadventures with injectable Teflon. Arch. Otolaryngol. 101:114–116.

Rubow, R. T., Rosenbek, J. C., Collins, M. J., and Celesia, G. G. 1981. EMG biofeedback in the treatment of hemifacial spasm and associated dysarthria: A case study. Poster session at Annual Convention of American Speech-Language-Hearing Association, Toronto.

Samra, K., Riklan, M., LeVita, E., et al. 1969. Language and speech correlates of anatomically verified lesions in thalamic surgery for parkinsonism. J. Speech Hear. Res. 12:510–540.

Shane, H. C., and Bashir, A. S. 1980. Election criteria for the adoption of an augmentative communication system: Preliminary considerations. J. Speech Hear. Disord. 45:408–414.

Wertz, R. T. 1978. Neuropathologies of speech and language: An introduction to patient management. In: D. F. Johns (ed.), Clinical Management of Neurogenic Communicative Disorders, pp. 1–102. Little, Brown and Co., Boston.

Westlake, H. 1951. Muscle training for cerebral palsied speech cases. J. Speech Hear. Disord. 16:103–109.

# CHAPTER 19

# Apraxia of Speech: A Neurogenic Articulation Disorder

*Frederic L. Darley*

*Apraxia of speech is an interesting but difficult disorder to treat. In this chapter Darley provides a thorough review of the cause, assessment, and treatment of this articulation disorder.*

1. *Provide a clinical description of the disorder apraxia of speech. Include in your description the common speech errors of the apractic patient.*
2. *What conditions seem to provoke articulation errors in apractic speakers? Conversely, what conditions show no effect on their speech?*
3. *Testing for apraxia of speech involves several considerations. How does apraxia differ from dysarthria? How is oral apraxia assessed? What method is used to assess the severity of apraxia for speech tasks?*
4. *What are the fundamental objectives for the treatment of apraxia of speech indicated by Darley? What particular procedures does Darley recommend are to be used to teach articulation of sounds to apractic speakers? In your answer cite the rationale for the attention given to suprasegmentals when teaching articulation.*
5. *What is developmental apraxia of speech? What evidence is there to indicate the validity of this speech disorder? How is it treated?*

---

Masculine pronouns are used throughout this chapter for the sake of grammatical uniformity and simplicity. They are not meant to be preferential or discriminatory.

A DISTINCTIVE ARTICULATION DISORDER attributable to dysfunction of the motor programming function of the central nervous system has long been recognized. Unlike articulation problems in dysarthria, it does not result from slowness, weakness, incoordination, or alteration of tone of the speech musculature. Unlike dysarthria, it does not have associated with it distinctive phonatory and resonatory deviations, and the prosodic alterations that sometimes accompany it are probably compensatory in nature. Unlike aphasia, it is not the result of impairment of the speaker's ability to decode or encode meaningful linguistic units; rather, it involves the programming of the elemental speech postures and sequences of them.

The disorder was first named "aphemia" in 1861 by Paul Broca, who recognized that it was separate from aphasia and dysarthria, that it represented the loss of "a particular faculty . . . for coordinating the proper movements of articulated language, or more simply the faculty of articulated language since without it articulation is not possible." It was later redesignated motor aphasia and Broca's aphasia, although Pierre Marie insisted that it was only one component of a Broca's aphasia; he redesignated that component "anarthria," "loss or disturbance of articulated speech, with more or less complete preservation of inner speech," "a defect in the coordination of the movements of phonation." This component came to be hidden in the concept of "predominantly expressive aphasia" (Weisenberg and McBride, 1935).

The dynamics of the problem came into sharper focus when Liepmann (1900) advanced the general concept of apraxia: an inability to perform at will and on command certain complex movements despite adequate muscle strength, sensation, attention, and volition. He considered "aphemia"/"anarthria" to be a particular form of apraxia of the glosso-labio-pharyngeal apparatus. Several variations of this terminology have been used: "apraxia of the speech musculature" (Wilson, 1908), "apraxic dysarthria" (Nathan, 1947), "articulatory dyspraxia" (Critchley, 1952), "cortical dysarthria involving a distinct apraxia of the articulatory muscles" (Bay, 1964), and "apraxia of vocal expression" (Denny-Brown, 1965). In recent years, the term *apraxia of speech* has come into fairly common usage and appears appropriate and useful, as Johns and LaPointe (1976) have pointed out, because the term "explicitly (1) directs one's attention to the motor aspects of speech; (2) emphasizes the volitional execution of articulation; (3) excludes significant weakness, paralysis, and incoordination of the speech musculature; and (4) indicates a discrepancy between execution of the speech act and relative linguistic intactness."

## ACQUIRED APRAXIA OF SPEECH

### How to Recognize It

After some sort of cerebral episode—whether a vascular accident, a brain tumor, trauma, an infectious process (encephalitis) or some inflammatory process—individuals who theretofore have had perfectly normal articulation may display this distinctive impairment. The speaker knows the words he wants to say, but he cannot say them efficiently. He appears uncertain as to how to position his articulators. He visibly gropes for correct articulation points but, failing to attain them, is frequently off target. More often than not he recognizes his error and tries to correct it, sometimes seeming to struggle effortfully to do so, even using his fingers to try to position his articulators. He may make several trials to produce the correct sound; he may succeed or he may in his successive trials mistakenly assume several different articulatory postures. Parts of his sentences may be fluent and well articulated; these islands of fluent speech make it clear that his problem is not due to inadequacy of innervation of any specific muscle group.

Here is how one patient read a standard paragraph demonstrating variable substitutions, additions, repetitions, prolongations, distortions, and omissions of sounds:

> You wiss to know all about my gwandfather. Well, he is nearly ninety-three years hold, yet he still thinks as chwiftly as ever. He dresses himself in an old black flock co—coat, usually sevrial buttons mit—missing. A long beers kins to his to—chin, giving who—those who obser—uh—observe him a pronounced feeling of the n—utmost ref—feh—respect. When he spuh—eaks, his v—voice is just a bit cratched and t—quivers a bick. Twice ea—each day he plays still—ful—ly and with t—zest upon a muh—small organ. Excep in the winter when the snow or ice pre—vents, he slowly takes an s—short walk in the open air each day. We have often hurged him to walk more and smoke less, but he always huh—answers, "Banana oil!" Grandfather like to be m—modern in his lain-dricks—hush—langwush—lang-gwiss—lang-chuh—lang-druss—It won't come out—langwish—langwicks. I don't think I can say it any better.

*Characteristics of Error Occurrence*    Studies of apractic speech errors have shown that they occur with certain lawfulness and predictability:

1. Speech sounds requiring complex motor adjustment of the articulators are most likely to be produced in error. Vowels evoke fewer errors than consonants. Of the singleton consonants, affricate and fricative phonemes evoke the most errors. Consonant clusters evoke the most errors of all. Palatal and dental sounds are signif-

icantly more frequently in error than other sounds classified according to place of production (Burns and Canter, 1977; Deal and Darley, 1972; Dunlop and Marquardt, 1977; Johns and Darley, 1970; LaPointe and Johns, 1975; Shankweiler and Harris, 1966; Trost and Canter, 1974).

2.  Errors are likely to occur in any position in a word. Some observers have reported that initial consonants tend to be misarticulated more often than those in other positions (Shankweiler and Harris, 1966; Trost and Canter, 1974), but others (Dunlop and Marquardt, 1977; Johns and Darley, 1970; LaPointe and Johns, 1975) have reported speech sound position to be unrelated to occurrence of error.

3.  On repeated performance in presenting the same content, whether in oral reading or in reciting well-learned material or in repeated presentation of self-generated material, apractic speakers demonstrate a consistency effect, tending to make errors at the same loci from trial to trial (Deal, 1974; Mlcoch et al., 1982). Less impressive than this consistency effect is a minor adaptation effect, as they tend to make fewer errors on successive presentations (Deal, 1974). Especially impressive is the variability of the errors at given loci on repeated trials (Mlcoch et al., 1982).

4.  Speech sounds that occur with relatively high frequency in the language are more likely to be articulated correctly than sounds that occur less frequently (Trost and Canter, 1974).

5.  When apractic speakers make substitution errors, the sounds they substitute are variably related to the intended target sounds in terms of distinctive features. Many errors are only one or two features away from target (Martin and Rigrodsky, 1974a,b), but a substantial proportion of the errors are more remote from target and bear little acoustic resemblance to the target sound (LaPointe and Johns, 1975).

How does apractic speech vary?

1.  As already mentioned, many apractic speakers display islands of relatively fluent speech punctuated by apractic errors. The fluent episodes usually occur on relatively automatic or reactive speech productions such as counting or reciting jingles, extending greetings, swearing, and making off-hand comments. Speech performance that might be described as more volitional or purposive is more likely to be characterized by apractic errors.

2.  The longer the word, the more likely the speaker will be to make articulation errors in it. Polysyllabic words are common sites of articulatory breakdown, as can be demonstrated by the patient's increasing errors as he produces a series of words with a common

syllable nucleus (sit, city, citizen, citizenship) (Johns and Darley, 1970).

3. Words that play an important role in communication are likely to elicit more apractic errors. For example, words that occur early in a sentence, that are longer, that are more abstract, that are nouns, adjectives, adverbs, or verbs, or that begin with more difficult to produce sounds are more likely to be misarticulated (Deal and Darley, 1972; Dunlop and Marquardt, 1977). Combination of these "weights" appears to determine occurrence of error more than single characteristics that occur in isolation.

*Influences That Seem Not to Affect Apractic Speech*    On the other hand, the appearance of articulatory errors does not appear to be significantly influenced by several other variables:

1. The number of articulation errors the speaker makes is not significantly altered by having the sound of his voice masked out by noise played into his ears (Deal and Darley, 1972).
2. When he is asked to delay an imitative response, the speaker does not typically perform better than in a no-delay condition (Deal and Darley, 1972).
3. Articulatory accuracy is uninfluenced by attempts to create certain instructional sets in the speaker. He typically performs equally well or poorly on an oral reading task whether told that the passage is easy, difficult, or undetermined with regard to degree of difficulty because of its articulatory characteristics (Deal and Darley, 1972).
4. Speech performance is not improved by imposing an external auditory rhythm such as by a metronome, whether to slow speech or to speed it up (Shane and Darley, 1978).
5. Accuracy of speech sound production and duration of the words produced is not influenced by imposing delayed auditory feedback (Lozano and Dreyer, 1978).
6. The frequency, consistency, and variability of articulatory errors seem to be generally impervious to conditions of stress imposed upon the speaker, both situational stress (performing before an audience) and communicative stress (doing the speaking or reading task as rapidly as possible) (Mlcoch et al., 1982).

*How to Test for Apraxia of Speech*    How can we determine whether the patient's articulation errors are on an apractic basis? It will be necessary to examine the oral speech mechanism to determine whether there is a significant degree of weakness, slowness, incoordination, or alteration of tone of the speech muscles. Absence of these suggests that the problem is not dysarthric in nature but possibly apractic. We can carry this examination a step beyond the usual inventory of tasks to determine whether the speaker can produce more complex volitional oral movements such as the following:

| | |
|---|---|
| Stick out your tongue | Bite your lower lip |
| Blow | Whistle |
| Show me your teeth | Lick your lips |
| Pucker your lips | Clear your throat |
| Touch your nose with tip of tongue | Move your tongue in and out |
| | Cough |
| Click your teeth together once | Puff out your cheeks |
| Smile | Wiggle your tongue from side to |
| Click your tongue | side |
| Chatter your teeth as if cold | Show how you kiss someone |
| Touch your chin with tip of tongue | Alternately pucker and smile |

Performance on these tasks can be scaled as follows:

| | |
|---|---|
| 8 | Accurate, immediate, on command |
| 7 | Accurate after trial and error, searching movements, on command |
| 6 | Crude, defective in amplitude, accuracy, or speed, on command |
| 5 | Partial, important part missing, on command |
| 4 | Same as 8, after demonstration |
| 3 | Same as 7, after demonstration |
| 2 | Same as 6, after demonstration |
| 1 | Same as 5, after demonstration |
| OP | Perseverative |
| OI | Irrelevant; some other oral performance, including speech |
| ON | Nil. No oral performance |

Some patients, but not all, who demonstrate apractic speech difficulty demonstrate an associated oral apraxia (DeRenzi et al., 1966), as would be indicated by a low total score on this test.

We can then use a series of tasks graduated in difficulty to determine at what levels and with what efficiency the patient can articulate in certain volitional speech tasks and where he breaks down:

1.  To get a sample of "automatic" speech performance, ask the patient to count to 10, list the days of the week, and repeat the Lord's Prayer or the Pledge of Allegiance or some other typically overlearned selection.
2.  Take the patient through an articulatory inventory, asking him to repeat after you each of the vowels, diphthongs, and single consonants, noting the nature of the errors if any.
3.  Moving on to a word level task, ask the patient to repeat consonant-vowel-consonant (CVC) monosyllabic words, again testing the various consonant singles but this time in context (mom, peep, bib,

nine, tote, dad, coke, gag, fife, sis, zoos, shush, church, judge, lull).

4.  Have the speaker repeat as rapidly and regularly as possible the syllables /puh/, /tuh/, and /kuh/, noting the rate at which these are produced; the regularity of their spacing, pitch, and loudness; and the ease with which the sequence is maintained. Then ask the patient to produce the overlapping sequence /puh-tuh-kuh/. Many apractic subjects can readily produce a single consonant repeatedly but experience inordinate difficulty in producing the overlapping sequence; they repeat parts of the sequence, omit parts, change the order, have difficulty initiating a syllable and maintaining the sequence smoothly.

5.  Ask the patient to repeat a number of polysyllabic words selected for phonetic complexity: animal, artillery, catastrophe, several, criminal, and phrases such as several umbrellas, statistical analysis, Methodist Episcopal Church.

6.  Have the patient repeat words of increasing length which share a common syllable core: zip—zipper—zippering; please—pleasing—pleasingly; door—doorknob—doorkeeper—dormitory.

7.  Ask the patient to repeat sentences laced with phonetically complex words: "There was criticism of the funeral ceremony"; "The municipal judge sentenced the criminal"; "My physician wrote out a prescription."

8.  Ask the patient to read a standard paragraph (My Grandfather, the Rainbow Passage) noting the frequency and types of articulatory error. Are the errors typically errors of simplification (omissions or distortions) or are there errors which constitute complications of the articulation act (additions, repetitions, substitutions, prolongations)?

*Analysis of Results*   The speaker who displays no impairment of strength, coordination, or tone of the speech musculature but who cannot readily produce single speech sounds in imitation of the examiner can be suspected of displaying a severe apraxia of speech. Other patients with less severe impairment demonstrate breakdown at some higher level of complexity of speech performance, perhaps at monosyllabic word level, perhaps at polysyllabic word level, perhaps only at sentence level. Better performance on automatic-reactive speech than on volitional-purposive speech suggests apractic involvement. The nature of the errors provides a further clue that the problem is apractic in nature: Are the errors inconsistent, in fact, highly variable as repeated trials are attempted? Are there frequent errors of substitution as well as additions, repetitions, and prolongations? Does the patient appear to be groping to find the correct articulatory postures? Is he aware that he is not on target? All of these behaviors suggest that the patient is unable at will and on command to perform complex motor speech tasks despite the integrity of the neuromuscular apparatus— that is, the patient is probably apractic.

***Remediation of the Problem***    What we do to help the patient will depend importantly upon how severe his apractic difficulty is and how much of a speech sound repertoire is available to him. But whether the severity is of greater or lesser degree, the core problem is essentially the same: when the speaker undertakes volitional speech movements to produce given sounds, he seems to have "forgotten" how to perform them. The goal in treatment is to help the apractic patient regain efficiency in voluntary accurate control in attaining the positioning of his articulators to produce speech sounds and sequences of them.

The approach to articulation treatment should be direct. Evidence is abundant that even though he may have an associated aphasia, as most apractic patients do, the patient's problem does not result from some imperception of the word he is trying to produce or the sound he is trying to articulate (Aten et al., 1971; Johns and Darley, 1970; Shankweiler and Harris, 1966; Square et al., 1981). Unless the associated aphasia is severe, these patients can demonstrate that they have clear perception of the target word and of the sounds comprising it. They do not need the general language stimulation that the aphasic patient needs, to be bombarded with the target word repeatedly in varying contexts, nor do they need training on auditory discrimination of sounds. Rather, we must help them relearn the crucial points for articulation of given sounds and how to put together a sequence of them.

Typically, auditory information alone is insufficient for the apractic patient to attain his target. The likelihood of his producing the target sound increases as he is able to use multiple kinds of information— visual, tactile, and kinesthetic, as well as auditory. Multimodality stimulation seems to help, as does working to heighten his awareness of all kinds of sensory feedback.

It seems that multiple opportunities to use this sensory information and get on target is more important to the speaker than multiple presentations to him of that sensory information. The speaker will more likely get on target if when he has heard a stimulus once, he undertakes repeated trials to imitate the stimulus than if we offer the stimulus several times and ask him to produce only a single trial of it.

We need to make clear to the patient the nature of the task he faces in treatment: he is trying to relearn some motor skills and there is no short-cut to relearning them. We will be engaging in drill, repetitious drill, during which he will develop a greater sensitivity for what his articulators are doing and how effectively he is programming their movements. His goal will be consciously and deliberately to perform movements that used to be automatic and easy. Drill will heighten his skill in monitoring his performance. He will learn to get better and better at listening to himself talk, observing precisely what his errors were, checking to see if he is doing what is required for production of a given sound, looking ahead and anticipating difficult sounds and words as they approach, learning to be watchful and learning from failure how to do better next time.

One of the first lessons we must teach him is to pace his speech so as to be able to make the necessary choices and get on target. A deliberate rate, slower than his former rate of speaking, is almost surely necessary.

The speaker will learn that his performance is noteworthy in its variability, and variability is a function of many influences. He will do less well when he is feeling sick or tired or when he is emotionally upset. His central nervous system experiences good days and bad days. He can learn to recognize these influences and their deleterious effect on his performance and learn not to struggle frantically and vainly. We can help the patient learn when his efforts are productive and when they seem to be counterproductive, when it is useful to keep on reaching for the target and when it is better to stop, rest, and begin over or wait until another day.

*Helping the Patient with Severe Apraxia of Speech*    The severely apractic patient is essentially speechless. He may perseveratively produce a small repertoire of unintended sounds such as "oh" or "I" or "ah." He has no spontaneous speech and demonstrates no repertoire of sounds that he can make at will. On the articulation inventory, he may have been able to imitate a vowel or two, perhaps a consonant or two.

It will be useful initially to try to get some kind of "automatic" speech going. We may ask the patient to count along with us or recite the days of the week or respond with everyday expressions, such as "hi," "fine," "thank you," "goodbye." Open-ended sentences that lead to essentially automatic completing words may elicit speech: "The American flag is red, white, and _____ "; "We wash with soap and _____ "; "Two and two are _____ ." Showing a picture: "I want a piece of _____ " or "I'll have a cup of _____ ." Perhaps the patient can hum along on a familiar song and begin to insert some words of the song together with the clinician.

Ultimately, we will probably have to move to the lengthy process of teaching the patient to produce the sounds to which he has no ready access (Dabul and Bollier, 1976). Recognizing the fact that phonemes fall in a hierarchy of difficulty for apractic patients, we may start with vowels, moving to nasals, glides, and semivowels. Plosives will probably be more difficult, fricatives and affricates still more difficult and therefore properly introduced later. One may well want to work early on sounds that provide visual cues /m, p, b, n, t, d, f, v/ and later work on those in which the articulation points are less visible. Probably the sounds worked on successively should be as dissimilar as possible; for example, after concentrating on /p/ one might prefer not to move to /b/ but rather to something as different as /f/ to obviate possible confusion and facilitate the patient's grasp of the unique character of the new sound.

As we teach each sound individually, we will provide not only auditory models but call the patient's attention to visual information about the production of the sound and tactile and kinesthetic feedback about it as well. Work can ordinarily best be conducted with clinician and patient seated in front of a mirror large enough to allow the patient to watch both the clinician's face as he speaks and his own face as he imitates the model. If the patient finds work before a mirror confusing, the clinician can face the patient.

Tell the patient how the sound is made—what position the tongue and lips are to take, how the air is to flow. Show the patient how to make the sound, asking him to listen carefully and watch (Rosenbek et al., 1973). Use phonetic placement and point out to the patient where the clinician's tongue and lips are, touching the patient's articulators, emphasizing the visual, tactile, and kinesthetic information at his disposal. Visual cues can be provided also by showing him frontal and cross-sectional diagrams of the position of the articulators for each sound. Each sound might be associated with something else—/p/ is a popping sound, /m/ is a humming sound, /ʃ/ is a shushing sound. One may go a step further and introduce a gesture to be associated consistently with a given sound—a closing of the fist, raising of the hand, tapping on the table. (Pairing of gesture and speech—an intact system with an impaired one—is an example of Luria's (1970) intersystemic reorganization, which seems to improve verbalization in some patients (Rosenbek et al., 1976).)

We may ask the patient first to assume the necessary articulatory posture for the target sound without actually producing the sound. Then he can produce the sound in isolation, prolonging it, carefully observing what is involved in making the sound. We know that it is harder for the patient to produce sounds in units of increasing length, so we begin with sounds in isolation and move successively to VC or CV syllables,

CVC syllables, strings of these syllables, and then words (Dabul and Bollier, 1976).

Using as an example the sound /p/, we produce and ask the patient to imitate the production of /p/ in isolation, silently then aloud. We add a vowel to produce pah, then in turn a series of vowels and diphthongs, practicing the production of each many times: pee, poo, paw, po, pow. We may use a visual layout with /p/ as a nucleus and a circle of vowels and diphthongs surrounding it, showing the patient how to make a quick adjustment in moving from one to another. Next we may double the syllable and practice a series of these bisyllables: papa, papa, papa; popo, popo, popo; poopoo, poopoo, poopoo; then the sequence papa—popo—poopoo. Next /p/ can be added as a final consonant in the syllable: pop, peep, poop, the patient repeating each many times.

We move to word level and practice a series of meaningful words beginning with and containing relatively easy phonetic elements: pie, pine, pat; then with the sound in both positions: pipe, pip, pope. Move to two-word sequences in which both words begin with /p/: pig pen, pie pan; then to words ending with /p/: wipe up, help chop; then to two-word combinations in which /p/ begins the first word and ends the second: put up, pull rope. Finally, we move to multiple word phrases and polysyllabic words, later incorporating these in sentences: a paper cap, deep dish apple pie.

After work has progressed successfully through several sounds, drills can contrast paired sounds. For example, if the patient has gone through the above sequence of drills on /p/ and also on /t/, we can help him practice making the transition from one sound to the other in successive words: pick-tick, sap-sat. At first, the members of the contrasting pairs should be well separated in terms of the articulation points involved, but gradually the distance between them can be reduced, progressing to cognate pairs identical with regard to position and manner but different with regard to voicing. In such work the patient may be helped by having him use such suprasegmental features as changes in loudness from the first to the second of the pair, changes in pitch, associated with changes in gesture and even in bodily position.

When the patient is able to produce several consonants with some facility, we may use a visual layout with a vowel or diphthong as a nucleus and a series of consonants surrounding it to practice moving quickly from one syllable to another (may, tay, kay, say, shay). Drill on consonant clusters can follow.

We progress through tasks of increasing length and complexity and work for carryover of articulation skills to conversational speech. Emphasis never ceases on the patient's watchful monitoring of what his articulators are doing, anticipation of sounds coming up, and careful planning of the necessary articulatory postures, with immediate self-correction of any error.

The speech pattern that results will probably be slow and seem over-deliberate, even stilted, too carefully articulated to sound normal. But as the patient continues to recover and incorporate his new skills into conversation, we can expect his rate to accelerate and the whole prosodic pattern to sound more natural and spontaneous.

*Helping the Less Severe Apractic Patient*    Less severe apractic patients will have more fluent speech interrupted periodically by articulatory lapses. The speech produced indicates that a patient has a wide repertoire of sounds but has inefficient access to it. He can produce all of the sounds at times, so it is not necessary to teach production of the individual sounds from the ground up as in the case of more severe patients. Rather, treatment is designed to improve his efficiency at accessing his speech sound repertoire, to facilitate correct production of sounds he is clearly capable of producing.

Again, we use the method of auditory and visual stimulation, resorting to phonetic placement as it seems desirable. It may help if at first the patient produces his response simultaneously with the clinician's presentation of the word or sentence stimulus. Later, after presenting a stimulus we may ask the patient to imitate it as we this time present only a visual cue, silently mouthing the stimulus: later we may ask him to wait after we have presented a stimulus and imitate it without further visual or auditory cues (Rosenbek et al., 1973).

A number of suprasegmental features may facilitate production of the correct sound. Sometimes it helps if the clinician increases his loudness and in turn asks the patient to increase his loudness in producing the response. Almost surely, rate must be slowed to permit more accurate imitation of the stimulus. We may exaggerate natural syllabic and word stress in presenting a sentence stimulus. Intonational patterns may be adopted as a facilitator—the clinical procedure called Melodic Intonation Therapy; one converts the prosodic patterns of spoken speech into intonational patterns using a pitch range of three or four whole notes (Sparks, 1981). Producing the utterance in a rhythmic pattern may also facilitate its production.

An extension of these procedures is the use of contrastive stress drills as suggested by Rosenbek (1978). We use the stress elements of pitch, loudness, and time to highlight a syllable or word and contrast it with another syllable or word containing the same or a different sound. For example, if we are concentrating on production of /s/, we may present the stimulus sentence "I saw the suit." The patient repeats it. Then we ask, "You *bought* the suit?" He responds with an exaggerated stress on the verb, "I *saw* the suit." Then we ask, "You saw the *coat*?'' and the patient responds with an exaggeration of the contrasting noun, ''I saw the *suit*.'' Or if we are working on more than one consonant at a time, for example, /b/ and /t/, the patient may imitate the presentation of a sentence like ''Bill hit Tom.'' We ask, ''Who hit Tom?'' and the patient responds with contrastive stress on the first noun, ''*Bill* hit Tom.'' We ask, ''Bill *kicked* Tom?'' and the patient responds with an exaggeration of the verb, ''Bill *hit* Tom.'' We ask, ''Bill hit *Bob*?'' and the patient responds with an exaggeration of the noun object, ''Bill hit *Tom*.'' Accuracy of sound production may be facilitated as we ask the patient to vary the presentation of a sentence to present alternative meanings: ''*Please* pass the salt; Please *pass* the salt; Please pass the *salt*.'' As with severely apractic patients, so with more mild patients, introducing associated gestures or bodily movements in the contrastive stress drills facilitates correct production.

Emphasis continues throughout on the need for the patient to monitor his performance, helping him grow in confidence in his ability to proceed less tentatively, more assertively.

### DEVELOPMENTAL APRAXIA OF SPEECH

It seems reasonable to believe that there may be a childhood form of apraxia of speech resulting from a congenital dysfunction of the speech programmer which inhibits the child's learning to produce consistently complex movement patterns necessary for speech. Morley (1965) has for years written about children with what she calls a developmental dyspraxia, and a scattering of other clinical workers have alluded to this possibility in patients they have seen and worked with. Yoss and Darley (1974a) carried the observations a step further in an attempt to determine what the characteristics of such a disorder might be and how some articulatory-defective children may be singled out as representing an apractic disorder requiring distinctive treatment. They administered a series of speech and nonspeech oral performance tests to 30 public school children with moderate to severe articulation problems, who were also given neurological examinations, audiometric tests, and psychometric tests. None of the children showed gross neurological impairment, but on 14 volitional oral tasks, including such things as blowing, licking their lips, puffing out their cheeks, showing how to kiss, whistling, and coughing, some children proved to be extremely poor, whereas others performed normally. The group was divided into two subgroups on the basis of how well they performed nonspeech oral tasks. Discriminant function analysis was used to determine what speech signs differentiated the two groups. It was found that those who performed poorly on the volitional oral tasks had more neurological signs than the others, sometimes being identified as generally dys-praxic, clumsy, awkward. These children also had slower rates of oral diadochokinesis, and when they tried to repeat the series puh-tuh-kuh they often produced an incorrect syllable sequence. They displayed greater difficulty in repeating polysyllabic words, often omitting, re-vising, or adding syllables. When their errors were analyzed with regard to distinctive features, these children presented more two- and three-feature errors, more prolongations and repetitions of sounds and syl-lables, more distortions, such as minimal nasalization or voicing errors, and more additions. They displayed more prosodic differences such as slowed rate and equalized stress. With the exception of some of the older children who had been in treatment for some time, the children did not typically display the highly variable trial and error groping behavior that adult apractic patients display in trying to produce a target sound. It seemed reasonable to conclude from the data that there was indeed a subgroup of children who behaved differently on oral praxis and in articulation, justifying the designation of developmental apraxia of speech.

Another feature that Morley has reported as identifying devel-opmentally apractic children is the general recalcitrance of their prob-lem to treatment. Many of the children studied by Yoss and Darley had been in treatment for a long time; the clinicians working with these children often reported that in desperation they finally abandoned the usual auditory approach in retraining and resorted to phonetic place-ment procedures, organizing their treatment so as to emphasize the use of visual, tactile, and kinesthetic cues (Yoss and Darley, 1974b).

*Testing for Apraxia of Speech*   The procedures described for eval-uating the oral and articulatory performance of patients suspected of having an acquired apraxia of speech can be adapted for use with chil-dren. The child's ability to produce volitional oral movements should be tested, and performance scaled in the manner described for adults. An articulatory inventory and production of CVC monosyllabic words should be done as well as putting the child through the oral diado-chokinetic manuevers. Polysyllabic words can be tested, using simpler words than those used with adults: snowman, animal, careful, um-brella, bicycle, handkerchief, tornado, accident. Words of increasing length with a common syllable core should be tested, and the child should be asked to repeat sentences, simpler than those used for adults: "Stars twinkle in the sky"; "Grandmother took a ride in an automo-bile"; "Those skates belong to Charles."

*Remediation of the Problem*   Unlike our practice with children with nonorganic articulatory problems, in our work with youngsters judged to be apractic in speech we will want to devote much time to heightening their sensitivity concerning the position and movements of their articulators. It may be necessary to spend many sessions simply observing and experimenting with the oral speech mechanism, playing follow-the-leader games as the youngster tries to imitate oral movements made by the clinician, learning to watch these movements in the mirror, getting the feel of the tongue as it is protruded between the lips, pressed between the teeth, raised to the alveolus, elevated to the palate, lateralized to the corners of the lips, alternately protruded and retracted. Similarly, heightened awareness of lip movements and jaw adjustments can be developed.

As we get around to working on sounds, we will use the phonetic placement approach predominantly. The techniques suggested for teaching the adult with an acquired apraxia can be adapted and the child can be led through a hierarchy of performance on the sound in isolation, in syllables, in words with the sound occurring initially, then finally, then in both positions, then in two-word combinations, and finally in multiple word phrases and polysyllabic words. Contrasting pairs to highlight the difference between articulation points can be used. We must continually emphasize the child's monitoring of what he is doing, helping him set a standard for production, check to see whether he has met it, and correct inadvertent errors. A deliberate rate of speech will be encouraged despite its at least temporary unnaturalness. Ultimately, the child will get to feel at home with his articulation, come to trust his tongue, and engage more boldly in the intricacies of articulation.

## REFERENCES

Aten, J. L., Johns, D. F., and Darley, F. L. 1971. Auditory perception of sequenced words in apraxia of speech. J. Speech Hear. Res. 14:131–143.

Bay, E. 1964. Principles of classification and their influence on our concepts of aphasia. In: A. V. DeRueck and M. O'Connor (eds.), Disorders of Language. Little, Brown, Boston.

Burns, M. S., and Canter, G. J. 1977. Phonemic behavior of aphasic patients with posterior cerebral lesions. Brain Lang. 4:492–507.

Critchley, M. 1952. Articulatory defects in aphasia. J. Laryngol. Otol. 66:1–17.

Dabul, B., and Bollier, B. 1976. Therapeutic approaches to apraxia. J. Speech Hear. Disord. 4:268–276.

Deal, J. L. 1974. Consistency and adaptation in apraxia of speech. J. Commun. Disord. 7:135–140.

Deal, J. L., and Darley, F. L. 1972. The influence of linguistic and situational variables on phonemic accuracy in apraxia of speech. J. Speech Hear. Disord. 15:639–653.

Denny-Brown, D. 1965. Physiological aspects of disturbances of speech. Austr. J. Exp. Biol. Med. Sci. 43:455–474.

DeRenzi, E., Pieczuro, A., and Vignolo, L. A. 1966. Oral apraxia and aphasia. Cortex 2:50–73.

Dunlop, J. M., and Marquardt, T. P. 1977. Linguistic and articulatory aspects of single word production in apraxia of speech. Cortex 13:17–29.

Johns, D. F., and Darley, F. L. 1970. Phonemic variability in apraxia of speech. J. Speech Hear. Res. 13:556–583.

Johns, D. F., and LaPointe, L. L. 1976. Neurogenic disorders of output processing: Apraxia of speech. In: H. Whitaker and H. A. Whitaker (eds.), Studies in Neurolinguistics, Vol. 1. Academic Press, New York.

LaPointe, L. L., and Johns, D. F. 1975. Some phonemic characteristics in apraxia of speech. J. Commun. Disord. 8:259–269.

Liepmann, H. 1900. Das Krankheitsbild der Apraxie. Monatsschrift für Psychiatrie und Neurologie 8:15–44, 102–132, 182–197.

Lozano, R. A., and Dreyer, D. E. 1978. Some effects of delayed auditory feedback on dyspraxia of speech. J. Commun. Disord. 11:407–415.

Luria, A. R. 1970. Traumatic Aphasia. Mouton, The Hague.

Martin, A. D., and Rigrodsky, S. 1974a. An investigation of phonological impairment in aphasia, Part I. Cortex 10:317–328.

Martin, A. D., and Rigrodksy, S. 1974b. An investigation of phonological impairment in aphasia, Part II. Distinctive feature analysis of phonemic commutation errors in aphasia. Cortex 10:329–346.

Mlcoch, A. G., Darley, F. L., and Noll, J. D. 1982. Articulatory consistency and variability in apraxia of speech. In: R. H. Brookshire (ed.), Clinical Aphasiology Conference Proceedings 1982. BRK Publishers, Minneapolis, MN.

Morley, M. 1965. The Development and Disorders of Speech in Childhood. 2nd Ed. Williams & Wilkins, Baltimore.

Nathan, P. W. 1947. Facial apraxia and apractic dysarthria. Brain 70:449–478.

Rosenbek, J. C. 1978. Treating apraxia of speech. In: D. F. Johns (ed.), Clinical Management of Neurogenic Communicative Disorders. Little, Brown, Boston.

Rosenbek, J. C., Collins, M. J., and Wertz, R. T. 1976. Intersystemic reorganization for apraxia of speech. In: R. H. Brookshire (ed.), Clinical Aphasiology Conference Proceedings 1976. BRK Publishers, Minneapolis, MN.

Rosenbek, J. C., Lemme, M. L., Ahern, M. B., et al. 1973. A treatment for apraxia of speech in adults. J. Speech Hear. Disord. 38:462–472.

Shane, H. C., and Darley, F. L. 1978. The effect of auditory rhythmic stimulation on articulatory accuracy in apraxia of speech. Cortex 14:444–450.

Shankweiler, D., and Harris, K. S. 1966. An experimental approach to the problem of articulation in aphasia. Cortex 2:277–292.

Sparks, R. W. 1981. Melodic Intonation Therapy. In: R. Chapey (ed.), Language Intervention Strategies in Adult Aphasia. Williams & Wilkins, Baltimore.

Square, P. A., Darley, F. L., and Sommers, R. K. 1981. Auditory and speech perception among patients demonstrating apraxia of speech, aphasia, and both disorders. In: R. H. Brookshire (ed.), Clinical Aphasiology Conference Proceedings 1981. BRK Publishers, Minneapolis, MN.

Trost, J. E., and Canter, G. J. 1974. Apraxia of speech in patients with Broca's aphasia: A study of phoneme production accuracy and error patterns. Brain Lang. 1:63–79.

Weisenberg, T., and McBride, K. E. 1935. Aphasia: A Clinical and Psychological Study. Commonwealth Fund, New York.

Wilson, S. A. 1908. A contribution to the study of apraxia with a review of the literature. Brain 31:163–216.

Yoss, K. A., and Darley, F. L. 1974a. Developmental apraxia of speech in children with defective articulation. J. Speech Hear. Disord. 17:399–416.

Yoss, K. A., and Darley, F. L. 1974b. Therapy in developmental apraxia of speech. Lang. Speech Hear. Serv. Schools 5:23–31.

# CHAPTER 20

# Cluttering: Its Diagnosis

*William M. Diedrich*

*Cluttering is an unusual and controversial speech disorder.
In this chapter, Diedrich thoroughly describes its distinguishing symptoms and recommends procedures for treatment.*

1.  *What are the five clinical signs that define the disorder
    of cluttering according to Diedrich? In particular, what
    are the speech and language behaviors that characterize
    cluttering?*

2.  *What related speech and language disorders may be con-
    fused with cluttering? Can a distinction easily be made
    between these disorders and cluttering? If the answer is
    no, what are the reasons?*

3.  *What procedures are recommended by Diedrich for the
    treatment of cluttering? What procedures are not rec-
    ommended? Is prognosis favorable?*

---

This chapter does not include a survey of the historical literature; however, the
interested reader can begin by reviewing 12 articles in *Folia Phoniatrica,* 1970, 22:247–
382. In addition, Luchsinger and Arnold (1965), and the classic monograph by Weiss
(1964) should be required reading.

THERE ARE NUMEROUS REFERENCES to cluttering in the clinical literature since it was formally described more than a century ago by European authors. In my opinion, the diagnosis of cluttering has functional implications. The purpose of this chapter is to suggest criteria for the differential diagnosis of cluttering from other developmental language and articulation disorders. Consideration also will be given to prognosis and issues in the management of cluttering.

## THE CLUTTERING SYNDROME

The diagnosis of cluttering can be made on the basis of a collection of signs and symptoms, therefore, it can be termed a syndrome. Grewel (1970) and Van Riper (1970), among others, have struggled to distinguish cluttering from other similar developmental language and speech disorders. So it is with trepidation that these criteria for diagnosis are presented. There appear to be five characteristic features that define cluttering: 1) age of appearance, 2) impairment in language formulation; 3) speech disorder(s); 4) lack of self-awareness about the disorder; and 5) hereditary or familial origin. Each of these features is summarized in Table 1 and is discussed here.

Table 1. Characteristic features of cluttering are indicated and contrasted with developmental apraxia of speech (DAS), learning disability (LD), and stuttering

| Cluttering | DAS | LD | Stuttering |
|---|---|---|---|
| Age of appearance (diagnosis usually confirmed after CA of 7 or 8 years) | Earlier | Earlier or later | Earlier |
| Impaired language formulation (dissociation between thinking and speaking) | [a] | [a] | [a] |
| Speech disorder (one or more) | | [a] | |
|   Articulatory indistinctness[b] | [c] | | No |
|   Dysfluency[b] | [a] | | [c] |
|   Monotonous melody-rhythm | [a] | | |
| Lack of self-awareness | [a] | [a] | No |
| Hereditary or familial | [a] | [a] | [d] |

[a] Sometimes discussed in the literature, but not a consistent symptom.

[b] Usually improves with attention (exaggerated speech).

[c] Usually does not improve with attention.

[d] Kidd (1980) has stated that transmission of stuttering exists in families which may be explained by a genetic hypothesis.

## Age of Appearance

It is of interest to note that among our patients, as well as those reported in the literature, a diagnosis of cluttering is usually made after the age of 7 or 8 years. Studies have indicated that the development of articulation (Sander, 1972) and spoken language (Lee, 1974) is essentially complete by this age. Also, by this time stuttering is recognizable as a disorder. Becker and Grundmann (1970) noted that by the ages of 7 or 8 years the symptoms of cluttering are identified. According to Luchsinger and Arnold (1965, p. 397) "cluttering is usually diagnosed at about the tenth year of life." Langova and Moravek stated (1970, p. 325) "Cluttering arises in childhood, worsens in puberty and persists as a rule throughout life." Thus, the appearance of the typical clinical features for cluttering is usually not clear until the formal maturation period for language and speech is essentially complete, and at a time when disorders of speech and language are clearly apparent.

## Impairment in Language Formulation

The common thread that emerges from the many descriptions of cluttering is an impairment in language formulation and dissociative thinking. Weiss (1964, p. 36–37) regarded cluttering to be a central language imbalance.

> One of the most basic characteristics of cluttering is a lack of clarity of inner formulation, and as a result, delivery is hackneyed, haphazard, and studded with moments when the clutterer seems to lose the thread of thought completely, or to forget what he has said or the next word to be spoken.

De Hirsch (1965, p. 315) agreed with Weiss when she stated that "Cluttering is basically a disassociation between thinking and speaking." Despite differences in the description of cluttering, Arnold (1970, p. 248) concluded that there is essential agreement that "cluttering is a hereditary and familial disorder which affects the highest level of linguistic formulation and integration." The disorder of cluttering involves impaired formulation in word finding, sound and word sequencing, and errors in syntax and morphology. Sometimes comprehension is impaired, but not always.

## Speech Disorder

A lack of coordination between breathing and phonation has been described, as well as a tendency for hypernasal resonance. As one listens to the speech of the clutterer, however, the most prominent features are articulatory indistinctness, dysfluencies, or monotonous melody and rhythm (prosody), which can occur singly or in combination. Furthermore, the degree of cluttering may be influenced by the psychological state, the environment (friends, strangers), or the stimulus situation (spontaneous speech, oral reading, etc.).

One useful diagnostic sign that distinguishes cluttering from other speech disorders is the use of slow and exaggerated movements of articulation. Volitional (versus automatic) speech generally results in improvement of intelligibility. Comparable articulatory improvement is not seen in dysarthria, apraxia, or functional misarticulation. When slow, exaggerated speech is used, dysfluencies decrease, which is not typical of the stutterer. Perkins (1979, p. 103) has suggested, however, that slowed phonetic rates decrease frequency of stuttering and coupled with "syllable prolongation practically eliminates stuttering." The observation is not new that concentration improves fluency, and slowed delivery improves articulation in the clutterer. Kussmaul in 1877 observed the former and Liebmann in 1900 the latter (cited by Weiss, 1964, p. 3 and 26).

*Misarticulation*   Two patterns of articulation errors may occur in the clutterer. First, speech often consists of imprecise, indistinct, or slurred articulation. Second, there may be consistent mispronunciation of one or more sounds, usually the liquids /r/ and /l/, and the sibilants. It is relatively easy to distinguish between these two types of errors in children beyond 8 years of age. When the clutterer speaks in a slow and exaggerated fashion, clarity is increased. This improvement stems from an increase in precision and distinctiveness of articulation for most sounds. The use of exaggerated speech generally does not significantly alter sibilant and liquid errors nor are these sounds easily stimulated in isolation or in consonant-vowel (CV) units.

*Dysfluency*   As the clutterer gropes to translate thought into words, and syntax into spoken speech, two kinds of dysfluencies may be observed. Neither typifies the dysfluencies found in stutterers. For most stutterers, dysfluencies consist of tense repetitions of initial sounds and syllables, and/or prolongations of sounds. The dysfluency in the clutterer is an easy repetition of whole words and phrases and/or frequent use of interjections, such as "and" or "uh." Conscious attention to speech or oral reading by the clutterer results in a markedly reduced number of dysfluencies not commonly observed in stutterers.

*Monotonous Melody-Rhythm and Rate*   Cluttering speech is monotonous and involves poor use of linguistic phrasing and inappropriate use of intonation and stress. There is a lack of normal variability in pitch and loudness and the typical suprasegmental features that distinguish a geographic region may be missing.

In the early descriptions of cluttering, rapid rate was considered to be one of its primary characteristics. In fact, the word *tachyphemia* (rapid rate) was often used interchangeably with the word *cluttering*

(Arnold, 1965a). Although the speech of the clutterer frequently may appear to be fast, when carefully analyzed the perceived rapidity is due, in part, to deletions of single consonants or entire syllables, for example, "PresenKendy" for "President Kennedy." These contracted utterances are usually perceived as rapid speech. Weiss (1964, p. 12) noted two types of deletions in the speech of clutterers. Interverbal acceleration is the shortening of pauses between words and phrases, and intraverbal acceleration is the contraction of longer words. Weiss (1964) noted also that there are clutterers whose rate of speech appears slower than normal or whose rate is not different from normal.

Hutchinson and Burke (1973) also found that clutterers pause time and phonation time were not different from normals. They reported that reading rates under normal auditory conditions were similar for normals and clutterers. Data provided by Rieber et al. (1972), however, suggested that pause time in clutterers was shorter than in normals. When discussing speaking rate in the clutterer, Arnold (1970, p. 248) modified his position by saying "even the established term, tachyphemia, may have to be replaced." Speaking rate appears too variable to provide meaningful diagnostic information at this time.

Another aspect of speech rate is diadochokinesis, which is the repetition of rapidly said syllables or sounds. Studies on the diadochokinetic rate of clutterers have not produced uniform results. Seeman and Novak (1963) found in a speed syllable test (repetition of "ta") that prepubertal clutterers performed similarly to normals. In postpubertal clutterers, however, the number of syllables strikingly increased over the normals, and reached a maximum after the age of 22 years. Becker and Grundmann (1970) found that 30% of the clutterers, 7 and 8 years old, produced "ta" faster than normals. Further comparison with other developmental speech disorders is necessary before diadochokinetic rates can be used as a diagnostic sign for clutterers.

## Lack of Self-Awareness

All authors have commented on the lack of self-consciousness that the clutterer exhibits about his or her language and speech disorder. Even after years of hearing stereotype phrases, such as "slow down," "think before you talk," "would you repeat that," clutterers remain seemingly oblivious to the listener's reactions to their spoken utterances. This lack of self-awareness is not typical of stutterers nor of adult apractics who are usually aware of their articulatory errors and will attempt self-correction. Yoss and Darley (1974a) found that children suspected of developmental apraxia of speech did not "appear to be aware of their errors unless they were older or had extensive therapy."

The lack of self-awareness about the disorder is a diagnostic sign that distinguishes adolescent cluttering from other speech disorders.

## Hereditary and Familial

The terms *hereditary* (genetic origin) and *familial* (uncertainty about genetic or nongenetic environmental origin) (Levitan and Montagu, 1977, p. 832) are applied when a trait occurs in several members of the same family (parents and children, siblings, grandparents, aunts, uncles, and first cousins). Many investigators have reported that cluttering appears in several generations of the same family (Luchsinger, 1970; Luchsinger and Arnold, 1965, p. 601; and Op't Hof and Uys, 1974). Careful inquiry about the occurrence of cluttering in family members should be made at the time the clutterer is examined. The clinician should question whether other family members exhibit imparied language formulation (thought processing), articulatory indistinctness, dysfluency (including stuttering), or monotonous melody-rhythm. For example, asking the parents: "Are there any other family members who have a language-speech problem?" in a perfunctory manner, commonly results in the nonreflective answer, "I don't know of any." The interviewer must specifically ask about both sides of the family, draw a family tree on paper, and take a personal interest in all the family members. At the same time, the interviewer should provide specific examples of behaviors, such as word finding difficulty, metathetic errors, and indistinct speech, so that a parent has something concrete with which to relate to the phrase "speech problem." When examples are provided the parent will often respond: "Oh yes, now that I think about it, Mom did say that Uncle Jim was slow to talk and sort of stuttered when he started school. As a matter of fact he still gets his words jumbled up. Is that what you mean?"

When there is evidence in the family of a general language disability indicated by the clinical disorders of mixed handedness, a written language impairment (reading, spelling, writing), or delayed speech development, it does not necessarily indicate a diagnosis of cluttering. In some families cluttering may occur along with a general language impairment (oral or written).

## OTHER RELATED DISORDERS

In the past, many different clinical findings have been associated with cluttering and are summarized in Table 2. The use of diverse descriptions has been one of the problems in the utilization of cluttering as a diagnostic label. Another is that many of the speech behaviors associated with cluttering are not easily described in writing. We are ac-

Table 2.   Common clinical findings reported for cluttering, developmental
apraxia of speech (DAS), learning disability (LD), and stuttering

|  | Cluttering | DAS | LD | Stuttering |
|---|---|---|---|---|
| Usually males | X | X | X | X |
| Mixed or left handedness | X | X | X | |
| General motor incoordination (dyspraxia) | X | X | X | |
| Written language disorders (reading, writing or spelling, but not arithmetic) | X | X | X including arithmetic | |
| Amusicality | X | | | |
| Resistant to previous speech therapy | X | X | | |
| Soft neurological signs | X | X | X | |
| Personality (extrovert aggressive, hasty, careless, untidy) | X | | X | |
| Delayed speech development | X | X | | |
| Poor concentration and short attention span | X | X | X | |
| IQ within normal limits | X | X | X | X |
| Family history of written language disorders | X | | X | |

customed to picture-frame diagnosis. When Perkins (1978) referred to cluttering as a microcosm of speech-language pathology, he meant that the many behaviors seen in different speech and language patients can be found in a single clutterer. Unfortunately, many of the same clinical behaviors may be observed in four different diagnostic groups: cluttering, developmental apraxia of speech (DAS), learning disability (LD), and stuttering. The classic issues in the differentiation of any two disorders which have similar clinical findings have been addressed by Van Riper (1970). The diagnostic problems of cluttering will not disappear with these discussions, but hopefully the reader will acquire some new insights from the comparisons to be made.

*Developmental Apraxia of Speech*   The term *congenital dyspraxia* is sometimes used to describe the general body motor incoordination of the clutterer, but only infrequently to describe the speech of the clutterer. Pearson (1965) concluded that clutterers have a general lag in motor development. She used such terms as *clumsiness* and *motor infantilism* to describe gross motor control. Pearson does not use the term *developmental dyspraxia* or *articulatory apraxia* as does Morley (1965), who in turn did not use cluttering or tachyphemia in her description of childhood speech disorders. Arnold (1965a, p. 7 and 1965b, p. 39) listed *congenital dyspraxia* (among others) as an etiologic factor regularly associated with the syndrome of cluttering. He also used the term *dyspractic articulation*, but general clumsiness and poor body coordination to refer to the clutterer's motor control. Roman (1965, p. 80) stated: "The dysgraphic and oral (tachyphemia) dysrhythmia manifested by clutterers are component manifestations of a basic psychomotor inadequacy, known as congenital dyspraxia." Weiss (1964) did not use the term dyspraxia to describe any of the symptoms or etiologic conditions of cluttering. Grewel (1970, p. 304) reported that "oral motorics are especially clumsy in some clutterers, to such a degree in some—rare—cases that one must consider the possibility of oral dyspraxia." It is not clear whether he was referring to speech or nonspeech oral dyspraxia.

There is little agreement on the clinical findings presumed to be associated with the diagnosis of DAS (Guyette and Diedrich, 1981). Williams et al. (1981) carefully replicated the frequently cited study of Yoss and Darley (1974a) and generally failed to support their findings. One explanation Williams et al. gave for their findings is that different clinical subgroups with articulation errors may exist. Before their investigation, Winitz (1975, p. 8–9) indicated methodologic problems of subject selection in the Yoss and Darley (1974a) study and concluded their results were an experimental artifact. It appears then that among children with misarticulations, different clinical subgroups and patterns of articulation errors occur and apraxia may be one of the reasons for their appearance (e.g., see McLaughlin and Kriegsmann, 1980).

The reader may ask: if a clutterer's speech reveals errors of articulation, how can these be distinguished from apraxia or dysarthria? In children beyond the age of 8 years, the best clinical evidence is obtained by requesting slow and exaggerated speech responses. The clutterer's speech will show a marked diminution in the number of inconsistent articulation errors, whereas the articulation errors of an apractic or dysarthric generally will not improve with mere instruction or by being asked to imitate stimuli spoken by the clinician.

Therefore, in my judgment, cluttering is to be regarded as a problem in self-monitoring of speech output. As such, it involves poor coordination among respiration, phonation, resonance, articulation, and prosody. Apraxia is a problem in the initiation of a specific consonant or consonant-vowel (CV) articulatory unit. Cluttering is a problem in maintaining sequential articulatory units with little self-consciousness about the difficulty. Unlike clutterers, apractic patients are aware of their difficulty in speech production. Some articulatory errors in the speech of clutterers may reflect dyspraxia; however, apraxia is not necessarily characteristic of the cluttering syndrome.

*Learning Disabilities*    Cluttering has also been compared with learning disability (Tiger et al., 1980). Therefore, it is instructive to provide the definition of a learning disability given by the National Advisory Committee to the Bureau of Education for the Handicapped, Office of Education, in 1968. Congress included this definition in Public Law 94-142, the Education for All Handicapped Children Act of 1975. A learning disability is

> a disorder in one or more of the basic psychological processes involved in understanding or in using language spoken or written, which disorder may manifest itself in imperfect ability to listen, think, speak, read, write, spell, or do mathematical calculations. Such disorders include such conditions as perceptual handicaps, brain injury, minimal brain dysfunction, dyslexia and developmental aphasia. Such terms do not include children who have learning problems which are primarily the result of visual, or emotional disturbance, or environmental, cultural, or economic disadvantage.

From the above definition, an LD could be described as a language learning disability or language disability rather than a learning disability because language is central to the handicapping condition.

A disturbance in language formulation is usually cited as a characteristic feature of cluttering. Other language impairments have also been described as part of the symptomatology of cluttering. This impairment includes reception as well as expression. Arnold (1965a, p. 4) and Grewel (1970) have discussed sensory and motor cluttering. Reading, writing, and spelling deficiencies also have been noted in clutterers. Arnold (1965b, p. 34) has indicated that arithmetic skills are generally good, and has observed that clutterers can be found among engineers and accountants. It would be of considerable interest to know why arithmetic skills are unimpaired in these individuals.

Many of the clinical findings associated with cluttering, as described in Table 2, fit the descriptions of DAS and LD. In fact, because the definition of a learning disability includes only "one" impairment of all the basic psychologic processes involving language, all clutterers could be classified as learning disabled.

Tiger et al. (1980) pointed to the interrelatedness of LD and cluttering. They identified four obligatory diagnostic categories of cluttering which represented a consensus among professional workers. One disorder within each category must be present for the diagnosis of cluttering. The categories are as follows:

1. Language disorders: reading, writing, speaking, and auditory comprehension
2. Speech disorders: fluency, prosody, articulation
3. Perceptual problems: visual-motor, auditory-perceptual disabilities
4. Lack of complete awareness of the above disorders

LD children have disorders of reading, writing, and spelling, but not all clutterers have written language impairments. A disorder(s) of speech is essential for a diagnosis of cluttering, but it is not obligatory for the diagnosis of LD, although individuals with learning problems frequently have speech problems. A clutterer's lack of self-awareness has parallels in the characteristic absence of social perception observed in children and adolescents with LD. These children demonstrate confusion in interpreting ordinary nonverbal communication conveyed through facial expression, gesture, or touch (Wiig and Semel, 1976, p. 297). The lack of self-awareness in the clutterer has commonly been ascribed to poor skills in auditory monitoring of speech, thus it is of interest to suppose that their visual modality may likewise be affected, but this aspect needs substantiation.

If one accepts the legal definition (PL 94-142), which states that a child with any language impairment apparently due to brain dysfunction is LD, then all diagnosed clutterers are also LD because of their impaired language formulation skills and presumed disrupted CNS due to genetic/familial reasons. Obviously, however, not all LD children are clutterers.

*Stuttering* In some descriptions of cluttering the primary emphasis in diagnosis was to distinguish cluttering from stuttering (Luchsinger and Arnold, 1965; Van Riper, 1970). The focus was on the speech rate and dysfluency of the clutterer. Efforts have been made to distinguish stuttering and cluttering on the basis of reading rates, more specifically, on measures of phonation time and pause time. We have pointed out that the data are not clear about the differences between normals and clutterers on pause time. Pause time was found to be significantly longer in stutterers than clutterers (Hutchinson and Burke, 1973; Rieber et al., 1972). According to Hutchinson and Burke (1973), phonation time was longer in stutterers than clutterers, but phonation time was shorter in stutterers than clutterers (although not satistically significant) in the Rieber et al. (1972) study. Clinically, it would be difficult to make a differential diagnosis between clutterers and stutterers on pause or phonation time variables.

In other descriptions of cluttering, attention was given to language and thought, and their influence on the spoken utterances. For example, Weiss (1964) presented the notion of central language imbalance in cluttering, and Arnold (1970) suggested that cluttering is the residual result of a congenital language disability. Weiss (1964) has stated that cluttering (and central language imbalance) was the "mother lode" of stuttering. There have also been efforts to demonstrate that stuttering is a language disorder (Hamre, 1978; Helmreich and Bloodstein, 1973; Sodderberg, 1967; Wingate, 1967).

A neurologic basis for stuttering has long been disputed. Rosenbek et al. (1978) have discussed striking similarities between developmental stuttering and acquired cortical stuttering. DeFusco and Menken (1979) have described linguistic symptoms, including syllable and word repetitions, in adults with acquired neurological disease(s) which are symptomatic of cluttering. Recently, Riley and Riley (1979) presented the viewpoint that there are four "neurologic" components which contribute to stuttering. They are attending, auditory-processing, sentence-formulation, and oral-motor production. Each component has been previously reported as associated with cluttering, so it is of interest to find that some authors now believe each to be associated with stuttering.

It would appear, then, that clinical similarities in dysfluent behavior exist for adult and developmental disorders, and organic and nonorganic nonfluent disorders, although there may be disagreement on the behavioral distinctivenss of the dysfluencies (i.e., tension versus nontension or initial sound/syllable repetition versus whole word/ phrase repetition). However, there is agreement on the issue of awareness. Stutterers are conscious of their dysfluencies, but clutterers exhibit no such self-awareness of their speech disorder.

In summary, the appearance of five characteristic features, as given in Table 1, indicates that cluttering is a clinical entity which can be distinguished from other related disorders, such as developmental apraxia of speech, language learning disability, and stuttering. Cluttering may be confused with LD or apraxia when the clinical findings common to each disorder are applied, as presented in Table 2. When a given patient has all five characteristic features and speech improves through conscious and exaggerated effort, a diagnosis of cluttering is suggested.

## Treatment and Prognosis

Because cluttering is a heterogeneous mix of language and speech disorders, its treatment is complex. Langova and Moravek (1970, p. 332) have stated that if the abnormal EEGs found in clutterers represent an organic condition "the patient would hardly be able to eliminate this disorder by his will." Yet, many have noted a marked improvement in articulation and fluency when clutterers attend to their own speech by using a slow and exaggerated pattern. Self-attention to speech does not seem to improve the clutterer's poor performance in language formulation. Perhaps volitional control has more affect on speech—a motor output behavior—than on inner language formulation.

Problems of language formulation and dissociated thinking found in older children and adolescents who clutter are usually subtle. Clutterers do not show an obvious difficulty in word finding often observed in the adult aphasic or an unreality in the use of language heard in the speech of the psychotic patient. To aid language formulation, Weiss (1964, p. 91–96) suggested exercises in telling stories that require accuracy in sequencing. Likewise, telling jokes requires semantic and syntactic precision, and an understanding of double meanings and innuendoes. The techniques described for adolescents with language disability would be appropriate (e.g., Wiig and Semel, 1976, p. 259–296).

A basic approach to the treatment of cluttering has been to improve speech intelligibility. To some this may mean teaching specific sounds such as /r/, /l/, and sibilants. More importantly, intelligibility means teaching clutterers volitional control over their total speech output. When the clutterer slows down and uses exaggerated movements of the articulators (lips, tongue, and jaw), immediate success is commonly observed across the speech parameters of articulation, fluency, melody and rhythm. As an example, one 14-year-old boy we saw had 30 articulation errors and 15 dysfluencies while reading a given passage. After practicing one time with exaggerated speech gestures, the second reading of the same passage contained eight articulation errors and two dysfluencies.

In addition to slowing and exaggerating speech movements, we work on intonation and stress patterns. Body movement, arm gestures, and finger tapping in conjunction with syllabic emphasis, phrasing of speech, and upward/downward intonation have been utilized. All of these procedures are reminiscent of the "melodic intonation therapy" frequently used over the past decade with adult apractics. Although these procedures may be helpful under special treatment conditions, there remains the nagging and persistent problem of generalization.

The crucial difficulty for the clutterer is to maintain highly controlled voluntary speech. The continuous self-monitoring required on the part of the patient is not usually maintained. Simkins (1973), using behavioral techniques with a 9-year-old female clutterer, demonstrated improved speech intelligibility in oral reading, but little generalization to conversational speech. Similarly, Marriner and Sanson-Fisher (1977) used a behavioral approach with a 26-year-old female clutterer, and reported a lack of generalization to conversational speech in the non-treatment environment. We have not experienced much success in teaching postadolescent clutterers to automate slow, conscious, deliberate speech. Despite various behavioral methodologies, our success at transfer, carryover, or habituation to conversational speech with the adult patient has been minimal.

Attempts by investigators to use auditory control in the clutterer have not been very successful. An automatic auditory feedback masking device improved stammering, but not cluttering (Dewar et al., 1976). Hutchinson and Burke (1973) found increased word production errors with clutterers under delayed auditory feedback (DAF) conditions. DAF, called *the Lee effect* by European writers, had a detrimental effect on the speech of clutterers (Langova and Moravek, 1970). They found that 85% of their clutterers became worse with DAF, whereas 82% of their stutterers improved. When chlorpromazine was administered, clutterers appeared to get better under DAF conditions. Sedlackova (1970) also noted that clutterers improved with chlorpromazine. In neither study was the long-term effect of the drug reported. Perhaps there is a general disruption in the clutterer's entire feedback system. The clutterer's lack of self-awareness about his speech may extend beyond auditory considerations into visual, tactual, proprioceptive, and kinesthetic feedback processes, as suggested by various investigators (Langova and Moravek, 1970).

The literature is inconsistent about the prognosis for cluttering. Some authors have stated that clutterers can acquire normal speech, others have observed cluttering to be resistant to treatment throughout adulthood. The prognosis for improvement appears to be age related. It would seem important to make the diagnosis before adolescence in order to maximize the effectiveness of intervention. I have observed that some children begin with a severe language and speech disorder and improve with treatment from 4 to 8 years of age, at which time they appear to be cluttering. Additional treatment, between the ages of 8 and 12 years, has resulted in relatively normal communication. None of the adults whom I have diagnosed as clutterers has ever achieved normal speech. Improvement may be noted in some speech behaviors which seem to justify a period of trial training for adults, especially if the clutterer has had little or no previous treatment.

It is of interest to examine the prognosis of DAS, LD, and stuttering. Children with DAS have been reported to be resistant to speech-language training (Aram, 1980; Blakeley, 1980; Yoss and Darley, 1974b). In the 12 cases Morley (1965, p. 244) reported, 5 had normal speech before 10 years of age; 4 cases were not normal by 10 years; and for 3 the final outcome was not stated. In our experience, school clinicians have reported few cases of DAS in their caseload of high school children, and we have seldom identified teenagers or adults with DAS in our clinic. Although DAS may be primarily a disorder of childhood, rarely occurring past puberty, it has been observed in adults (Macaluso-Haynes, 1978; Morley, 1965; Saleeby et al., 1978). Learning disabilities have also been reported in adolescents and adults (Blalock, 1981; Tiger et al., 1980; Wiig and Semel, 1976). Stuttering is well known to persist for some into adulthood (Boberg, 1981). The conclusion appears to be that some childhood language and speech disorders that have different diagnostic labels (cluttering, DAS, LD, or stuttering), but similar clinical findings, may continue throughout adulthood regardless of treatment.

## CONCLUSION

There are many clinical findings observed in cluttering which are also found in other disorders, such as developmental apraxia of speech, learning disability, and stuttering. The characteristic features of the cluttering syndrome are age of appearance, impairment in langauge formulation, speech disorder(s), lack of awareness about the disorder, and hereditary or familial origin. In addition, there is one useful indicator that distinguishes cluttering from the other related disorders. Conscious, slow, and exaggerated movements of speech generally results in transient improvement of intelligibility in the clutterer, but not in disorders of speech and language which show some of the same symptoms as cluttering. Prognosis is difficult to predict, but intensive treatment in preadolescence seems to result in better outcomes than in postadolescence. We also know that there will be difficulty in generalization of new speech responses to conversational use in the non-treatment environment for the adolescent and adult clutterer.

## ACKNOWLEDGMENTS

The author is indebted to the following persons for the many hours of stimulating discussion and constructive criticism of this manuscript: Tom Guyette, Bimla Arora, and Mary Ann Carpenter.

## REFERENCES

Aram, D. M. 1980. Developmental apraxia. Paper presented at the Annual Convention of the American Speech-Language-Hearing Association, November, Detroit.

Arnold, G. E. 1965a. Present concepts of etiologic factors. In: G. E. Arnold and M. A. Snyder (eds.), Studies in Tachyphemia: An Investigation of Cluttering and General Language Disability. Speech Rehabilitation Institute, New York.

Arnold, G. E. 1965b. Signs and symptoms. In: G. E. Arnold and M. A. Snyder (eds.), Studies in Tachyphemia: An Investigation of Cluttering and General Language Disability. Speech Rehabilitation Institute, New York.

Arnold, G. E. 1970. An attempt to explain the causes of cluttering with the LLMM theory. Folia Phoniatr. 22:247–260.

Becker, K. P., and Grundmann, K. 1970. Investigation on incidence and symptomatology of cluttering. Folia Phoniatr. 22:261–271.

Blakeley, R. W. 1980. Screening Test for Developmental Apraxia of Speech. C. C. Publications, Inc., P. O. Box 23699, Tigard, OR 97223.

Blalock, J. W. 1981. Presistent problems and concerns of young adults with learning disabilities. In: W. M. Cruikshank and A. A. Silver (eds.), Bridges to Tommorrow, Vol. 2: The Best of ACLD. Syracuse University Press, Syracuse, N.Y.

Boberg, E. (ed.). 1981. Maintenance of Fluency. Elsevier, New York.

DeFusco, E. M., and Menken, M. 1979. Symptomatic cluttering in adults. Brain Lang. 7:25–33.

De Hirsch, K. 1965. Diagnosis of developmental language disorders. In: G. E. Arnold and M. A. Snyder (eds.), Studies in Tachyphemia: An Investigation of Cluttering and General Language Disability. Speech Rehabilitation Institute, New York.

Dewar, A., Dewar, A. D., and Barnes, H. E. 1976. Automatic triggering of auditory feedback masking in stammering and cluttering. Br. J. Disord. Commun. 11:19–26.

Grewel, F. 1970. Cluttering and its problems. Folia Phoniatr. 22:301–310.

Guyette, T. W., and Diedrich, W. M. 1981. A critical review of developmental apraxia of speech. In: N. Lass (ed.), Speech and Language: Advances in Basic Research and Practice, Vol. 5, pp. 1–49. Academic Press, New York.

Hamre, C. 1978. Stuttering as a language disorder: Four heuristic models. Paper presented at the Annual Convention of the American Speech-Language-Hearing Association, November, San Francisco.

Helmreich, H., and Bloodstein, O. 1973. The grammatical factor in childhood disfluency in relation to the continuity hypothesis. J. Speech Hear. Res. 16:731–738.

Hutchinson, J. M., and Burke, K. W. 1973. An investigation of the effects of temporal alterations in auditory feedback upon stutterers and clutterers. J. Commun. Disord. 6:193–205.

Kidd, K. K. 1980. Genetic models of stuttering. J. Fluency Disord. 5:187–201.

Langova, J., and Moravek, M. 1970. Some problems of cluttering. Folia Phoniatr. 22:325–336.

Lee, L. L. 1974. Developmental Sentence Analysis. Northwestern University Press, Evanston, IL.

Levitan, M., and Montagu, A. 1977. Textbook of Human Genetics. 2nd Ed. Oxford University Press, New York.

Luchsinger, R. 1970. Inheritance of speech defects. Folia Phoniatr. 22:216–230.

Luchsinger, R., and Arnold, G. E. 1965. Voice—Speech—Language. Wadsworth, Belmont, CA.

Macaluso-Haynes, S. 1978. Developmental apraxia of speech: Symptoms and treatment. In: D. F. Johns (ed.), Clinical Management of Neurogenic Communicative Disorders. Little, Brown, Boston.

Marriner, N. A., and Sanson-Fisher, R. W. 1977. A behavioral approach to cluttering: A case study. Aust. J. Human Commun. Disord. 5:134–141.

McLaughlin, J. F., and Kriegsmann, E. 1980. Developmental dyspraxia in a family with X-linked mental retardation (Renpenning Syndrome). Devel. Med. Child Neurol. 22:84–92.

Morley, M. E. 1965. The Development and Disorders of Speech in Childhood. 2nd Ed. Williams & Wilkins Co., Baltimore.

Op't Hof, J., and Uys, I. C. 1974. A clinical delineation of tachyphemia (cluttering): A case of dominant inheritance. South Afr. Med. J. 48:1624–1628.

Pearson, M. A. 1965. Summary. In: G. E. Arnold, and M. A. Snyder (eds.), Studies in Tachyphemia: An Investigation of Cluttering and General Language Disability. Speech Rehabilitation Institute, New York.

Perkins, W. H. 1978. Human Perspectives in Speech and Language Disorders. C. V. Mosby Co., St. Louis. MO.

Perkins, W. H. 1979. From psychoanalysis to discoordination. In: H. H. Gregory (ed.), Controversies about Stuttering Therapy. University Park Press, Baltimore.

Rieber, R. W., Breskin, S., and Jaffe, J. 1972. Pause time and phonation time in stuttering and cluttering. J. Psycholing. Res. 1:149–154.

Riley, G. D., and Riley, J. 1979. A component model for diagnosing and treating children who stutter. J. Fluency Disord. 4:279–293.

Roman, K. G. 1965. The interrelationship of graphologic and oral aspects of language behavior. In: G. E. Arnold and M. A. Snyder, (eds.), Studies in Tachyphemia: An Investigation of Cluttering and General Language Disability. Speech Rehabilitation Institute, New York.

Rosenbek, J., Messert, B., Collins, M., and Wertz, R. T. 1978. Stuttering following brain damage. Brain Lang. 6:82–96.

Saleeby, N. C., Hadjian, S., Martinkosky, S. J., and Swift, M. R. 1978. Familial verbal dyspraxia: A clinical study. Paper presented at the Annual Convention of the American Speech-Language-Hearing Association, November, San Francisco.

Sander, E. 1972. When are speech sounds learned? J. Speech Hear. Disord. 37:55–63.

Sedlackova, E. 1970. A contribution to pharmacotherapy of stuttering and cluttering. Folia Phoniatr. 22:354–375.

Seeman, M., and Novak, A. 1963. Über die Motorik bei Polteren. Folia Phoniatr. 15:170–176.

Simkins, L. 1973. Cluttering. In: B. B. Lahey (ed.), The Modification of Language Behavior. Charles C Thomas Publishers, Springfield, IL.

Sodderberg, G. A. 1967. Linguistic factors in stuttering. J. Speech Hear. Res. 10:801–810.

Tiger, R. J., Irvine, T. L., and Reis, R. P. 1980. Cluttering as a complex of learning disabilities. Lang. Speech Hear. Serv. Schools 11:3–14.

Van Riper, C. 1970. Stuttering and cluttering. Folia Phoniatr. 22:347–353.

Weiss, D. A. 1964. Cluttering. Prentice Hall, Englewood Cliffs, NJ.

Wiig, E., and Semel, E. 1976. Language Disabilities in Children and Adolescents. Charles E. Merrill, Columbus, OH.

Williams, R., Ingham, R. J., and Rosenthal, J. 1981. A further analysis for developmental apraxia of speech in children with defective articulation. J. Speech Hear. Res. 24:496–505.

Wingate, M. 1967. Slurvian skill of stutterers. J. Speech Hear. Res. 10:844–848.

Winitz, H. 1975. From Syllable to Conversation. University Park Press, Baltimore.

Yoss, K. A., and Darley, F. L. 1974a. Developmental apraxia of speech in children with defective articulation. J. Speech Hear. Res. 17:399–416.

Yoss, K. A., and Darley, F. L. 1974b. Therapy in developmental apraxia of speech. Lang. Speech Hear. Serv. Schools 5:23–31.

# Index

chlorpromazine for, 319
controlled voluntary speech in,
    318–319
delayed auditory feedback for,
    319
diadochokinesis in, 311
diagnosis, 308–312
disorders related to, 312–317
    developmental apraxia of
        speech, 313–315, 319–320
    language learning disabilities,
        313, 315–316, 320
    stuttering, 313, 316–317, 320
dysfluency in, 310
generalization in, 318–319
hereditary and familial, 309–312
as impairment in language
    formulation, 308–309
intelligibility improvement and,
    318
intonation and stress patterns in,
    318
lack of self-awareness in, 309,
    311–312, 316, 319
misarticulation in, 310
monotonous melody-rhythm and
    rate in, 309, 310–311
prognosis, 319–320
as speech disorder, 309–311
tachyphemia in, 310–311
treatment, 317–319
Coarticulation, for articulation
    training, 106–114
    baseline diagnosis in, 106–108,
        113
    coarticulation drills in, 101,
        108–109, 111–113, 113–114
    order for, 108
    parallel transfer in, 109, 110, 114
    probe testing in, 109–110,
        110–111, 114
    spontaneous conversation and,
        113, 114
    training stimuli, 108–110
Communication, young child's
    success in, 154–155
Communicative intent, articulation
    errors and, 155–157
    semantic conflict approach and,
        157–159

Computers
    demographic data from, 201
    for individualized educational
        programs, 197–201, 317–323
Congenital craniofacial anomalies
    (CFA), velopharyngeal
    dysfunction and, 213
Congenital dyspraxia, 313–314
Congenial palatopharyngeal
    incompetence (CPI), 212–213
Consonant clusters
    multiple articulation deviations
        and, 101
    severely unintelligible children
        and, 84
    unintelligible children and, 77, 79
Consonant singletons, unintelligible
    children and, 77
Contextual generalization, 132
Contrastive stress drill
    apraxia and, 300–301
    dysarthria and, 256–257, 258
Coordinative structures, 57
Counseling, dysarthria and, 250
CPI, see Congenital
    palatopharyngeal
    incompetence
Cronzon disease, velopharyngeal
    dysfunction and, 213
Customary production, variability
    in, 125
Cycles
    phoneme targets for unintelligible
        children in, 80–81, 85–87
    unintelligible children and, 78

DAF, see Delayed auditory
    feedback
DAS, see Developmental apraxia of
    speech
Day care workers, carryover
    enhanced by, 189
Deep Test of Articulation, individual
    variation in speech sound
    acquisition and, 127
Degenerative processes, articulatory
    deficits resulting from,
    242–243, 244–245